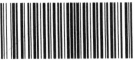

"Joe Lisa does not write a word without the hard documentation to back it up. Many other authors have drawn on his expertise and documentation. . .He is no 'ivory-tower' author speaking loftily. . .He is a determined and staunch advocate of the rights of individual doctors of alternative medicine in the ever-present face of 'big brother.'"

—The late Donald M. Peterson, D.C.

THE ASSAULT ON MEDICAL FREEDOM

P. Joseph Lisa

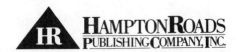

HAMPTON ROADS
PUBLISHING COMPANY, INC.

I dedicate this book to
Nico, Gio, Sierra, Donovan, and Marla.
The future is in the hands of our children.
What we do today determines the quality of their tomorrow.

Copyright © 1994 by P. Joseph Lisa

Cover art by Francine Barbet

Cover design by Matthew R. Friedman

For information write:

Hampton Roads Publishing Company, Inc.
891 Norfolk Square
Norfolk, VA 23502

Or call: (804) 459-2453
FAX: (804) 455-8907

If you are unable to order this book from your local
bookseller, you may order directly from the publisher.
Quantity discounts for organizations are available.
Call 1-800-766-8009, toll-free.

ISBN 1-57174-003-1

10 9 8 7 6 5 4 3 2 1

Printed on acid-free paper in the United States of America

Contents

Preface

Nowhere in this country will you find any publication that delves into the medical/pharmaceutical connections as this book does. It presents what the problem is and who is responsible for the problem. It gives many examples of how a campaign against medical alternatives has been applied (from A to Z—Acupuncture to Zen) in an attempt to destroy them. It also addresses:

1. What the solutions to these problems are.
2. What individual practitioners can do about the problem.
3. What consumers/patients can do about the problem.
4. What manufacturers can do about the problem.
5. What can be done overall to undo the harm that has been done.
6. How the government can "save face" with regard to its part in this travesty of justice that has been perpetrated against the free-enterprise system and the alternative health-care industry.

There are even outlets for the medical, insurance and pharmaceutical industry to use to redeem themselves for their part in this massive propaganda campaign.

The damage has been done, and it continues to get worse every day. In June 1993 there was a raid on an internationally recognized nutritionist's place of business in Southern California. His business records were seized, his computers and disks taken, his bank accounts frozen, and anyone doing business with him targeted. I even have reports of the FBI *going into Mexico* and working with the Mexican federal government to close down all of the alternative clinics below the border. In February 1994, FDA agents, with guns drawn, raided a little "mom and pop" health-food store in a Detroit suburb, seizing supplements and records.

Will it ever stop? Quite frankly, no. It will not stop until the practitioners, patients, consumers, manufacturers, their families, and friends of alternative health care join together and fight back. There are solutions, very workable ones, which, if done through the right channels, could bring an end to this war.

In this book I will show you the weapons with which to fight back, how to use these weapons, and on whom to use them in order to end this health war. As Sun Tzu says in *The Art of War*, ". . .one able to gain the victory by modifying his tactics in accordance with the enemy situation may be said to be divine."

Our entire free-enterprise system in health care is at stake. This is no game. They are playing for keeps.

Consumers: Do not wait for some doctor to tell you, "Your mother is dead. We did all we could do to save her. There was nothing more we could do. She had the best treatment medicine could give her. Sorry!" That is the Big Lie. They *didn't* do everything they could have done, because they never gave you or her a chance to find out if an alternative treatment could save her life. There was something more that they could do, but they wouldn't dare send you to their competition. They have too many dollars to lose. They didn't give her the "best treatment medicine could offer." Other treatments out there that are *much less expensive* might have saved her life. They would never tell you about them.

Practitioners: Don't wait until it's too late. Don't wait until your license to practice medicine (or chiropractic or homeopathy or acupuncture or naturopathy or osteopathy, etc.) is gone before you do something. Don't wait until no insurance company in the country will pay you for your services, treatments, or products. Don't wait until government agents come busting through your front office to seize products, records, and bank accounts. It can destroy your practice, your life, and your family's future. The same warning applies to manufacturers of alternative products.

It is really happening, and it's no joke. This book could be the key to your survival and the survival of the free-enterprise system in health care. I invite you to read it and use the data in it to do what you can to help save our freedom of choice in health care.

No one can just sit by and let this happen. To emphasize this point, I quote a Lutheran minister, Martin Niemoeller, who said the following about the Nazis:

> In Germany they came first for the Communists, and I didn't speak up because I wasn't a Communist.
> Then they came for the Jews, and I didn't speak up because I wasn't a Jew.
> Then they came for the trade unionists, and I didn't speak up because I wasn't a trade unionist.

Then they came for the Catholics, and I didn't speak up because I was a Protestant.

Then they came for me, and by that time no one was left to speak up.

Each of you has a responsibility to speak up on behalf of alternative medicine. Make sure you do, before it's too late to make a difference.

Acknowledgements

I would like to acknowledge the following people for their support and belief in what I have been doing over the past eleven years, putting together the research and documentation that has now resulted in this book being published. First and foremost, I would like to acknowledge and thank my wife Susi for her undying support and loyalty over the year that it has taken me to complete this book. I appreciate her especially for always being there for me during the eleven years it has taken me to collect this information from around the United States. I spent too many days away on the road seeking out the truth, and without her at my side I could have never completed such a massive undertaking.

I would also like to thank Frank DeMarco and Robert Friedman for their courage in publishing this work, and for their support and faith in my ability to piece together a very complex and challenging story. I would like to thank Susi, Frank, and Kathy Grotz for their work on the manuscript. They have turned it into a smooth-flowing, understandable, and intelligently presented final product, which was a long way from the coffee-stained, error-filled first draft they had to work with at the start.

I started more than twenty-five years ago on a career of documenting wrongs in certain sectors of society. A lot of the research and investigation that resulted in this book started back in 1968 and was picked up again in 1983. I would have never bothered had I not seen first-hand the injustices that continue to this day with regard to the persecution of the drugless alternatives. It is my life's hope to attempt to balance the scales, and my readers give me the motivation to do so. Thank you for your positive comments and encouragement.

Lastly, I would like to thank all of those practitioners, manufacturers, and individuals who are working within the alternative health-care system to make life a little bit better for their patients and the consumers in this country. These practitioners, their staff, and the people who manufacture the products necessary for patients and consumers to achieve the goal of better health are sticking their necks out on a daily basis. They do so despite the opposition they are confronted with for their practices and beliefs. Perhaps now they can breathe a little easier knowing something can be done to right the wrongs that they have suffered.

Introduction

My introduction to the seedy world of medical politics began in the fall of 1968, when I conducted an investigation into the American Medical Association's sponsorship of a series of media attacks directed against what they called "mental health quackery" the previous summer. I began my investigation by visiting several groups in the New York and the Washington, D.C., area that had been involved with this media campaign. Each place I visited, I explained that I was working on a book on "mental health quackery" and asked the "experts" for help. In each place I was provided with files and records on the subject being investigated.

I repeated this successful action over and over again, for about six months. When I had enough background data under my belt, I proceeded to my main objective, the American Medical Association.

It was my policy then, as it is now, that when something good was under attack, I simply asked myself this question: "Who has the most to gain by this action?" In this way I compiled my investigative leads.

I then proceeded to schedule and plan my visit to the American Medical Association's headquarters in Chicago in April 1969. Spokesmen for the AMA and the American Psychiatric Association had come out in an article published in *Life* magazine attacking religion and faith healing as forms of "mental health quackery." This term *quackery,* I was to later find out, was a label that orthodox medicine attached to anything they wanted to discredit in the public's eye. I soon found out to what extent they were involved in a massive propaganda campaign, against every aspect of what has become known as "alternative medicine."

When I arrived at the AMA headquarters I entered into the world of medical politics. Not knowing what to expect, and armed only with the investigative ability that had gotten me that far, I started on my fact-finding journey with some uncertainty as to where it would take me. Today I am still on that road searching for the truth.

As I stood in front of the revolving doors of the building known by medical insiders as "535" (the street number of the AMA's building on North Dearborn Street), I was not prepared for what I was confronted with once I entered into the halls of orthodox medicine. With a strong Chicago wind coming off Lake Michigan at my back, I pushed through the revolving doors. A gust of wind propelled me, along with dust from the streets of North Dearborn, into the large open lobby.

The first thing I noticed were the security surveillance cameras pointing at the entrance. I walked across the marble floor to the reception desk. A uniformed security guard looked up from his paperwork and suspiciously asked who I was there to see and if I could produce identification. I stated my purpose, which was an appointment with the head of the AMA's Department of Investigation, Doyl Taylor. I then produced my identification, whereupon he picked up a phone and called up to the sixth floor where Taylor's office was located. He told someone I was in the lobby to see Taylor, got a reply, and hung up.

His expression of distrust faded slightly as he looked me over. He said that someone was coming down to the lobby to escort me up to the sixth floor. I was given a VISITOR name tag to pin on my suit while I waited for my escort. I could still feel his steel-cold stare as he stood measuring me up and down, making judgments about this outsider standing before him. It was as if I were some trespasser infringing upon the turf which he had been entrusted to guard. He did so with the glare of a zealot.

The elevator doors slid open a few minutes later and a tall lanky man dressed in a dark pin-striped suit stepped authoritatively toward me. With a stern expression on his face, he droned, "I'm Doyl Taylor." I introduced myself, we shook hands, and he turned around without saying a word. I followed him into the elevator, which took us up to the sixth floor.

As I walked behind Taylor through a maze of offices, hallways, and partitions, I noticed a huge room that contained hundreds of file cabinets. I was soon to find out that these filing cabinets contained the most comprehensive collection of misinformation, correspondence, memoranda, propaganda, and reports on "quackery" in the world, bar none. In fact, Taylor was so proud of his files that he quickly pointed out that the FBI, the FDA, the IRS, and even foreign countries came to him to extract data and collect information on "quacks." Taylor assigned me a large table in the conference room, where for three days I combed through hundreds of these files, hand-delivered to me by Taylor's personal secretary.

The conference room was adjacent to the massive file room which was the composite mind of the ruthless Department of Investigation. This was my first exposure to organized medicine's propaganda machine, headed by Taylor and his staff. They had gathered up misinformation, propaganda, and lies about organized medicine's economic competitors from all over the world, and had spread their fabrications on a global basis.

At first he was very leery of me, and checked out my background with phone calls to the officials I had previously interviewed. He made it a point to tell me that if it were not for my impeccable credentials he never would have allowed me access to his records. He said this with the same pompous air that a high priest would use with a commoner who was being allowed into the sacred cave for the first and only time in history.

After the first few hours of talking with him, I won his confidence by playing on his ego. I deliberately positioned myself in the subordinate position of a neophyte having to rely on his expertise and direction in my quest to expose "mental health quackery." Seeing himself grandly as the molder of ideas to place in my impressionable head, he placed in my hands hundreds of files on "quacks" he felt I should know about and expose. Of course, he hoped to use me as a medium to spread AMA propaganda about "quackery" to the general public.

He said that he had to leave town on a trip to New Orleans and he wouldn't be back for three days, but that I would have *carte blanche* access to his files in his absence, and that his secretary would copy whatever I felt I needed for my book on quackery. Of course I took advantage of such an opportunity. My initial goal was more than accomplished, as I accumulated hundreds of documents from inside the AMA's files proving that there was an organized campaign to discredit religious groups and faith healing as forms of "mental health quackery."

I was also given access to other targets of the AMA's propaganda campaigns over the years. The files included psychic healing, faith healing, acupuncture, cancer and arthritis "cures," chiropractic, homeopathy, naturopathy, vitamins, herbs, and more. There was more in those files than I could ever copy and take with me. I picked the best documents related to my main objective and had them copied per Taylor's instructions. I left Chicago with a feeling of great accomplishment.

In viewing the files that were made available to me I not only found that there was a major campaign against every single aspect of alternative medicine, I also was able to analyze the data for a common denominator that would explain why organized medicine felt compelled to attack these entities. My common denominator, back in 1969, still holds true today. Each and every one of the targets that the AMA went after was in some way a form of drugless-healing arts. These methods did not use pharmaceuticals in their approach to healing diseases. I made a mental checklist as I looked through the files, and in almost every case my common denominator held true.

There were a few exceptions, such as a case where a licensed orthodox medical doctor broke away from established medicine after having developed or becoming aware of a drug produced in Europe or Asia that was effective in curing certain diseases. But even in such cases, the common denominator was that these were not pharmaceuticals produced in this country and therefore were in competition with American drug companies.

In a large number of cases, orthodox medical doctors, after years of practice, one day happen upon alternative treatments that makes what they have been doing all those years a waste of time. A transformation takes place and the orthodox medical doctor "converts" to alternative medicine. This happens frequently. There are more "alternative" doctors out there than is commonly thought. Many of them operate "in the closet" for fear of losing their licenses or coming under attack in the press. Such doctors are an embarrassment to the medical establishment. Some are even considered by their orthodox peers to be traitors.

In all instances of the information-gathering process involving the AMA and other groups or organizations I visited and copied files and collected information from, everything that I did was done in a legal fashion, so that the legal integrity of the evidence collected could be used in a court of law. The techniques employed included what is known in law enforcement as "pretense calls" or "pretense visits," using a cover story to shield one's true mission. Using references above suspicion, I was able to gain the trust of the opposition or target area so that they would openly and willingly turn over their files to me. Other techniques included using data from whistleblowers (people inside the "enemy camp") who courageously gave me information about targeted subjects of the investigation. At times, reams of documents have been sent to me anonymously in the mail from sources inside an area under investigation.

No illegal breaking and entering was ever employed. No rifling of desks or file cabinets ever took place. Originals were never taken. Copies were always made of the originals.

About two years after my initial visit to the AMA's Department of Investigation, I found myself confronting thousands of documents that were copied from their files on "quackery." Most notable were the files on chiropractic. By reviewing these files over a ten-month period and studying the United States antitrust laws and trade cases dealing with violations of these laws for several months, I was able to analyze what points of law the AMA had violated regarding chiropractic and others they campaigned to destroy. I "lived and breathed" AMA documents for almost a full year. I knew what they were doing better than some of their own staff. I certainly had a better overview than the government agencies the AMA officials were misusing and directing in their campaign against "quacks."

Along with the files on the "quacks" came files from inside the AMA's Committee on Quackery. This Committee was entrusted with a chilling, unethical, and illegal mission. According to their own statements made by the Committee's lone layperson, H. Doyl Taylor (the Committee's secretary), in a memorandum dated January 4, 1971:

> Since the AMA Board of Trustees' decision at its meeting on November 2-3, 1963, to establish a Committee on Quackery, your Committee has considered its prime mission to be, first the containment of chiropractic and, ultimately, the elimination of chiropractic.

This document and hundreds of others that were selected from the thousands to choose from were then used by William Trever to write a exposé on the AMA's propaganda campaign against chiropractic. The book was self-published and titled *In the Public Interest*. This book was sold to chiropractic associations and the documents included in the book clearly proved that the AMA was involved in illegal activity in its efforts to "contain and eliminate" the profession of chiropractic.

More than a hundred pages of documents were assembled and given to key chiropractors around the country. This was done with the hope and expectation that they would *do* something with them. During 1972-73 the documents were in fact used to defeat legislation that was introduced by the medical establishment in over eleven different states. The legislation was designed to adversely impact the practice of chiropractic in these states. The documents served a good purpose in that regard.

The AMA's current campaign is driven by the same motivation as the campaign back then. The bottom line is that greed is the driving force perpetuating this illegal propaganda campaign against all the alternatives, not just chiropractic. This book shows why the free-enterprise system in health care is under attack, what the covert war being waged against alternative medicine is all about, who is funding this campaign, who the spokesmen are for the campaign, what their actual plans are, and how they are carrying out these plans. The problem becomes very clear. The solutions are also presented for use by practitioners, consumers, patients, and the manufacturers of alternative products, treatments, services, modalities, therapies, and clinics.

What is going on today in America is nothing less than an enforced totalitarian medical-pharmaceutical-police state. It is being shoved down the public's throat. It is "their way or no way—your money or your life." However, it doesn't have to stay that way.

Part One of this book, *The Problem*, outlines the history of organized medicine's campaigns against the alternative health-care movement in America. The campaign that is currently being actively pushed against alternatives (1983 to the present) is covered in great detail, based on hard documentation obtained over a ten-year period of investigation. Part One includes information from personal interviews, data obtained from the pharmaceutical industry, the insurance industry, the medical establishment, and state and federal agencies involved in this massive anti-competitive campaign. This campaign is directed against the *economic competitors* of the pharmaceutical industry, which is funding this campaign.

Part Two covers case histories of this campaign against the targeted alternative practitioners, clinics, products, treatments, therapies, modalities, and manufacturers. In essence, this section of the book is *The Implementation of the Campaign*. It shows how the plans have been applied to the alternatives.

Part Three presents *Solutions* to the many problems with which the alternative health-care movement is confronted. These include solutions for the practitioners, professional groups, the manufacturers, and the general public—patients and consumers—who are the real victims of this campaign. We can *all* do something about preventing the death of medical freedom, by stopping the assault.

Knowledge is the light at the end of mystery's tunnel. It is also power, but having it is only one step toward a solution. It must be *used* to bring about the change that is needed. I invite you to use the information in this book to make others aware of the existing scene in health care. It is my hope that we may all work toward a more ideal scene for everyone concerned with the future of health care in this country.

Part One

The Problem

Chapter 1

The Clash of Medical Philosophies

"Gullible America will spend some $75 million in the purchase of patent medicines. In consideration of this sum it will swallow huge quantities of alcohol, an appalling amount of opiates and narcotics, a wide assortment of varied drugs ranging from powerful and dangerous heart depressants to insidious liver stimulants and, far in excess of all other ingredients, undiluted fraud."
[Samuel Hopkins Adams, "The Great American Fraud," *Colliers*, October 7, 1905.]

The History of Medical Propaganda

When the American Medical Association was established in 1847, the idea was to form an organization that would improve at least two things: the ethical conduct of practitioners and the quality of education in medicine, according to a book entitled *The AMA and U.S. Health Policy Since 1940* (Chicago Review Press, 1984), written by Frank Campion, head of the AMA's Department of Communication. However, detractors of organized medicine have a different view of why the AMA was formed and what it represented. Some say it was simply a way to control competition in health care back in the 1800s and continues to be that today. The association has been criticized as simply being a trade union for doctors. It has been said to be the political arm of organized medicine, with one of the strongest political action committees in the country. It has been said that everything that the AMA does is to maintain the status quo in the health-care system today. Organized medicine has been cunning and ruthless and has systematically worked to eliminate its competition from the very start.

Back in 1847, allopathic (orthodox) medicine was really just coming into being. Homeopathy was on equal footing with the allopathic practice of medicine and was widely accepted and used. During the early formation of the medical establishment, the powers within its structure apparently planned the elimination and control of their competition. The first step was to establish universal licensing boards in all states. This was accomplished by 1883. It is common knowledge in economics that one can not have a monopoly without having laws on the books to perpetuate such anti-competitive controls. These laws were passed and remain in effect today. They also put together a Commission to investigate and inspect all medical schools operating in the United States. The Council on Medical Education conducted a survey in 1905 of some 162 medical schools. This included surveys of competitive schools of allopathic medicine. They didn't publish their findings, but instead took them to Henry S. Pritchett, president of the Carnegie Foundation. As history tells it, the officers of the AMA asked if the Carnegie Foundation would undertake a similar evaluation and make the findings public. An "independent" study? Following this visit, Pritchett and the Carnegie Foundation set up a study group headed by Abraham Flexner to do a tour of medical schools in the U.S.

Flexner was not a physician, but an educator. His brother, Simon Flexner, M.D., directed all medical research into disease cause and prevention from 1903 through the 1930s at the Rockefeller Institute. With regard to the widespread economic impact of the study that has been uncovered in this book, it is a fact that is of interest. Abraham Flexner went on to study with Dr. Nathan P. Colwell of the AMA, who conducted the AMA's earlier study. Funded by the Carnegie Foundation for Advancement of Teaching, Flexner completed the inspection in 1910. By then there were 131 medical schools, including non-allopathic centers of medical education. One of the criteria used in his "inspections" was whether the professors at the various medical schools were capable of teaching "modern scientific medicine." This was no doubt a euphemism for Rockefeller pharmaceutical science, considering that during this same period of time the pharmaceutical industry was coming into vogue. The Rockefeller empire during this same time period had made its mark in oil and its by-products.

Using Dr. Simon Flexner to work on developing new uses for pharmaceuticals in treating diseases, it is little wonder that medical schools were pushing "scientific medicine" as a criterion for what constitutes a good medical school. These "good medical schools" were financially supported with money from the Rockefeller empire. To this day the pharmaceutical industry gives billions to medical education and research.

In existence, then, was a vested interest, not to mention a fixed study by the AMA, designed to have the appearance of originating from outside of medicine. Since the 1910 study, the AMA has always been quick to state that Flexner was an educator, not an M.D. His report could more aptly be named "the Rockefeller study." It greatly reduced the numbers of medical schools (particularly non-allopathic schools) in the country. Flexner made no official distinction between "allopathic medical schools" and "non-allopathic" medical schools, but it was very clear that homeopathic colleges would never meet the standards expected of a "modern" medical school. According to orthodox standards, a good medical school should be capable of teaching "modern scientific medicine." It was no mere coincidence that homeopathic schools did not use "modern scientific medicine" a la Rockefeller pharmaceuticals. It was good that allopathic medical schools wanted to raise their own standards. However, allopathic "inspectors" had no right being inside schools of homeopathic medicine or osteopathic medicine. These inspectors were simply not qualified to sit in judgment of their economic competitors in the health-care system. This can be likened to asking the devil, "Which way to heaven?" For research purposes this was the first of several fixed studies mentioned in this book. All such studies have adversely affected the competitors of allopathic medicine.

In the case of organized medicine, one might ask what preceded the AMA's decision to inspect all of the medical schools in America? In doing an investigation, or a statistical analysis, one always looks for what took place just prior to any significant change. In locating the incident which preceded the change, one can get a better under-standing of what was behind the scene, what the motivation was, and why it took place.

One would also ask, "What interests were being served by the survey of these medical schools?" At a glance one can clearly see that the pharmaceutical industry was certainly being served. How-ever, there was more. Ever since its formation, the AMA has been accused repeatedly of seeking to maintain a scarcity of medical doctors for economic reasons. There are several ways to accomplish this. One is by passing licensing laws and setting up licensing boards to control the number of licenses issued for medical doctors. Another way is to control the number of graduates coming out of medical schools. Another way is to control the number of medical schools issuing degrees in medicine. Still another way is to control one's existing competition by putting them out of business. Lastly, future projected competition can be nipped in the bud by regulating schools of competing medicine out of existence.

Just prior to the 1905 decision to "survey" medical schools, several things occurred which influenced the AMA to "purge" medical schools in America and reduce the numbers of doctors practicing in this country. The issue of "overcrowding" in the profession of medicine was addressed in 1903 by the then-president of the AMA, Dr. Frank Billings. In an article published in the *Journal of the American Medical Association (JAMA)* entitled "Medical Education in the United States," Billings denounced shameful conditions in the schools and "the evils of an overcrowded profession, which reduced the opportunities of those already in the profession to acquire a livelihood." Here we can clearly see economics as the motivation. In the book *The AMA and U.S. Health Policy Since 1940*, Frank Campion defends Dr. Billings' statement about the "overcrowding" issue by stating that over-all Billing's speech was idealistic. Campion claims that Billings was reflecting more on higher standards for education rather than a practitioner's complaint about competition. Perhaps he was, but it is extremely difficult to accept this interpretation of Billings' comments if one considers what took place the very next year.

In 1904 Dr. George H. Simmons, editor of *JAMA* since 1899, gave a speech while dedicating a new building for the Drake University Medical Department in Des Moines, Iowa. He said, "Our profession is enormously overcrowded. . .We have twice as many physicians, in proportion to the population, as England, four times as many as France, five times as many as Germany, and six times as many as Italy." Evidently he considered that something had to change.

It was also a fact that during this same period of time pharmacology became the mainstay of organized medicine. Without allopathic medicine, pharmacology would not have survived. The pharmaceuticals which medical allopaths dispensed to patients kept the drug companies in business. It was not the homeopaths, naturopaths, eclectics, or chiropractors who were pushing pharmaceuticals. It was the allopaths. Only the allopathic medical schools were funded with money from the drug interests. The Rockefeller Foundation and fledgling drug companies had an obvious vested interest in supporting the allopathic schools. It was to serve this vested interest that the medical establishment purged the competition's medical schools, while at the same time doing something about the "overcrowded" profession that so concerned the AMA's leaders. A balance had to be reached. The medical establishment sought to reduce the competition by releasing adverse findings on the standards of their competitors' schools. At the same time, reducing the numbers of medical doctors licensed in the country, they addressed and handled the problem of making sure that their own doctors would "acquire a livelihood."

In 1904 there were 5,747 medical school graduates. By 1919, following the Flexner Report, there were only 2,658. There was a 50% reduction in the number of medical schools in the U.S. from 1904 to 1919, from 162 down to 81. By 1970 there were only 107, and ten years later there were 142. The amount of money spent on health care and on drugs has risen proportionately since the turn of the century. It was a matter of economics in 1904, and it is still a matter of economics 90 years later.

The AMA asking the Carnegie Foundation to re-do the evaluation on medical schools it had previously done was apparently part of its strategy against the economic competition at that time. Having the Carnegie Foundation conduct and publish this study gave the appearance of independence from the vested interests of allopathic medicine, thus attempting to avoid accusations of a tainted study. It would seem that the outcome of such a study could have been predicted, considering the association between Flexner and his brother at the Rockefeller Institute. Allopathic medicine stood in the way of the AMA doctors making a good living. This competition also stood in the way of the pharmaceutical industry's profits. This was true at the turn of the century and it is true today. What the competition was and how these competitors approached disease clearly demonstrates why the AMA and the drug companies were interested in eliminating them from the competitive playing field in health care, then and now.

A good example of why organized medicine and the pharmaceutical industry considered homeopathy an undesirable economic competitor is demonstrated in an advertisement that ran in the 1902 Edition of the Sears, Roebuck Catalogue (reissued in 1986 by Crown Publications). Listed among the many remedies that were freely available to the American public through the catalogue were homeopathic formulas. On page 451, the ad stated in part:

> Every one of the following specifics is a **special cure** for the disease named on it.
>
> If you have them near at hand, we *guarantee* they will **save you many a doctor's bill,** and what is of more consequence, quickly relieve any suffering member of the family and ward off more serious sickness.
>
> A **12-Box case** will save you many dollars in doctor's bills in a year and may save your life. **No family should be without a case of our Homeopathic Remedies.**

The remedies listed were priced from 15¢ to 60¢, and a 12-box case ran $3.00. It was a known fact in 1902, as it is today, that homeopathic remedies were both effective, harmless, and a lot more economical than pharmaceutical medicine or surgery. Sears, Roebuck openly advertised that with the use of homeopathic remedies one would save on doctor's bills, while at the same time helping to cure family members of various diseases and illnesses. For a few pennies you could get a home remedy, save the expense of seeing a doctor, and apply homeopathic remedies to cure illnesses at home. Was this so terrible? Was this an economic threat to the allopathic medical establishment and the drug industry? Was this reason enough to attack homeopathic colleges and schools? Was this justification to campaign against the homeopaths in the United States? It must have been, because the relentless campaign against homeopathic practitioners continues even today.

Homeopathic physicians approached disease with the philosophy that "like cures like." They postulated that a person with an illness should be treated with a medicine that would induce the same symptoms in a healthy person. The doses that were administered were infinitesimally small, and therefore harmless. Today organized medicine employs this same basic philosophy in administering vaccines to children all around the world. A marked difference between vaccines and homeopathic remedies, however, is that vaccines may contain lethal amounts of active disease agents in serum. The Center for Disease Control reports thousands of deaths directly linked to deadly reactions to such vaccines.

Today, throughout the world, homeopathy is practiced and accepted as a valid choice in the health-care systems of many countries including England, Germany, and Sweden. In these countries homeopathy is recognized and paid for by health insurance plans. The Queen of England has her own personal homeopathic physician. It has been this way for more than 150 years in Europe. However, the numbers of homeopathic practitioners working in the United States has been significantly reduced, as a direct result of the early campaign by the AMA to rid the country of its competition. Homeopathy is making a strong comeback today and is sought out by many patients. Notwithstanding, organized medicine is still on the warpath, actively seeking to destroy what is left of this growing competition.

At the time allopathic medicine came into being as an organized body under the AMA, other schools of medicine existed which also represented economic competition, including:

Eclectics. They applied single remedies to pathological illnesses. Following the principles of Wooster Beach, a medical doctor who popularized eclectic medicine in the 19th century, practitioners of eclectic medicine worked mostly with herbal remedies. By 1906 there were only ten eclectic schools in the United States. Today there are none.

Osteopaths. Founded on the theories of Dr. Andrew Still, the practitioners of osteopathy believed that a normal body could defend itself from disease and illness. It was Still's theory that disease and illness arose from derangements within the musculoskeletal system, which required manipulation of that system to correct.

Chiropractors. Started in 1895 by David Palmer in Davenport, Iowa, chiropractic postulated that diseases could be cured by the adjustment of vertebrae. It was theorized that if a vertebra was "out," resulting in a nerve being "pinched" or the flow of blood being interrupted to any part of the body, that part of the body would not function correctly. Once the vertebra was adjusted, the "flow" opened up to that part of the body, and it would function better.

Naturopaths. This school of medicine relied on natural remedies. Such things as water, heat, sunlight, and massage were used to cure disease. Naturopaths did not employ drugs or surgery, unlike allopathic medicine. Many practitioners of this method strongly believe that this approach to healing has its roots in the Bible.

The one thing that all of these approaches had in common was that, for the most part, they were non-pharmaceutical applications of the healing arts. The other thing they had in common was that they posed *direct economic competition* to established allopathic medicine and the pharmaceutical industry.

There were other schools of medicine on the scene, but these were the most common. In 1847 the AMA's approach to medicine and disease was simply one of treating the symptom and not the cause. This holds true today. The bottom line is that allopathic medicine's roots are in the philosophy and theory that the body has been invaded by some "evil entity" or germs which must be named, located, and then "called out" or cut out (surgery). Some opponents of allopathic medicine refer to orthodox medicine as representing a cult based on the tenets of "cut, burn, and poison" (surgery, radiation, drugs).

Certainly, there are times when allopathic medicine should be applied to various extreme, acute, or emergency conditions. For example, if your arm were severed at the elbow, you would definitely want a specialized surgeon to put it back together. If your baby were premature, you would want the advances in neonatal care applied to save the baby's life. If you were wounded by gunfire, you might justifiably want a pain killer such as morphine to help get relief.

However, even the United States government has reported that *only 15% to 20%* of allopathic medicine is effective. A report by the Congressional Office of Technology Assessment said that the rest of allopathic medicine is basically a hit-and-miss situation, that allopathic medicine's effectiveness lies in emergency medicine (trauma) and neonatal. The rest of it (80%-85%), according to the study, *is not effective.* Yet America is paying out hundreds of billions of dollars for something that is only 15% to 20% effective!

While today more and more Americans are seeking alternative health care as a valid approach to their health problems, the powers that be within the structure of organized medicine have not changed their political views of the competition in nearly 150 years. The tactics have changed since the turn of the century, but the goal of eliminating all competition has not.

In order to maintain more control over its competition, the American Medical Association in 1906 created the Propaganda Department. Dr. Arthur Cramp, an editorial assistant at *JAMA*, ran this Department from 1906 up until he retired in 1935. The AMA set up a system to monitor and investigate the efficacy and claims of therapeutic values of various treatments, modalities, and services. This analysis was done by a subcommittee set up by the AMA's Council on Pharmacy and Chemistry. The allopathic physicians would review and analyze the targeted treatment to determine what they considered wrong with it. They would then report their findings to the Council, which in turn would have the findings published in JAMA. This was propaganda at its best.

One has organized medicine reviewing the therapies that exist in positions of direct competition. Then, while sitting in judgment of the economic competition, organized medicine determines whether or not it works. (They did this same thing again in 1987 with a study on the alternatives. This is covered in later chapters.) They then have their critical review and analysis published in *JAMA* to spread the obviously slanted findings to the whole country. This is an almost-perfect propaganda machine.

Dr. Cramp's targets included what the AMA referred to as "nostrums." These nostrums were described as "remedies for which the ingredients were kept secret." Homeopathic remedies would have fallen into this category. Since homeopathic remedies were in direct competition to the pharmaceutical remedies of the AMA, the Propaganda Department's findings could have been nothing more than a tainted analysis of allopathic medicine's number one economic competitors.

Other targets of the Propaganda Department's program included patent medicines (which supposedly had patented formulas) and non-approved proprietary medicines (whose names were registered). What these two had in common was that they were not manufactured by the pharmaceutical companies which were supporting allopathic medicine and medical schools during this time period.

This is not to say that there weren't nostrums, patent medicines, and other remedies that were questionable products. This is not to say that from 1847 to 1935 there weren't quacks or false miracle cures and medical scams. There most certainly were, and they are still around today. However, under no circumstances could the analyses and reviews that were being performed by the AMA and its Council's subcommittee and the Propaganda Department *ever* be considered independent studies free of vested interests. To the contrary, they were studies that for all practical purposes were carried out with a preconceived prejudice and with a vested interest in the outcome. This alone constitutes an inherent flaw.

It would have made more sense to form a panel of valid experts from each of the disciplines of the day, to oversee and analyze the various remedies and formulas, rather than have one discipline reviewing its competitors' products and remedies and passing judgment on them. This would have been a fairer and more logical approach.

Alternative medicine should complement allopathic medicine. In some cases there is a need for allopathic medicine. In other cases it would be best to employ some form of alternative (or complementary) medicine. In some instances, a patient may require a combination of approaches to healing. However, for any one discipline to sit in official judgment of its economic competitors and to distribute propaganda to the public about how bad its competitors' remedies and treatments are is not only unethical, it is bad medicine. It is unfair and illegal, in that it violates the Sherman Antitrust Act which forbids such anti-competitive activity. Regrettably, restraint of trade, unfair trade practices, anti-competitive activity, and conspiracy to eliminate the competition have been hallmarks of American medicine. It has been this way from its conception and blatantly continues to this day.

Chapter 2

Dirty Politics and Dirty Tricks

"WASHINGTON June 30, 1975. A series of confidential memorandums revealed the American Medical Association (AMA) has been heavily involved in political and other non-medical activities for years."
[Dan Thomasson and Carl West, "Secret Memos Show AMA Deeply Involved in Politics," Alburquerque *Tribune*]

This headline appeared at a time when the media was attacking the AMA and exposing its behind-the-scenes activities. Investigations revealed violations of federal laws dealing with several issues, including taxes, political influence, unethical funding from drug companies, questionable lobbying activity, violations of postal privileges by its medical journals, and more. Not a week went by between June and September 1975 without some sort of new document leaking out from AMA headquarters in Chicago. There were also leaks from the Washington, D.C., office of its Political Action Committee (AMPAC), resulting in embarrassing newspaper articles exposing the AMA's questionable, unethical, or illegal activities. Many of the non-medical activities the AMA was involved in included its relentless propaganda campaign against its economic competitors. What was exposed in the press in 1975 was just the tip of the iceberg. Much of what the AMA did against its competitors has never been known until now. For the past thirty years, the American Medical Association and its allies in and out of government have waged war against their economic competitors in alternative medicine. They have not been above using covert operations, dirty tricks, "fixing" government studies, adversely influencing government policy and insurance company coverage, and much, much more.

Following in the tradition of the old Propaganda Department, the American Medical Association continued its campaign against its economic competitors all through the 1950s. It changed the name of the Propaganda Department to the Department of Investigation. It was a clearinghouse of information and propaganda on every aspect of the alternative health-care movement in the United States.

The AMA's Board of Trustees meeting, held November 2-3, 1963, established the Committee on Quackery, to look into targeted alternative treatments, modalities, services, products, manufacturers, and practitioners. The Committee on Quackery was headed by its secretary, H. Doyl Taylor, who was also the head of the Department of Investigation.

Following the formation of the Committee on Quackery, Doyl Taylor organized a tightly knit group of governmental and non-governmental organizations which worked behind the scenes to destroy alternative medicine. This group, formed in 1964, was known as the Coordinating Conference on Health Information (CCHI). The CCHI paralleled what the AMA's Committee on Quackery was doing. The main difference between these two arms of the AMA's propaganda war was that the Committee on Quackery was usually open about its anti-competitive activities. The CCHI operated entirely behind the scenes, working behind closed doors, with the minutes of its meetings hidden from public view even though government agencies were involved. It is important to understand which groups were members of the CCHI in order to better comprehend the scope of the AMA's propaganda campaign.

The following are the groups that were members of the CCHI:

Non-Governmental Members

American Medical Association
American Cancer Society
American Pharmaceutical Association
Arthritis Foundation
Council of Better Business Bureaus
National Health Council

Governmental Members

Food and Drug Administration
Federal Trade Commission
U.S. Postal Service
Office of Consumer Affairs

The group wanted to maintain a low profile from the start. According to the minutes of one of its first meetings, in November 1964, one of the members referred to the group as a "committee."

The representatives from the U.S. Federal Trade Commission said that they ". . .could not participate as members of any committee without very specific and direct authorization of the Commission" — that they "could attend meetings but could not be members of a committee." Dr. Milstead said that this was true, also, of the staff of the FDA.

It was determined at that point that the group would be referred to as the Coordinating *Conference* on Health Information. In this way there would be less "red tape" and the individual members of the governmental agencies could in effect keep their involvement and activities with the CCHI hidden from the public. With the group being a private-quasi-governmental organization, there would be less exposure to the public and the media about what the group was doing behind the scenes.

The actual working structure of the CCHI was such that the AMA's representative, H. Doyl Taylor, chaired the CCHI's meetings. The role that the AMA played was actually a lot more influential than just chairing the group's semi-annual meetings (usually held in May and November each year in different cities). In fact, the AMA and other medical groups dictated to the government agencies what they wanted the government to take action on. The meetings usually consisted of the AMA and the others outlining what they felt were priority targets, and the governmental agencies reporting the actions taken on the various priority targets.

The direction and priorities were almost always set from the viewpoint of what the medical vested interests of the CCHI wanted the government to do about the "quacks." For the entire time that this group was in existence, from 1964 to 1975, the medical interests influenced the government agencies into investigating, seizing, embargoing, and prosecuting their economic competitors. The adverse propaganda laid down during this time period is still present in each of the governmental agencies today. As a matter of fact, what was going on back then is *still* going on today.

Each governmental agency had a different role to play in their zealous efforts to comply with the wishes of their medical masters. For example:

> The U.S. Food and Drug Administration (FDA) would inspect, seize, send Regulatory Letters, and get injunctions against and prosecute targets given to them in the form of priority targets from the AMA and other medical vested-interest groups in the CCHI.

The Federal Trade Commission (FTC) would get injunctions against advertisements, file complaints, and also seek prosecution against designated targets.

The U.S. Postal Service (USPS) would work with the FDA and sometimes Customs in tracking products going through the U.S. mails. They would put "mail watches" on certain clinics, practitioners, and manufacturers to gather up "evidence" of mail fraud, and then prosecute.

Although the Council of Better Business Bureaus is not a government agency, it played a large role as the outlet for the propaganda directed against the priority targets. It was a perfect outlet. A person calling in about a targeted practitioner or company could easily be told that it/they were not recommended. It could be hinted that the subject was being "looked into by the government."

These actions continue today, only with some new players. This is covered at length in Chapter Three.

In effect, the CCHI and the AMA were acting as a national clearinghouse and a task force on quackery. Made up of the government agencies which were empowered to take actions against the "quacks" (economic competitors of the AMA) they were effective in carrying out that mission. Some examples are presented here to highlight this point. According to the minutes of their May 1975 meeting, the following took place:

The AMA said it was interested in having something done about the following:

Chiropractic
Psychic Surgery
Cellular Therapy
Acupuncture
Homeopathy
Naturopathy
Vitamin Therapy

The American Cancer Society (ACS) stated its priorities:

Koch Vaccine
Japanese Cancer Vaccine
Books on Cancer Treatment (Unproven methods)
All alternative cancer treatments/modalities

The Arthritis Foundation considered these priorities:

Leifmann Methods
Radon Mines
DMSO
Honey and Vinegar Treatment
Burbank Serum
Foot Reflexology

As they sat around the table, these three groups relayed their concerns to the FDA, the FTC, and the Postal Service. In an apparent effort to please the medical vested interests, the governmental agencies reported on the following items as they related to the targets they were working on for the medical interests. The following are some of the actions which were reported:

One of the specific items on the AMA list—"Dr. Fairweather's book—*How To Cure Cancer in Two Months or Less*"—had a hand-written note next to it, stating, "P.O. [Post Office] ACTION SUCCESSFUL—Newark."

An item under the Arthritis Foundation's priorities also had a hand-written note which indicated that the Federal Trade Commission took action against Radon Mines. The note stated, "CONSENT ORDER AGAINST MINES."

Another item, "Solarama Board—Elifetron," under Arthritis Foundation also had a hand-written note, stating, "VITALATOR SEARS—Santa Barbara. FDA CALIFORNIA LOOKING INTO IT."

Still another indication of the AMA dictating actions against its economic competitors was found under the heading "Acupuncture needles." A hand-written entry stated, "INJUNCTION BY FDA AGAINST IMPORTATION FROM HONG KONG."

According to the minutes of all of the meetings that the CCHI held for ten years, similar scenarios took place at each meeting. These were not isolated incidents. Also, according to a source who attended these meetings, there was absolutely no doubt that it was the AMA that supervised, dictated, and ran the CCHI. There was no doubt that the government agencies carried out actions that were dictated to them by the medical vested interests. If the CCHI hadn't existed, these actions would have not taken place.

Once again, each of the priority targets had two things in common. They did not use pharmaceuticals in healing, and they were *direct economic competition* to both medicine and pharmaceuticals. This type of anti-competitive activity is clearly in violation of the antitrust laws of the United States. Not only are the perpetrators in violation of these laws, but there are strong indications that they are engaging in criminal conspiracy to deny the practitioners of the alternatives their civil rights to practice their profession. It has also been theorized by some very sharp activist attorneys that this may all come under RICO (Racketeer Influenced and Corrupt Organizations Act) laws. There is strong evidence to support a RICO case due to the fact that the evidence clearly shows a long-standing (and apparently on-going) conspiracy to violate federal laws.

The AMA's illegal anti-competitive activities started to be exposed to the public and the media in 1972 with the release of the book *In the Public Interest*, by William Trever. This book exposed documents from inside the Department of Investigation's files which clearly exposed the AMA's criminal activity directed against its chief competitors in the alternative health-care field—chiropractic. Key documents were listed and published at the end of each chapter. These were used to fight, in more than a dozen states, AMA-sponsored bills which the AMA was pushing to adversely affect chiropractic. This is covered fully in the chapter on Chiropractic in this book, but is mentioned here because it was the beginning of the end of the Department of Investigation, the Committee on Quackery, and the Coordinating Conference on Health Information.

Between 1972 and 1975, a series of incidents occurred which adversely affected the AMA's standing with government agencies such as the Internal Revenue Service, the U.S. Postal Service, the Federal Election Commission, and Congress. The documents that were used to publish the Trever book were anonymously sent to chiropractic leaders around the country. Dr. Gustave Dubbs in New York, Dr. Sid Williams in Georgia, Dr. McAndrews in Iowa, and Dr. William O. Day in Washington state all received copies of the documents and the book. At that time, nothing was done in the courts using these documents. What did take place was that the AMA leaders became aware that these damaging documents were in the hands of their "enemies" and were being used to expose the AMA.

At this time a group of disgruntled AMA employees were circulating anti-AMA pamphlets and memos protesting AMA policy.

The main area of discontent was the paranoid tactics that were put in place in an attempt to seal the security leak that had resulted in the documents from Taylor's Department of Investigation files ending up in "enemy hands." The Department of Investigation, working with building security personnel, had set up an elaborate camera surveillance system. Security cameras were set up in hallways, in the lobby, in the parking lot, and in the alleyways of the building. Spot checks and searches of employees' briefcases and purses and "pat downs" of their bodies were reported. There was an air of paranoid suspicion in every department and cubicle. There were even reports of lie detectors being used on employees in an attempt to find the source of the leaks. The morale of the employees was at an all-time low. People suspected of copying documents were investigated and put under surveillance. Some people were fired. Others quit. It was not a safe place to work.

Doyl Taylor and his department came under fire from the Board of Trustees and other officials of the AMA because their image had been tarnished and his department was ultimately held responsible for the leaks.

In 1975, the ultimate violation took place. Someone was copying memoranda, reports, and documents from inside the very core of medicine's most closely guarded files. From the sanctuary of the office of the Executive Vice-President in Chicago and the American Medical Association's Political Action Committee in Washington, D.C., the most highly guarded secrets started to show up in the media. This time the documents were not only an embarrassment, they were a legal liability. Headlines exposing the AMA's illegal, unethical, and immoral activities were spread across the United States in dozens of newspapers. Damaging documents got into the hands of the media, resulting in such headlines as:

> Secret Data Reveals AMA Schemes for Health Jobs.
> Secret Memos Show AMA Deeply Involved in Politics.
> Drug Firms Gave AMA $851,000.
> Secret AMA Link to Nixon Disclosed.
> AMA Official Let Company Use Name.
> AMA Asks Probe for Theft of Data Used in News Stories.
> FBI Refuses to Probe AMA "Theft."
> Single IRS Blow Could Knock AMA into Fiscal Tailspin.
> AMA Magazine Buying Draws Postal Scrutiny.
> Postal Service Targets AMA in Fraud Check.
> AMA Takes a Publicity Beating Others Have Escaped.
> Justice Department Starts Probe of Alleged AMA Fraud.

AMA Hit For $1-Million Postage.
Journals Face IRS Squeeze.

In the end the AMA had to pay the U.S. Postal Service $1 million, and the IRS demanded more than $15 million. According to the AMA's annual audit report, in as late as 1986 the AMA was still paying the IRS several million dollars dating back to the 1975 IRS probe based on these leaked documents.

The AMA had to do some serious budget cutting in order to prepare for the onslaught of penalties and fines which the federal government planned to levy against them. At one point, the officials at the top of the AMA were seriously considering cashing in their liquid assets. They assessed how much real property they owned and its net worth. Raising membership dues was also considered and done. During this same period the AMA's journal advertising revenue took a drastic dive. The AMA lost membership. More importantly, income from drug advertising declined.

The AMA oversees ten different medical journals, the largest being the *Journal of the American Medical Association (JAMA)*. A large part of the AMA's income is pharmaceutical companies' advertising in these journals. For example, in 1967 the AMA received $13.6 million from drug ads. That figure represented 43% of its total income that year. In 1968 this figure went down $1 million. In 1969 it went down another $1.3 million from 1968. By 1974 they were in deep financial trouble. The income from drug advertising was anticipated to be only $8.3 million, an all-time low.

At its annual meeting in Oregon in 1974 some drastic changes were plotted out. These included the dissolving of some of the AMA's committees and councils and departments. The Department of Investigation and the Committee on Quackery were among the sections slated for extinction. By the time the 1975 annual meeting was held in Atlantic City, New Jersey, the sweep was completed.

H. Doyl Taylor had seen the writing on the wall. At the May 1974 meeting of the Coordinating Conference on Health Information (CCHI) he took several actions which seemed odd at the time. When a group is formed one of the first things done is to outline the group's goals and objectives. One would also detail the structure of the group, its operating procedures, and the membership, including organizations they represent. A priority, as well, would be setting up the criteria for membership, where meetings would be held, etc.

This was never done with the CCHI—until *after* Taylor knew that the group was going to be disbanded. According to the May 10,

1974, minutes of the CCHI's meeting held at the AMA headquarters in Chicago, Taylor laid out the CCHI's goals, objectives, membership, and operating procedures at one of the CCHI's *last* meetings. The stated GOAL of the CCHI was:

> Protection of the public by gathering and disseminating by all means possible any and all information involving health quackery to each member (of the conference), particularly, those agencies involved in law enforcement.

Under OBJECTIVES, Taylor instructed that the CCHI should:

1. Encourage each member organization [of the conference] to maintain a fund of up-dated information on all forms of health quackery for which they each have a responsibility.
2. Encourage each member organization [of the conference] to maintain contact and stimulate activities by other agencies (when appropriate) concerned with health quackery at national, state, and local level.
3. Encourage each member organization to develop model strategies (e.g. the California anti-cancer quackery law) that can be used at the state and local level.
4. Encourage member organizations [of the conference] to disseminate to consumers by all means possible information on health quackery.

Under OPERATING PROCEDURE, Taylor made a point of maintaining secrecy surrounding the CCHI's meetings. He dictated that:

> Proceedings of the Coordinating Conference on Health Information are for information of members of the Conference only and *shall not be formally recorded.* However, member organizations may provide information at the meetings which can be used for general distribution.

It was known at this meeting that Taylor's department was slated for purging from the AMA, which would put Taylor out of a job. (This did in fact occur following the dissolution of his department.) In retrospect one can clearly see that Taylor was laying out the design, structure, and operation of the CCHI as groundwork for the *rebirth* of his group following the AMA hierarchy's purge. There is no other logical conclusion as to why Taylor was laying out a blueprint for the *creation* and *continued operation* of the CCHI, if not to create a new one, or simply continue to operate the old CCHI under another name or cover.

What Taylor may have had in mind, and what was apparently created following these events, is covered in the following chapter. What can be said about all of this is that the propaganda machine that was created by organized medicine to defame and destroy its competition apparently still exists today. Under a different name, but with some of the same players, they are still going after the same old economic competitors. One might say that organized medicine *did* learn something from the embarrassments suffered between 1972 and 1975. They went underground with their campaign. The campaign was still intact; it was just a lot harder to find. It has, however, been found and is now being exposed.

Chapter 3

Rising Out of the Ashes

"Really, we're a bunch of guerrillas. . . "
[Dr. Stephen Barrett referring to the Lehigh Valley
Committee Against Health Fraud, *AMA News*, August
1975.]

Research shows that during the first one hundred years of the
AMA's existence it formed councils and committees which sat in
judgment of its economic competitors. These committees would
"investigate" the various alternative health-care systems and would
then report on their findings and make determinations and recommendations that the public should stay away from such "quackery."
The CCHI and the AMA's Committee on Quackery continued to
serve this function from 1963 to 1975. However, when the writing
was on the wall, Doyl Taylor saw that his propaganda department
was "going down for the count." He apparently took steps to see that
his work continued even if he weren't around to supervise the
AMA's campaigns against the "quacks."

In his description of what the CCHI should be, he took steps to
maintain its secrecy by dictating that no minutes of their meetings
should be taken. This made finding the new CCHI (or "shadow"
CCHI) a lot more difficult. However, even those most careful to
cover their tracks often leave clues for determined investigators to
find. In the case of the CCHI, Taylor left one big clue. In the
OBJECTIVES and GOALS of the CCHI, he stated:

> Protection of the public by gathering and disseminating by
> all means possible any and all information involving health
> quackery to each member [of the conference], particularly
> those agencies involved in law enforcement.

By itself it isn't much of a clue. But when one dissects this stated
GOAL of the CCHI and looks closely, one can clearly see several
good leads to follow in unearthing this "shadow CCHI." To find such
an organization, one needs to find a group who:

First, is pretentious and arrogant enough to espouse the principle that the public needs to be "protected" in the health-care marketplace. From what are we being "protected"? Health "quackery" of course. Exactly what is health "quackery"? Apparently it's simply anything that the medical and pharmaceutical industry cannot control. Interestingly, it is also the *economic competition* to drugs and medical treatment.

Second, claims to be "protecting" the public by "gathering and disseminating any and all information involving health quackery." One would have to find a group that has a large storage of information on "health quackery."

Third, is connected to the government and whose members are "gathering and disseminating" information on "health quackery," particularly to "those involved in law enforcement."

Fourth, has a *vested interest* or is doing the work of or for a vested interest. It was proven that the AMA had a vested interest in the original CCHI.

Fifth, consists of most of the same members of the CCHI, or at least is connected to the members of the CCHI.

Sixth, serves the same or similar function as did the CCHI in terms of spreading the propaganda through Congresses on Quackery or some similar type of "conference" on "quackery."

With these leads in mind, I began the search for the link between the old AMA campaign and the current one. I began to build the bridge between the two with information I had come across over the years, as well as information I obtained during my current investigation, which began in earnest in 1984.

Looking back at my visits with Doyl Taylor, I began to assemble the pieces of the puzzle using information he had bestowed upon me regarding activities the AMA was involved in regarding its fight against "quackery."

For some years prior to the 1975 dissolution of his Department, Taylor worked to get groups outside the AMA to take an active role in their campaign against "quackery." One of Taylor's tactics had been to get other groups to take a stand against quackery, to develop position papers on quackery, and to parallel what the AMA was doing in this area. Quite often these groups would simply duplicate the AMA's position on the issue. The AMA would help that group develop their statements, and then the AMA would tout that group's position as being independent of the AMA's. In this fashion the AMA used the other group's statements to strengthen its own campaign. In the seedy world of intelligence this is known as "multiple reports." One creates outlets from outside one's immediate area, and then points to these reports as evidence that there is a "national movement" or "public opinion" against one's target in a campaign.

Another way of doing this is to create either a front group or a cover organization to carry on one's campaign. In the case of a front group, one simply helps to start up a group which parallels one's own organization. One then can feed that group money or information or both. The front group usually has a different name, but its function is the same. It is always run by someone who knows what the group is all about. This leader is usually in direct communication with the group that helped set it up, so as to continue to receive support from the originating organization. An example of such an operation would be the Central Intelligence Agency (CIA) setting up a front group such as Radio Free Moscow to transmit propaganda into the USSR. Radio Free Moscow would receive funding covertly, and the people who would run the operation would also be CIA operatives or employees. The role and mission would be known to all who work there.

However, the function and mission of a cover organization or group would be totally different. Upon cursory inspection it would appear to be just what it was held up to be. The employees of a cover group would not necessarily know what the group was really all about. The person heading the organization would know, but the link between this person and the organization he or she was truly working for would be totally hidden. Usually the group would be a self-supporting entity and no money trail would ever be found going back to the original group that set it all up.

For example, a public relations firm set up in New York during World War II headed by a third-generation German-American could serve as a cover group for a German spy. He or she would go about doing the normal business of a public relations firm. In actual fact, the head of this cover group would be using his firm as a cover to obtain information for the German cause. Upon inspection of the office files and operation, it would appear to be what it seemed to be, when in fact it is only a cover group.

The AMA was not beyond setting up such groups. The Department of Investigation was itself a front group, in a sense. It appeared to function as a clearinghouse of information on quackery, when in fact it was much more than that. It was a propaganda machine involved in effecting the destruction of medicine's competition. It didn't just collect, organize, and disseminate information on quackery. In its attempts to adversely influence government reports and studies on medicine's economic competition, it was directly involved in working behind the scenes to get insurance plans to exclude its competition. This was an anti-competitive activity.

As far as helping to set up front groups, this apparently came into play in the early 1970s. Doyl Taylor made it known that there was a psychiatrist in Allentown, Pennsylvania, a Dr. Stephen Barrett, who was a crusader against "quackery." Taylor encouraged me in 1970 to make contact with Barrett, as he was very involved in the same issues as the AMA, especially in the area of chiropractic. Taylor said that he had given Barrett full access to the "quackery" files in the Department of Investigation between 1969 and 1975. Barrett's group was known as the Lehigh Valley Committee Against Health Fraud. (*Health Fraud* is a euphemism for *quackery* which is still used interchangeably today.) The group was incorporated in Harrisburg, Pennsylvania, on April 19, 1970.

In reviewing published statements by the AMA and Dr. Barrett, I was able to find some of the pieces of the puzzle in the *AMA News,* as well as in the minutes of the CCHI. These pieces pointed to the distinct possibility that organized medicine may have very well been involved in setting up, or helping to set up, the first group outside the AMA to fight "quackery" or "health fraud."

The following are Dr. Stephen Barrett's own words, published in the *AMA News* on August 25, 1975, describing the Lehigh Valley Committee Against Health Fraud. This was five years after it was incorporated.

Several of the professional societies endorsed our group and donated money to help the Lehigh Valley Committee Against Health Fraud, Inc. The medical society allowed us to use its office equipment until we obtained our own.

. . .By working "undercover" using assumed names and box numbers, we've gotten all sorts of information and publications other groups, like the medical societies, haven't been able to lay their hands on.

. . .Really, we're a bunch of guerrillas—we're not a large group, there are about 40 members, but we're the only such group in the country.

Here we have, in Barrett's own words, the apparent link between organized medicine and his group's operation. Although he didn't name the specific "professional societies" that endorsed and donated money to his group, he did state that such organizations as medical, dental, osteopathic, and pharmaceutical groups did help him set up his operation.

In an apparent attempt to be free of the taint of being directly linked with the medical establishment that helped fund his set-up, Barrett said, "We incorporated to make it clear that we were independent of sponsoring organizations." He goes on to state, "As we attracted publicity we received financial support from individuals— mainly health professionals." These "health professionals" were most likely from the medical society.

Another piece of the puzzle came to light in the minutes of the May 4, 1973, meeting of the Coordinating Conference on Health Information. Lois Smith reported, "Dr. Steven Barrett, psychiatrist, Lehigh Valley, Pennsylvania, is writing a book entitled *The Deadly Deceivers,* covering all phases of quackery."

Doyl Taylor was quick to add that "Dr. Barrett is zealously opposed to medical quackery," and Taylor suggested that members of the CCHI cooperate with Dr. Barrett in his quest to attack "quackery." There is little doubt as to why Taylor would want the members of the CCHI to cooperate with Dr. Barrett in his quest to attack "quackery." Barrett's specialty was attacking chiropractic, and, as the *AMA News* pointed out, Barrett's group was instrumental in helping to defeat legislation "requiring chiropractic coverage under Blue Shield."

This was one of the many connections between Barrett and members of the CCHI that have been uncovered over the years. However, this was the first *published* link that I could find. As will be seen later, Barrett's relationship with the governmental members (U.S. FDA, FTC, and U.S. Postal Service) continues even today.

His group was touted by the *AMA News* as providing the media with "one of the country's most complete clearinghouses of information on quackery." As Barrett had been given access to Taylor's files over the years, it is little wonder that Barrett has such a file of information on the AMA's economic competition. His group apparently parallels the AMA's anti-competitive campaign in many ways. Chiropractic was at the top of his list, as it was on the AMA's. At the time Taylor wrote his infamous memorandum to the AMA's Board of Trustees in 1971 stating that the Committee on Quackery's prime mission was first "the containment of chiropractic, and ultimately, the elimination of chiropractic," he was also feeding his files to Barrett, and apparently had been doing so for more than a year.

Among the targets that Barrett's group went after, in addition to chiropractic, were vitamins, "organic food fads," megavitamins; arthritis and cancer "quackery," naturopathy, acupuncture, and alternative "health promoters." Each of these alternative entities were also on the AMA's priority list. Considering the source of Barrett's "clearinghouse of information on quackery," it is not surprising that he pursued the same targets as those chosen by the AMA.

Here we see that a group, the Lehigh Valley Committee Against Health Fraud, was set up to act as a clearinghouse of information on "health fraud and quackery," probably using as a data base the AMA's Department of Investigation's files, as well as information that Barrett was able to assemble on his own. This group dedicates itself to attacking the same targets that the AMA has been going after for years. The AMA then uses this group's statements and press articles as a means to strengthen its own campaign against alternatives by pointing to this group and touting its work in the area of anti-quackery as being another source "outside of organized medicine" which feels the same way about alternatives. At one point the AMA reportedly turned over thousands of anti-chiropractic books to Barrett's group to sell and distribute around the country as part of its anti-chiropractic campaign.

It is obvious that the campaign by Taylor and the AMA against the alternative health-care system was destined to continue after the Department of Investigation, the Committee on Quackery, and the CCHI were dissolved. The AMA had invested too much money and time in this anti-competitive campaign. Barrett's group could easily function in place of the AMA's Propaganda Department, but there would have to be another entity to replace the CCHI. This was to come into the picture later.

In 1975, Barrett stated that his group was the only one of its kind in the United States. However, this was soon to change. In December 1977, a new group came into being in Southern California. It called itself the Southern California Council Against Health Fraud, and it was headed up by a man named William Jarvis, headquartered at Loma Linda University in Loma Linda, California. The group formed several years after the AMA's Department of Investigation disbanded. It is unlikely that Jarvis' group had the same access to the AMA Department of Investigation's clearinghouse on "quackery" that Barrett had. However, the two apparently did hook up. In December 1984, Jarvis changed the name of his group to the National Council Against Health Fraud (NCAHF). This group included Dr.

Stephen Barrett on its Board of Directors, and Barrett's group is an affiliate of the NCAHF to this day.

It is probable that the NCAHF used Barrett's data base as its own in setting up its "clearinghouse" on "quackery." This most likely took place just prior to Jarvis's group going "national." The similarities between the Barrett group, the Jarvis group, and the AMA's anti-competitive campaign are many. In one of the first newspaper articles on the Southern California Council Against Health Fraud in the Los Angeles *Times,* Jarvis was quoted as attacking vitamins, minerals, raw milk, and laetrile. Each of these was a target of the AMA's campaign from the past.

Soon after the NCAHF came into being, another group entered the scene. This was the Kansas City Council Against Health Fraud and Nutritional Abuse. It was headed by Dr. John Renner. His group also became an affiliate of the National Council Against Health Fraud. The Kansas City group changed its name a few times, also calling itself the Mid-West Council Against Health Fraud. Today Dr. John Renner heads up the Consumer Health Information Resource Institute, in Kansas City. Renner was also on the Board of Directors of the National Council Against Health Fraud (NCAHF), and his group is an affiliate member.

Each of these groups attacked the very same targets that the AMA had been attacking from 1963 to 1975, as well as many new ones. The difference was that on the surface they had no known connections to the AMA, even though they were apparently continuing the AMA's "quackery" campaign. It would appear that these groups are paralleling the old anti-competitive campaign that the medical establishment initiated with the help of the pharmaceutical industry in the name of "consumer protection." Each group claims to be independent of any medical association or the drug industry. However, this may not be the case. There is a very strong indication from documentation obtained over the years that these groups have been acting in the capacity of mouthpieces for orthodox medicine. This adds a new twist to the old anti-competitive propaganda campaign, and has been going on since 1983.

This campaign has been found to be financed by the vested interests within the pharmaceutical industry. Additionally, there are direct links between these groups and the AMA, the Federal Trade Commission, the United States Postal Inspectors, the United States Food and Drug Administration, and the Council of Better Business Bureaus. Each of these groups was at one time a member of the old Coordinating Conference on Health Information (CCHI). Their function today is apparently the same as it was when they were dictated to by the AMA at the CCHI meetings.

Although these groups claim to be independent of any vested interests, in doing their work to "protect the public" from "quackery and health fraud" there is every indication that this may not be the case.

What the AMA was to the earlier conspiracy and anti-competitive campaign these groups are to the current propaganda campaign. The differences are (1) who is fronting the campaign, and (2) who is openly financing the current campaign.

The people bearing the message are different than in the earlier campaign, but these new messengers are singing the same tune. They are apparently carrying forward an older campaign to restrain and eliminate the competitors of organized medicine and the pharmaceutical industry. These groups claim that they have no financial interest in conducting such anti-competitive activities. However, although they are not the direct beneficiaries of such a campaign, it is possible to benefit in several other ways. These groups and their spokespersons stand to gain (1) publicity, (2) public exposure, (3) increased membership, (4) funding for their activity, (5) financial rewards from the insurance industry in the form of consulting fees for "peer review work" and evaluation of insurance claims, and (6) honorariums paid to these "expert" speakers at conventions and conferences.

Who would stand to gain the most today from such an anti-competitive campaign? Upon inspection the answer would be (a) the medical establishment, and (b) the pharmaceutical industry. If the campaign against the alternative health-care system were successful, one might see the following:

1. More than 20 million patients who are currently going to chiropractors for back problems would be forced to go to medical doctors. This is a conservative estimate.
2. Instead of a chiropractic adjustment, these patients would now be confronted with surgery or drugs or both for their pain.
3. The pharmaceutical industry would stand to gain a tremendous additional income from the drugs that the medical doctors would prescribe.
4. The patients seeking chelation therapy would be forced to undergo heart-bypass surgery or other risky surgical procedures. In addition, they would be put on heart medication and

other drugs. In this way both the medical profession and the drug companies would profit.

5. The overall dollar amount spent on health care in 1992 was $817 billion. Of this amount, drugs sold to the public totaled $56.8 billion. The medical and pharmaceutical establishment would control all of the health-care pie. The bottom line is profit.

6. The people taking vitamins, minerals, supplements, and herbs would be forced to either get these through an M.D. by way of a prescription or resort to pharmaceuticals instead of these supplements and/or herbs. There is currently a push in Congress that, if successful, could result in herbs and certain supplements being taken off the market (some have already been taken off the shelves of health food stores) and put into the hands of M.D.s. These items would be made available only through prescriptions, or, worse, would be no longer available at all. At the very least, a charge for an office visit to obtain these supplements by prescription would substantially raise the cost to the consumer.

Additionally, this campaign has targeted vitamins, homeopathy, naturopathy, and many others. The removal of these options would represent many billions of dollars in new drug sales.

The increase in drug sales is good reason in itself to conduct a campaign directed at one's economic competitors. The earlier campaign and the current one have *dollars and profits* as one common denominator. The other common denominator is that both campaigns are in blatant violation of antitrust laws, as well as RICO conspiracy laws. There can be little doubt that the current crusade is just an extension of the earlier campaign.

The current campaign has several elements in it that were not seen as frequently in the old AMA campaign. These include such illegal acts as breaking and entry, unauthorized phone taps, the theft of files from practitioners offices, intimidation and harassment of patients, violations of search-and-seizure statutes, physical violence and threats of violence, and break-ins into attorneys' offices involving the theft of case records. In most cases, the perpetrators of these illegal acts have not yet been identified or prosecuted. However, these crimes *are* being committed against alternative practitioners, manufacturers, and distributors.

The one thing about the current campaign that is very different from the old AMA campaign is that the funding lines have been discovered. It is clear who is behind this campaign, and it is not a shock to anyone familiar with the vested interests in the pharmaceutical industry.

The old campaign and the current campaign have this in common: *the vested interests want the whole pie and thus more of the profits available in the health-care marketplace.* Unfortunately, they have been very successful in their attempt to accomplish this end.

Chapter 4

The Current Campaign

"STRATEGY—To utilize public service announcements (PSAs) in public service media channels in electronic and print media, and a public relations program, backed by volunteer effort and funding, sponsored by both the PAC (Pharmaceutical Advertising Council) and the FDA."
[From the 1983 PAC/FDA Public Service
Anti-Quackery Program.]

The current campaign's strategy is much more complex in its efforts to exclude the alternative health-care system from mainstream America. It involves a network of people using many seemingly different organizations and groups. However, this complex web may in fact constitute what is known as an "interlocking directorate."

It began in 1983 when the Pharmaceutical Advertising Council (PAC) and the United States Food and Drug Administration (FDA) signed an agreement to enter into a *joint campaign* which they called a Public Service Anti-Quackery Campaign.

PAC and the FDA officially signed this agreement in March 1984. However, plans were developed and actions were taken for almost a year prior. This entire campaign continues to be financed jointly by the FDA and the drug companies. Using the cover of a "health-care coalition," the parties involved have been directing their anti-competitive campaign directly at those entities that are in *economic competition* with the pharmaceutical and medical industries.

The economic competitors who have been targeted by this campaign are referred to only as "quacks" or "health frauds." These labels position the competitors (in the eyes of the government, the media, and the public) as something less than desirable.

The most chilling and bizarre aspect of this unholy alliance between the FDA and the pharmaceutical industry is that the very industry the FDA should be looking into, the drug industry, is instead the FDA's partner in a campaign designed to direct the FDA at the drug industry's economic competitors. Instead of policing the drug industry, the FDA is going after targets *the drug industry says* need to be investigated and prosecuted. The result of such an anti-competitive alliance is, of course, the destruction of the economic competitors of the pharmaceutical houses. Thus, billions of dollars in profits are redirected into the pockets of the drug companies that are dictating this campaign to the FDA.

According to documents obtained from the FDA and from PAC, representatives from the FDA and PAC worked out the initial funding for out-of-pocket expenses to get the campaign started. The person who headed up this campaign for the drug industry was Paul Chusid, then president of the now-defunct Grey Medical Advertising firm in New York City. Grey Medical was one of the largest medical advertising firms in the world, with offices all over the world. Chusid was also a member of PAC at the time the campaign was initially developed. Chusid's client list at Grey Medical included Lederle and Syntex pharmaceutical companies. Also on the Board of PAC was a representative from Hoffman-LaRoche drug company. These three drug houses put up an initial $105,000, while Chusid put together a grant request and received another $55,000 from the FDA. The whole campaign was put together on a small budget of $160,000. However, there are indications that much more than this has been put into this campaign over the years. Some speculate that tens of millions have been poured into the campaign over the past ten years.

In a letter dated May 27, 1983, to Paul Chusid, Joseph Hile, then Associate Commissioner for Regulatory Affairs of the FDA, stated, "The press release as drafted leaves out mention of the $160,000 total out-of-pocket cost of the program. This was done intentionally as we believe that the $160,000 doesn't *begin to tell the true expenditures that will eventually be involved.*" [Emphasis added.]

On March 20, 1985, Roger Miller, Director of Communications Staff, of the Public Health Services Department of Health and Human Services, wrote FDA Commissioner Frank Young. He stated, "Chusid has collected $50,000 for production work on the campaigns. That is not a lot of money for the three campaigns, but it should carry us for some time. FDA's obligations are to reproduce and distribute the campaign materials. I estimate that will cost the agency about $30,000 per campaign."

What was possibly meant by the "three campaigns" was that they would put on three "Conferences on Health Fraud." Each would be in a different city, and each would have speakers, booths, materials, slide shows, videos, and so on. By 1988 they had conducted more than 20 such campaigns in as many different cities. To date, the number is estimated to be more than 40 such campaigns across the country.

Assuming that Miller's figures are correct, keeping in mind the original $105,000 from three drug companies and the $55,000 from the FDA, this is about a 2-to-1 ratio between the two funding sources. In addition, there was the reported $50,000 Miller said that Chusid collected "for production work." This $50,000 was collected almost two full years after the initial funding was received from the three drug companies. Even if each campaign cost only $50,000 (and it could be closer to $80,000), a conservative estimate of the cost of the 40+ campaigns would run anywhere from $2 million to $3.2 million. This does not include the television and radio ads that were produced. These were projected to be produced on a "volunteer" basis. If one contracted at going industry rates for such a media campaign, it is estimated that the cost would be in the tens of millions over a ten-year period.

It is also possible that the three campaigns referred to were advertising campaigns, and the $50,000 collected for production costs was related to a media campaign, or television/radio advertising. If that's the case, then the expense for such a media campaign would be *in addition to* putting on the National Health Fraud Conferences around the country. The conference expenses would include travel, lodging, and speaker expenses, plus printing costs for pamphlets, brochures, and programs for distribution by the FDA.

Chusid sought money, volunteer time, and creative ideas for an ad campaign from more than 4,000 advertising and public relation firms. He also sent letters to solicit funds from more than 200 pharmaceutical companies. Within the first year, he got positive responses from no fewer than another 23 pharmaceutical houses. This meant that a total of 26 drug companies were involved in the funding by November 1985. When requested, he sent me the list of contributors up to that time. The letter, dated November 15, 1985, had a joint logo of PAC and the F.D.A.

In a letter to Paul Chusid as President of Grey Medical International, dated November 29, 1984, Roger Miller, Director of Communications Staff of the FDA, stated, "Enclosed is a draft press release on Jim Miller, the FTC chairman, joining the panel of experts who will judge the health fraud submissions. [Note: These were the ads for the campaign submitted by various ad companies.] I sent a copy to FTC for comment. I figure you can release it on our joint letterhead. Of course, we could release it from here but then we would have to get approval all the way up to the [Health and Human Services] Secretary's office, so let's not bother with that."

The red tape to which Miller refers is exactly the type that the FDA and FTC knew they would run into, and that Taylor had earlier envisioned avoiding when he suggested the CCHI be called a "conference" and not a committee.

Miller's letter to Chusid also points out the fact that the FTC "is anxious to help us with the project and be identified as closely as possible with it, so we ought to take advantage of that."

There are many points of similarity between the old AMA campaign and the current PAC/FDA campaign. One vehicle that the AMA used during the 1960s in its campaign was to hold conferences called Congresses on Quackery. These were jointly sponsored by the AMA, the FDA, the U.S. Postal Service, and the U.S. Federal Trade Commission. They were held in several cities around the country and were used to launch propaganda directed at those alternatives targeted in the AMA's campaign.

The AMA would have "experts" on various forms of "quackery" speak on their subject of expertise. The programs always included speakers from the FDA, the U.S. Postal Service, the FTC, and the Council of Better Business Bureaus. The AMA also helped fund booklets, pamphlets, and brochures which were jointly sponsored by the FTC, the FDA, the Postal Service, and the Council of Better Business Bureaus. Usually, whatever the CCHI (Coordinating Conference on Health Information) was targeting at their secret meetings also made it onto the program. The guests and audience usually consisted of hundreds of officials from the government agencies that the AMA was trying to influence against the alternatives. The invited guests also included key Congressional leaders the AMA was attempting to influence against the alternatives.

Targets at these Congresses on Quackery almost always included chiropractic, vitamin therapy, homeopathy, naturopathy, and alternative cancer, heart, and arthritis treatments.

The private-sector groups and governmental agencies involved in the old AMA campaign included:

Private Sector:

American Medical Association
American Cancer Society
Arthritis Foundation
American Pharmaceutical Association
Council of Better Business Bureaus (CBBB)
National Health Council

Government Sector:

U.S. Postal Service
U.S. Food and Drug Administration (FDA)
U.S. Federal Trade Commission (FTC)

The *current* campaign includes all of these entities except the National Health Council, plus the following:

HIMA (insurance industry representative)
Pharmaceutical Advertising Council (PAC)
National Council Against Health Fraud (NCAHF)
National Health Care Anti-Fraud Association (NHCAA)
Emprise Inc.

Instead of calling the current meetings Congresses on Quackery, those currently involved call them Conferences on Health Fraud.

In a letter dated February 7, 1985, Roger Miller sent Paul Chusid information about the "Roper poll on quackery." This was a survey of the general public that the PAC/FDA campaign had commissioned in October 1984, in order to identify targets for the campaign. An inspection of the survey is most revealing.

Judging from the survey questions asked, it appears that those surveyed would get the impression that they were being asked these questions to solicit how *effective* these treatments were. However, the survey results apparently were used to identify what the public *considered most effective* in order to determine top-ranking priorities for the "anti-quackery" campaign. The following is a sampling of the survey:

How effective do you think (read item) is/are?

	Heard of	Very Effective	Moderately Effective	Not Very Effective/other
a. Vitamins for improved health	95%	29%	49%	9% / 8%
b. Chiropractors for back problems	85%	25%	40%	8% / 12%
g. Psychological Counseling for improved mental health	68%	25%	32%	4% / 8%

The category that "scored" fourth-highest was alternative cancer treatments. Others that appeared in the survey were weight reduction, body wraps for slimming, electrical muscle stimulators for body toning, creams to eliminate cellulite, DMSO for aches and pains, air ionizers for feeling healthier, laetrile for cancer, pills for a better sex life, pills to sober up, and creams to grow hair. The Big Three targets for the campaign became *(1) vitamins, (2) chiropractic, and (3) alternative cancer treatments.* All of the others named have been targeted in this campaign as well.

In putting together this campaign, officials of the pharmaceutical industry stated that they would not identify specific products or specific manufacturers by name. However, according to documents obtained from the FDA and PAC, they did in fact name specific products, manufacturers, treatments, modalities, services, clinics, and practitioners. A list of specific targets was drawn up but not released to the general public. The list was circulated within the PAC/FDA campaign and was considered to be *the* priority target list for the campaign.

The priority list of targets was attached to the document "Backgrounder on PAC/FDA Public Service Campaign Against Quackery." Apparently this list was made up *before* the Roper survey was sent out; in looking over the list one can see that most items in the survey apparently came from the list that was made up for the campaign. What apparently happened is that the FDA gathered up reports from all of their field and district offices on various products and companies that were of interest to the pharmaceutical industry. The campaign list was then made up based on this information. Entitled "Health Fraud Products," the list was four pages long and was divided into three categories. The following is a duplication of the target list made up for the campaign:

Health Fraud Products

Health frauds are listed in two categories: Fad Diets and Drug and Device Claims. The products listed are those in which consumers expressed the most interest, or on which FDA initiated action.

FAD DIETS

Herbal Life
Primarily a diet product, made with unproven herbs. It is marketed by Herbal Life International Inc., Culver City, CA., and it is quite often a pyramid operation. The CAO (Con-

sumer Affairs Office, FDA) in St. Louis says it is being
promoted for arthritis. The Nashville CAO reports the product
is gaining momentum.

Shaklee
Variety of food supplement and diet products. In the past
FDA has taken action because of false and misleading
therapeutic claims. Although the firm has revised its literature,
some promoters give false claims. There have been many
consumer inquiries to OCA (the Office of Consumer Affairs),
and six OCAs have reported interest by consumers.

Spirulina
A blue-green algae which can be legally marketed as a
food, is being promoted as a quick way to lose weight and
rejuvenate the body. Sales soared when National Enquirer
promoted it last year. It is primarily sold in health food stores.
CAOs still report consumer interest.

DRUG AND DEVICE CLAIMS

Aloe Vera
A common houseplant that has been promoted in recent
years for curing a variety of medical problems, including
arthritis, heart disease, and cancer. The FDA Dallas District
Office reported expanding sales and types of uses. For example, genital herpes, skin cancer, heart disease. Products are
distributed through pyramid operations and health food stores.
Manufacturers are careful to make no health claims on product
labels.

Herpes Cures
CAOs report consumer interest is growing in a variety of
fraudulent treatments: L-Lysine tablets, Herp-L supplements,
BHT food additives in high dosage, Gossypol (cotton seed)
and LSO lithium succinate. The Kansas City CAO reports
items are sold in health food stores. The CAO in San Francisco
reports it is a "burgeoning drug quackery topic. . ."

Starch Blockers
Tablets prepared from raw beans, are claimed to block
starch digestion and help weight control. In July 1982, FDA
stated they are an unapproved drug. More than three hundred
manufacturers and distributors were told to halt production.

Although some CAOs report interest has waned, the St. Louis CAO reports interest is still high. There have been three FDA seizures between January and March 1983.

Laetrile
Although proven ineffective as a cancer treatment, many states have legalized this substance. In January 1983, a bill was introduced in Congress to permit introduction of laetrile into interstate commerce without approval of NDA (New Drug Application) under the Act. Also, 215 consumers commented to FDA for approval of Laetrile (through the National Health Federation).

DMSO
The chemical compound dimethyl sulfoxide is a liquid residue of wood pulp. Its major use is as an industrial solvent. Although it has only one accepted medical use, for a rare bladder condition, it has been promoted as a cure for arthritis. FDA has moved against the manufacturer with a number of seizures. However, there continues to be interest in and use of DMSO. Since January 1983, the NCDB Consumer and Professional Staff has received 15 letters on this product.

Gerovital
This product is a solution of procaine, better known as Novocain. Dr. Anna Aslan of Rumania has used it to combat aging. It is an unapproved and misbranded drug. Since January 1983, the NCDB Consumer and Professional Staff has received 38 letters on this product.

Negative Ion Generators
These are small electrical appliances which project ions (charged particles in the air). Promoters claim they create a sensation of well-being. In the past, FDA has taken regulatory action for misbranding. However, in the past few years ads have appeared in national magazines and on TV promoting these products.

EMS
Electrical Muscle Stimulators, used for weight loss, contract muscles by passing electric currents through electrodes applied to the skin. They are used in health spas and figure salons. In 1981-82, FDA ordered 15 seizures and sent 25 regulatory letters. An import alert has also been issued.

Sexual Rejuvenation

NSP-70, Corazine-DL and Bio-Gene 81 are products promoted to restore or improve sexual potency. However, the ingredients in these products are ordinary vitamins and minerals. These products are promoted primarily through advertisements.

Hair Restorers

Eleven CAOs in the past eighteen months reported consumer interest in various products to cure baldness. An Advisory Review Panel on OTC Miscellaneous External Drug Products has concluded all hair grower and hair loss prevention active ingredients are reviewed as safe, but none are effective.

POSSIBLE FUTURE

Glucomman

A product promoted as a dietary supplement for weight loss, is said to consist of a powder extracted from the roots of the konjac plant. Promoters claim it absorbs liquid and swells in the stomach to form a gel which reduces hunger. (FDA Talk Paper 8/12/82.) CAO Qtr. Act. Rprts. (Quarterly Activities Reports) for 1st Qtr. FY 83 report the following information: Don Aird, Dallas District said there are 2000 investors in Manin Slim, a possible pyramid scheme, which promotes Glucomman. General Nutrition Centers are promoting Super Manin. Vera Lina, a combination of Spirulina and Aloe Vera is also very popular. These products are being advertised in two leading Dallas newspapers. Chicago CAO had 20 calls on Glucomman. Some consumer inquiries were also made to the CAOs in New York, Kansas City, Cincinnati and New Orleans.

Laser Face-Lifts and Laser Acupuncture

Mainly used by chiropractors, and sometimes called "biostimulation." In non surgical face-lifts, the laser beam is directed at certain acupuncture points on the face, or is scanned across the entire part of the face to be treated. In laser acupuncture, a low power laser beam instead of needles is applied to traditional acupuncture points. (FDA Talk Paper, 4/23/82.) CAO Qrt. Act. Rpt. 1st Qrt. FY 83 from Dallas reports item on it in Austin newspaper.

Vitamin A
CSPI Petition of 3/31/83 urges FDA to require warning
labels on all vitamin supplements containing more than 10,000
International Units (IU) of Vitamin A. It discusses the hazards
of Vitamin A toxicity resulting from excessive use of Vitamin
A for all population groups but particularly pregnant women
and children. CSPI is also urging FDA to investigate the
labeling of Vitamin A in baby foods.

In looking over this list, it becomes clear that many of the
products targeted are in direct economic competition to products
made by the pharmaceutical industry. In terms of categories of types
of products targeted by the Anti-Quackery Campaign paid for by
drug company dollars, the following comes to light:

Weight Loss/Diet Products—Products used for these purposes were mentioned seven separate times. This category of
product represents billions of dollars in lost drug sales to the
pharmaceutical industry.

Products for Treating Arthritis—Products used for arthritis
were mentioned three times on this priority list and represent
hundreds of millions of dollars, if not billions, in lost sales by
the drug companies involved in this campaign.

*Products for Treatment of Heart Problems/Cancer/Her-
pes*—Products which address these areas of concern by consumers each received two mentions in the target list. Again,
these alternative remedies represent a loss of billions of dollars
in sales to the very same drug companies which helped finance
this campaign against these products which are their economic
competitors.

In addition to these facts, other indicators contributed to these
products and companies making the priority list of the Anti-Quackery Campaign. At least three products or manufacturers on the list
were mentioned as "pyramid schemes" or "possible or suspected
pyramid schemes." According to information assembled during this
investigation, none of the companies mentioned as pyramid schemes
was ever cited or found to have been involved in pyramid schemes.
Another of the criteria seems to be that a product or company had
received inquiries from the public/consumers. This does not specify
if these inquiries or letters were complaints. As a matter of fact,

nowhere in the four-page list is there a mention of any consumers complaining about a product or company. To the contrary, using the FDA's own words, there were instances where the products or companies were the subject of "consumer interest." This is not the same as a "consumer complaint." In some cases, consumers wrote letters in support of a product or wrote letters asking about a product.

The items on the FDA's list, which was turned in to the Pharmaceutical Advertising Council and used as a guideline of priority "quack" products to go after, seem to have drawn the notice of the FDA because these products and companies were "gaining momentum," "expanding sales," or attracted reports of "interest by consumers." They also received attention by the FDA because they advertised in national newspapers, national magazines, or large metropolitan newspapers.

This brings one to question why the FDA would go after a product or company that the general public/consumer wants to use or is interested in. It also raises the point that it appears that the FDA has selected products and companies which are being successful. If sales were up, or the product was found to be "gaining momentum," it is apparent that the FDA considered this to be a very bad indicator.

Examination of the FDA's policy, activity, and criteria regarding products and manufacturers who are in direct economic competition to the FDA's pharmaceutical-industry allies raises some serious ethical questions about the FDA's alliance with the drug industry in this Anti-Quackery Campaign.

The FDA's Office of Enforcement, Division of Compliance Policy, Associate Commissioner for Regulatory Affairs, adopted a new policy on "Health Fraud." The policy established that:

> In evaluating regulatory actions against indirect health hazard products, the following factors should be considered by district and centers. . .
> Point 6—The source of the product, size of the industry distributing the same or similar products, and the impact of the action on that source or industry. . .
> Point 7—The cost of the product, the economic impact of this cost on the target user group, as well as the profit (per sale) realized from the sale of the product. . .
> Point 8—The amount (dollar and volume) of product sold, and the geographical scope of its distribution.

Additionally, the FDA outlined its criteria for taking action against a product that is new on the market, its dollar volume in sales not yet having been established. It stated, "We recognize that when a product with unproven therapeutic claims is first introduced, it is difficult to predict its economic impact because, whether or not a regulatory action is taken, the product may not be accepted in the marketplace."

And finally, the bottom line on FDA actions against any of these alternative products is really measured in this statement in its policy: "Regulatory Actions should be considered for products of limited health significance when it appears there is a growing national or substantial regional market for them."

In the end, the FDA's actions against any and all health products, usually those which are in direct economic competition to the pharmaceutical interests that the FDA serves, is determined by:

First: Dollars in total sales of a product
Second: Volume of sales nationally
Third: A growing geographical market for a product
Fourth: Acceptance of a product in the marketplace

In other words, the FDA will go after only those products that are popular, successful, receiving profits from sales, and recognized nationally in the marketplace by the consumers who buy the product.

In the free-enterprise system, the consumer is the ultimate judge of whether a product is good or not. If a product does not produce results, then the simple fact is that consumers will not buy that product any more. The result is that the product will not stay on the market very long. Even the FDA recognizes this fact, because it uses this law of economics as a guideline for its policy on products.

We see here further evidence that the FDA is working for its allies in the pharmaceutical industry. If a product which happens to be in direct competition with the drug industry does well in sales, is popular with the general public, and receives national attention in the marketplace and in the news media, then it is a threat to the drug industry and should therefore be attacked by the FDA.

Using this logic as a measuring stick against the actions of FDA over the years against alternative products, treatments, services, modalities, practitioners, and manufacturers, one can see that there is a *direct cause-and-effect relationship* between the alternatives that have been targeted and the fact that they are all in direct *economic competition* with the pharmaceutical industry.

The chapters that follow examine this campaign as a direct result of the pharmaceutical industry's quest to eliminate its economic competition from the health-care marketplace by using the FDA and others. The analysis of this relationship should leave no doubt in anyone's mind as to why this campaign is going on and who is benefiting from it.

The following is a very quick comparison of the earlier campaign headed by the AMA and the current FDA/PAC campaign. These similarities between the two campaigns are not by coincidence, but by design.

PARALLELS IN CONSPIRACIES

Earlier Campaign	Current Campaign
TITLE OF MEETING	
Congress on Quackery	Conference on Health Fraud
GROUP BEHIND CAMPAIGN	
Coordinating Conference on Health Information	PAC/FDA Anti-Quackery Campaign
GOVERNMENT MEMBERS OF GROUP	
FDA	FDA
FTC	FTC
USPO	USPS
Office of Consumer Affairs	Office of Consumer Affairs
NON-GOVERNMENTAL MEMBERS OF GROUP	
Council of B.B.B.	Council of B.B.B.
Arthritis Foundation	Arthritis Foundation
American Cancer Society	American Medical Association
American Medical Association	Pharmaceutical Advertising
American Pharmaceutical Assn	Council
SPOKESGROUP FOR CAMPAIGN	
American Medical Association	National Council Against Health Fraud
FUNDING FOR CAMPAIGN	
American Medical Association	Pharmaceutical Companies

SPONSOR FOR CONFERENCES

AMA	PAC/FDA
FDA	FTC
FTC	USPS
USPO	NCAHF

DICTATING GOVERNMENTAL ACTIONS

AMA	NCAHF & PAC

PRIMARY SOURCE OF DATA ON QUACKERY

AMA	NCAHF & PAC

SECONDARY SOURCES OF DATA ON QUACKERY

Arthritis Foundation	Emprise Inc.
American Cancer Society	American Cancer Society
Council of B.B.B.	Council of B.B.B.
FDA	FDA
FTC	FTC
U.S.P.O.	U.S.P.S.

GOVERNMENT TASK FORCE MEMBERS

FDA	FDA
FTC	FBI
U.S.P.O.	U.S.P.S.
	FTC
	Justice Dept.
	DHHS

INSURANCE INDUSTRY REPRESENTATIVES

Health Insurance Assoc. of America	NHCAA
Blue Cross/Blue Shield	Blue Cross/Blue Shield
Medicare	Medicare/HIAA

The two campaigns are similar in other ways, but these are the major items that parallel these two anti-competitive campaigns. The following chapters will clearly define the interests behind this campaign, and who the victims are.

PAC/FDA CHART

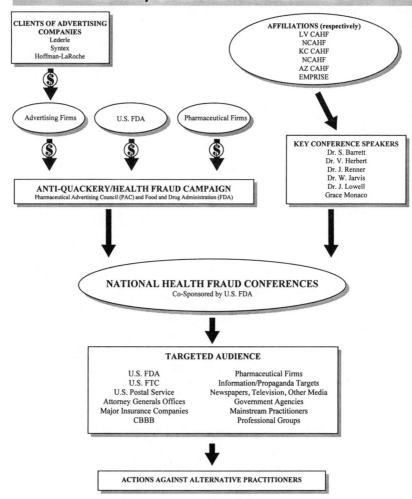

CLIENTS OF ADVERTISING COMPANIES
Lederle
Syntex
Hoffman-LaRoche

AFFILIATIONS (respectively)
LV CAHF
NCAHF
KC CAHF
NCAHF
AZ CAHF
EMPRISE

Advertising Firms

U.S. FDA

Pharmaceutical Firms

KEY CONFERENCE SPEAKERS
Dr. S. Barrett
Dr. V. Herbert
Dr. J. Renner
Dr. W. Jarvis
Dr. J. Lowell
Grace Monaco

ANTI-QUACKERY/HEALTH FRAUD CAMPAIGN
Pharmaceutical Advertising Council (PAC) and Food and Drug Administration (FDA)

NATIONAL HEALTH FRAUD CONFERENCES
Co-Sponsored by U.S. FDA

TARGETED AUDIENCE

U.S. FDA
U.S. FTC
U.S. Postal Service
Attorney Generals Offices
Major Insurance Companies
CBBB

Pharmaceutical Firms
Information/Propaganda Targets
Newspapers, Television, Other Media
Government Agencies
Mainstream Practitioners
Professional Groups

ACTIONS AGAINST ALTERNATIVE PRACTITIONERS

Chapter 5

The October Plan

"Sharing information is lawful, unless it reduces competition."
[Timothy J. Muris, Director of the Bureau of Competition, Federal Trade Commission.]

In October 1986, a plan was made to form a group called Public Issues in Health Care Choices (PIHCCO), later known as Emprise, Inc. The following quote from the plan describes the group's purpose:

> Unfortunately, no organization currently serves as a clearing house for the names of the defrauders; their products and services, and descriptions and formulations of these products and services. The proposed new organization would assume this function.

The concept of a clearinghouse on quackery is as old as the American Medical Association's campaign against its competitors. The AMA served as a clearinghouse for many years. However, in doing so it also opened itself up to lawsuits for libel, slander, and conspiracy to restrain trade. This new group proposed a way around such liabilities. It stated that it would act as a "neutral organization with no vested interest in [the] outcome, focusing only on facts that are needed by patient, provider and insurer to make sound medical choices."

This sounds like a logical and sound proposal, until one looks at the entire plan and sees who is involved. The PIIHCCO, referred to hereafter as Emprise, was initially made up of three individuals: attorney Grace Powers Monaco, attorney Ron Schwartz, and Dr. John Renner, a well-known anti-alternative spokesman and member of the board of the National Council Against Health Fraud.

One of the plan's more Orwellian aspects was outlined as follows:

Development of position papers to support the need for any physician or health-care provider using certain modalities in their practice to *register* with the state, indicate the representations they make about the role of that product/procedure in their practice *and provide the names of patients receiving such care with a summary of their medical history to the appropriate state agency for follow-up.* [Emphasis added.]

For example, some of the modalities that a state or state regulatory agency might require that information on are: hair analysis for vitamin and mineral prescribing; chelation therapy for any use but the treatment of lead poisoning; DMSO for any use but interstitial cystitis; dental amalgam testing and cytotoxic testing. This data would permit the state agency to follow and assess the value of the therapy as well as providing, with patient consent, a pool of persons undergoing the therapy, at the option of the state, [who] could talk to others who are considering the therapy.

This is nothing less than a massive tracking system to keep tabs on the economic competitors of the pharmaceutical industry. This group proposed, in addition, to basically "analyze" various forms of alternative treatments, services, products, and modalities, then put together "papers" on these subjects which could then be used for a variety of purposes. According to the plan:

It [the group] would provide "white" papers which could be used to support a variety of proposed initiatives:
- legislation or regulatory proposals on a national or state level dealing with credentialling
- public safety hazards of some treatments
- drug or biologic regulation
- registration of products and claims
- registration of practitioners who offer certain modalities together with a listing of the claims made by the practitioner for them,
- insurance coverage/reimbursement issues including the potential for fraud, abuse and misrepresentation on insurance claims, and informed consent.

It stated that these same white papers could be "used to support patient and professional education efforts and media focuses." They could also be a basis of reliance by insurers for change in "insurance coverage and policy definition issues."

They proposed to form clusters of professionals allegedly with no vested interest in these studies, to sit in judgment of these alternative treatments, modalities, products, and services. These "experts" would then publish white papers which would be used for the stated purposes. What one sees here is the opposition to the alternatives putting together a group of "independent experts" who would sit in judgment of the very treatments they have made careers out of attacking. Some of the people involved in the proposed review process, which was funded by a federal grant, were:

Grace Powers Monaco, Attorney. She has been at the forefront of this anti-competitive campaign since at least 1984. She is a key contact with the insurance industry, an industry that has been directed against the various forms of alternative health care. She was also the attorney for the American Cancer Society at the time PIHCCO/Emprise started up. (It has been rumored that her client, the American Cancer Society, provided some of the funding to get her group off the ground in 1986.) She is on the Board of the National Council Against Health Fraud (NCAHF), and is on the Advisory Board of the National Association for Chiropractic Medicine (a group which will receive closer examination in the following chapters). She is also very well-connected in the federal government.

John Renner, M.D., of Kansas City, MO. He has risen in the anti-alternative campaign and movement and is one of the most outspoken critics of anything to do with alternative medicine. He had his own group, the Midwest Council Against Health Fraud, which was an affiliate of the NCAHF. He is reportedly the custodian of the data base on the alternatives and is a Board member of the NCAHF.

Victor Herbert, M.D., of New York City. He is another key spokesman for the pharmaceutical industry's anti-competitive campaign against the alternatives.

Stephen Barrett, M.D., of Allentown, PA. A psychiatrist, he is the first spokesman who set up a anti-alternative group, the Lehigh Valley Committee Against Health Fraud. He is also a key spokesman for the FDA/PAC Anti-Quackery Campaign.

William Jarvis, Ph.D., of Loma Linda, CA. He is president of the National Council Against Health Fraud and also a key spokesman for the FDA/PAC campaign against alternatives.

Ronald Schwartz, Attorney, of Washington, D.C. He was one of the founders of the PICCHO and was formerly the Deputy Assistant Inspector General of the Department of Health and Human Services. He was formerly Attorney Advisor to the Chairman of the Federal Trade Commission and is listed as an "expert in health fraud and abuse."

Michael Botts, Attorney, of Kansas City, MO. Formerly with the Iowa Attorney General's Office Task Force on Health Fraud, he is also the attorney for the NCAHF and has represented some of the other key spokesmen in lawsuits directed against writers and publishers involved in exposing this campaign.

It is important to note that most of these individuals have been working aggressively over the past ten years to condemn almost every aspect of the alternative health-care system. They have actively spoken out against various forms of the alternatives. They have worked actively to legislate against alternatives. They have been key spokesman at Congressional hearings directed against the alternatives and have been media contacts for quotes against the alternatives. In addition, most of these people have acted as key spokespersons for the pharmaceutical industry's anti-quackery campaign from the start.

The campaign has adversely influenced insurance carriers and providers against alternative health care, in some cases resulting in those aspects of alternative care not receiving coverage or reimbursement by insurance companies. The campaign has grossly affected the economic potential of thousands of practitioners around the country who are involved in alternative health care.

Each of these people has played a key role in the PAC/FDA anti-competitive campaign. They are by no means impartial, neutral, or without vested interests in the outcome of this "anti-quackery" campaign. They apparently form the nucleus of the Interlocking Directorate, which is allegedly the core group of those "inside the loop." Simply stated, an interlocking directorate is a group of individuals who continually show up on the boards of several groups and who have similar purposes. These key directors on each of these boards carry with them common goals from one group to another. Such people wield a vast amount of influence and control within the structure of each of the various groups they are involved with. In some cases an individual can adversely influence a group simply by advising that group or speaking at a conference put on by a group or acting in an unofficial capacity by supplying a group with information that adversely affects that group's decision about alternatives.

Apparently, this has been the case over and over through the past ten years.

Investigation and study of each of the groups that have been involved in this massive campaign against the alternatives reveals a common denominator throughout the campaign. No matter which group is involved, the same people repeatedly appear as key antagonists against the alternatives. The main groups that have been involved in one aspect or another in the campaign against the alternatives are as follows:

> Pharmaceutical Advertising Council (PAC/FDA Campaign)
> National Council Against Health Fraud (and affiliates)
> PIHCCO/Emprise
> National Health Care Anti-Fraud Association
> National Association for Chiropractic Medicine

The individuals involved in some way with each of these organizations are the key people, the movers and shakers, in this anti-competitive campaign. They have also apparently influenced several government agencies to take actions against the alternatives.

The fact is: *If the pharmaceutical industry had not initiated and paid for this campaign, the alternatives would not be in the economic struggle they are currently in.*

The fact is: *If the pharmaceutical industry did not have the FDA taking actions against the alternatives, and spokesmen attacking the alternatives as "quacks," the alternatives would not be fighting for their very survival today.*

There isn't one single aspect of the alternative health-care system that is not currently under attack from this massive campaign to eliminate competition from the health-care marketplace. Some targets are receiving a higher priority than others, but in the end they are all being targeted by this complex web of vested interests.

The modalities, treatments, products, services, practitioners, and manufacturers being used in the practice of health alternatives are in fact slated for extinction by the very nature of this campaign. The many lists of alternatives that are in circulation are being used to direct attacks upon them by government agencies. These lists have been put together for the sole purpose of targeting those listed for elimination.

Interviews conducted with officials of various government agencies around the country clearly show that the FDA, the Department of Health and Human Services, the Office of Inspector General, the U.S. Postal Inspectors Fraud Division, the Department of Justice, the U.S. Attorney's office, and the FBI, along with other agencies, all have taken actions directed against those named by the vested interests as "quacks" or "health frauds." In most cases the government agencies involved took action against the alternative targets only because they are influenced by the fact that those directing them to attack these targets are the "authorities" and "experts" on "quackery and health fraud." This is all part of a joint effort on the part of government and the private sector.

There is no doubt that state government agencies involved in this campaign were directed toward specific targets to investigate, indict, and prosecute as a direct result of the anti-alternatives campaign being pushed and financed by the drug industry. Extensive investigation into this campaign against the alternatives reveals this bottom line: This is all being done for the sake of profits for the pharmaceutical industry and orthodox medicine.

There is no question as to why the government has attacked the alternative product manufacturers, practitioners, clinics, treatments, modalities, and services. The targeted professions of chiropractic, homeopathy, naturopathy, acupuncture, alternative cancer, heart and arthritis treatments, and vitamins/herbs all came under fire as a direct result of this anti-competitive campaign.

It is well-known that monopoly cannot exist without the agreement and assistance of government, whether it be through the legislature or through regulatory and enforcement agencies of the federal and state governments. In some cases the government officials are really dupes who are simply doing their jobs. It has even been theorized that no government official ever takes action without being influenced by some non-governmental vested interest. This is historically the case with the "anti-quackery" campaign.

The government agencies caught in this web of influence include, but are not limited to, the following:

U.S. Department of Health and Human Services (DHHS)
Office of the Inspector General
Food and Drug Administration
U.S. Postal Service (U.S.P.S.)
U.S. Postal Inspectors, Fraud Division
U.S. Federal Trade Commission (FTC)

Bureau of Consumer Affairs
U.S. Department of Justice
U.S. Attorney's Office
Federal Bureau of Investigation
Federal Task Force on Health Fraud (FDA and others)
Federal Task Force on AIDS Fraud (FDA and others)
U.S. Drug Enforcement Agency (DEA)
U.S. Customs Service
Internal Revenue Service
Offices of State Attorneys General (50 states)
National Association of Attorneys General (NAAG)

All of these have played major roles in carrying out the work of the Anti-Quackery Campaign, either directly with the pharmaceutical industry, or indirectly through one of the many arms of this campaign against alternatives.

The following people have been found to be involved in one way or another with the main groups that comprise the campaign against the alternatives:

John Renner, M.D.
NCAHF—Board member
Emprise Grant Project
NACM—Advisory Board
ACSH—Advisory Board/contributor
NHCAA—member/speaker
PAC/FDA Campaign—key spokesman
NCAHF Affiliate—Director
Insurance advisor
Key media contact for campaign

Grace Monaco, Esq.
Emprise Grant Project
NCAHF
NACM—Board of Advisors
ACSH
NHCAA—Speaker
PAC/FDA Campaign—Speaker
Insurance industry contact
Key media contact

William Jarvis, Ph.D.
Emprise Inc./Grant Project
NCAHF—President
ACSH—Contributor
NACM—Advisory Board
NHCAA—Speaker
PAC/FDA Campaign—Speaker
Key media contact

Stephen Barrett, M.D.
Emprise Inc./Grant Project
NCAHF
ACSH
NACM—Advisory Board
PAC/FDA Campaign—Speaker
NCAHF Affiliate—Director
Insurance industry contact
Key media contact

Jim Lowell, Ph.D.
Emprise Inc./Grant Project
NCAHF
ACSH
NHCAA—Speaker
PAC/FDA Campaign—Speaker
NCAHF Affiliate—Director
Key media contact

Victor Herbert, M.D.
Emprise Inc./Grant Project
NCAHF
ACSH
PAC/FDA Campaign—Speaker
Key media contact

It's important to note that these individuals are members, speakers, Board members, Advisory Board members, or key spokespersons for many of the same groups involved in the "anti-quackery" campaign.

When the PICHHO, later Emprise, first laid out its October Plan to study the alternatives, it proposed to report its "independent" findings to the insurance industry and federal and state government agencies. It didn't reveal *exactly* what vehicle it would use. It wasn't until Emprise submitted a grant request to the Department of Health and Human Services, Public Health Service, National Institute of Health, that the exact mechanism was revealed. These FOIA Grant documents were obtained by attorney Michael Evers of Texas, who represents alternative practitioners.

Emprise had proposed that several "expert panels" would be put together. The assignment would be the independent evaluation of various forms of alternative medicine, treatments, modalities, services, and products. These experts not only provided their talents to evaluate the alternatives, but also provided most of the data base upon which the study was based.

The first three proposals in the Grant request were:

(1) *Generalize evaluation strategy to major unproven and questionable therapies.* We propose to evaluate the 29 major and unproven therapies and cover inactive therapies and emerging therapies in overviews.

(2) *Assess for Validity and Accuracy.* Use panels of experts to review each writeup to insure it is complete, current, valid, accurate, and objective. Consensus panels will be established by discipline and will review all writeups falling within their subject matter. The panels will be: DIAGNOSTIC TESTS; DIET, NUTRITION AND DETOXIFICATION; DRUGS, BIOLOGICALS AND IMMUNE APPROACHES; ETHNIC, FOLK, HERBAL, BOTANNICAL AND ROOT MEDICINES; AND PSYCHOLOGICAL/PSYCHO-NEUROIMMUNOLOGICAL APPROACHES.

(3) *Refine the consensus panel strategy.* In the process of writing up the therapies, evaluate the dual use of experts [to write and to critique] to develop a system which can be used in Phase 3 to maintain the files.

The Grant request highlighted why there was a need to critically evaluate the alternatives, stating that:

Purveyors of questionable therapies seem to hold the view "that it is the job of science to disprove crazy ideas." Dwindling research funds should not be utilized to disprove the fads, frauds, and fancies of alternative medicine. However, the medical profession needs to be adequately prepared to educate the public on those issues lest *disappointment in us will surely drive many into the hands of the magicians.* [Emphasis added.]

The plan was to do "specially tailored, critical evaluations of these therapies, their rationale, literature relied upon, claims made, and anecdotal evidence presented. . ." It stated that such evaluation was essential to "filling in the knowledge gaps" without wasting funds on "expensive clinical trial procedures for unproductive therapies."

If the data to be used in this study and evaluation of the alternatives did not include clinical studies or clinical trial procedures, then where was this data to come from? The information uncovered in this investigation determined the following disturbing facts.

According to the Grant report dated June 1, 1988, the FDA had "pledged its efforts to continue working with other organizations to form coalitions which are aimed at sharing information and at providing consumers, health professionals and the news media with the information they need to avoid health fraud." At this point one must ask: *Who* is providing the FDA with the information that it is using as a guideline to what is or isn't 'health fraud and quackery'?

The Grant report further stated, "The societal impact of this program, referenced by the FDA, (see Health Fraud Status Report, Office of Consumer Affairs, February 1987), is confirmed by Dr. Jarvis, President of the National Council Against Health Fraud: 'we feel that this type of program is essential if the present meager anti-quackery resources of the nation are to be made more effective . . . we can be very effective if we can organize the data base, communicate and make our resources available to those who need it.'" (Letter of April 16, 1987, from Dr. Jarvis to Mrs. Monaco.) The appendices to the Grant included the full letter from Jarvis, which "pledged data base support."

The Report goes on to state, "Leaders in efforts against health fraud (including Dr. Barrie Cassileth, University of Pennsylvania, James Lowell, President, Arizona Council Against Health Fraud, Charles Moertel, M.D.,Dr. Benjamin Wilson, M.D., Oregon, Dr. John H. Renner, activist against health fraud in Missouri, Stephen Barrett, M.D., President of the Lehigh Valley Committee Against Health Fraud, and William Jarvis, M.D., National Council Against

Health Fraud) have pledged access to their materials and their efforts
to this project."

Considering that the members of the National Council Against
Health Fraud have been the key spokesmen for the Pharmaceutical
Advertising Council/FDA's Anti-Quackery Campaign from the
start, it is predictable that they would jump into this study, offering
their services and their data base to help "evaluate" the alternatives.

The report also revealed that the Grant study would include more
than just alternative cancer and AIDS treatments. It stated:

> Many of the unproven treatments for cancer are claimed to
> work on other diseases. For example, proponents of metabolic
> therapy claim that the removal of mercury amalgam fillings
> for the cure of allergies should also be undertaken by cancer
> patients to reduce the burden of metal toxicities in order to free
> the immune system to focus on eliminating cancer. Similar
> rationales are articulated for cytotoxic testing, hair analysis,
> vitamin supplementation and the like.
>
> This crossover of therapies for many different disease
> usages presents a unique opportunity for the use of a central
> data base that references what other diseases these treatments
> are claimed to ameliorate or cure.

The concept of including other diseases into the data base for the
study on alternatives received support from the Arthritis Foundation
and the National Multiple Sclerosis Society, to name two.

The uses to which these expert critiques would be put included
". . . offering a consulting service utilizing the data base and the
support core working group professionals to review and evaluate
insurance claims based on unproven and questionable cancer
therapies from a legal and scientific basis." They also planned to
"lease access to the data base and computer program to insurers for
use in evaluating claims submitted by patients for questionable and
unproven cancer therapies. This would also include lease to fiscal
intermediaries handling Medicare and Medicaid claims, and for use
in investigations of fraud and abuse."

As we have established, the working data base was put together
from the resources materials and libraries of some of the most
anti-alternative people in the country. The Grant Report revealed the
following regarding this library of information on "quackery and
health fraud": "One charge of the project managers was to obtain
permission to locate and to use the data bases of the major consumer
activist organizations who were already on a routine and continual

basis collecting materials. This has been accomplished." It went on to list the organizations agreeing to provide access:

The National Council Against Health Fraud
The University of Pennsylvania Cancer Center
The Arizona Council Against Health Fraud
The personal library of Benjamin Wilson (Oregon)
The Family Library (questionable therapy segments) of St. Mary's Hospital, Sisters of St. Mary System, John Renner, M.D., custodian
Lehigh Valley Committee Against Health Fraud, Inc.

It was noted that the Lehigh Valley Library is "one of the oldest anti-health fraud libraries in the country."

There is little doubt that any study undertaken by such a group (undoubtedly using the worst press articles, magazine stories, and established medical journal articles on alternatives in the country) would come up with a tainted analysis and report on the alternatives being studied and evaluated.

By itself, the October Plan appears to be just that. . .a plan. The Plan, however, became action in combination with the Emprise Grant Study. The Plan included what could be interpreted as questionable and anti-competitive activities:

(a) The proposal focused on setting up a project within an "established health information organization" in order to address public issues in health care that "are not addressed by existing consumer groups." Considering who was involved in this initial plan and the subsequent Grant Progress Report Summary (dated June 1, 1988, although work on the Study was done earlier), most likely the "established health information organization" referred to was Emprise, which incorporated officially in Washington, D.C., on April 25, 1988, or Dr. Renner's group in Kansas City, MO.

(b) It states that other groups have tried to take actions in this area in the past and have been sued, and that these groups have a vested interest and are hamstrung "by fears of successful legal challenge to their activities based on competition, self-interest, libel or slander." Was Emprise saying here that it would "front" anti-competitive activities so that these vested interest groups (such as the AMA or the pharmaceutical industry) would not have to risk lawsuits?

(c) In an apparent move to further ensure there would be no lawsuits against it for its planned activity, it proposed a "model immunity act which would protect from suit organizations having as one of their purposes the detection or prevention of fraudulent insurance acts or persons or associations furnishing information to such an organization or association." Something like this would certainly open the door to widespread reporting about targeted alternatives without fear of reprisals in the form of lawsuits.

We see that a group was set up for the purpose of evaluating health and insurance fraud and reporting on these entities, while at the same time being immune from lawsuits over what it reported. This might not seem to be so bad, except for the fact that it would eventually be reporting on the economic competitors to the pharmaceutical and medical industries. Whether by plan or by happenstance, the effect is that it would be doing what the pharmaceutical industry would like to see done. . .clearing the health-care playing field of economic competition from the alternatives.

(d) It then refers to this new health information organization as an "impartial group" that would be set up as a "neutral organization" so as to develop "reporting arrangements for information it receives through the National Association of Insurance Commissioners and state government offices dealing with insurance fraud." This puts this group into a position of reporting on insurance frauds to the Insurance Commissioners and state and federal government agencies involved in these issues. Who are the people that are going to sit in judgment of the "health and insurance frauds?"

Part of this plan included the "registration of practitioners" and their treatments, as well as filing the names and records of all of their *patients* with the government. The plan also provided for putting together white papers that could be used by the insurance industry. It stated that these reports would be the "basis of reliance by insurers for change in insurance coverage and policy definition issues." It further stated, "Those therapies with immediate undisclosed health hazards could be proposed as subjects for exclusion from use in the state/country or exclusion from reimbursement on public policy grounds."

The danger in all of this is simply this: Through whose eyes will this evaluation of what is a health hazard, what is a fraud, what is good, and what is bad for the public be made?

Most of the people involved in this scheme and the study of the alternatives have expressed their bias against the alternatives. Most of these same people are apparently involved in forwarding an anti-competitive activity directed at these very same alternative therapies, treatments, products, services, and practitioners. Yet they propose to sit in judgment of the very same alternative entities they have been attacking. They call this a fair or impartial study? By whose definition?

They have already demonstrated their bias in statements that have been published about various forms of alternative health care. These "impartial" experts doing these studies have claimed:

- That "nutritional scams often emphasize: megavitamin therapy, herbal therapy and natural or organic foods."
- That chelation therapy (considered at one point on the FDA's "Top Ten Health Frauds," and a target in the campaign against alternatives) is dangerous and that there are "recorded cases of deaths caused by it."
- That acupuncture is "unproven, based on primitive concepts that are totally out of step with present scientific knowledge."
- That vitamin and mineral therapy, especially the use of megavitamin therapy, is dangerous to a patient's health, and produces nothing more than "expensive urine."

The Plan also stated:

One aspect of the project will be to provide data on coverage. Another aspect will be to provide information on Potential Insurance Fraud or abuse and misrepresentation in billings to appropriate state, federal and private agencies to permit the government and insurers to take appropriate actions against documented health fraud.

It's important to note that throughout the documentation on this study there is no mention of talking to, interviewing, or obtaining data from any of the people within the alternative movement on their products, treatments, therapies, services, or modalities. The authors of the study do make mention that they planned on using papers and published articles on various alternatives. However, they never gave the people in the alternative movement an opportunity to present their case regarding what was being studied. They certainly weren't represented on any of the "expert panels."

What the Flexner study was to the AMA at the turn of the century, this study appears to be to the medical-pharmaceutical complex in the 1990s. Although the earlier study dealt with schools of medicine, it had a major impact on allopathic medicine's chief economic competitor at the time, homeopathy. The current study is also having a major impact on the economic competitors of orthodox medicine. There are other similarities between the Emprise study and the Flexner study besides the impact on competition. First, the pharmaceutical industry had a major interest in the outcome of both studies and stood to gain financially with the chief competitor of medicine out of the way. Second, the medical establishment also stood to gain from both studies with their competition eliminated.

The Emprise Grant Progress Report Summary outlined which alternative products, treatments, therapies, services, and modalities they planned to evaluate and report on. The list includes hundreds of alternative entities that have been and are still being used today—and which are also under attack today.

With the Flexner study, we saw that Flexner's brother worked for Rockefeller, whose empire included the pharmaceutical industry. With the current study we can see that many of the people involved in it were directed linked to the pharmaceutically-financed anti-"quackery" campaign. It would appear that this study was designed to target the very economic competitors that the pharmaceutical industry wanted out of the way. If this weren't planned this way, then the outcome and product of this study certainly has had such an effect on the alternatives.

The Report stated, "Each participant has been involved with the critical evaluation of questionable and unproven methods of cancer management in their professional and volunteer lives." The Consensus Panels were put together, and each one was assigned a specific area according to their expertise. The following is a verbatim account of what they were to study and evaluate and report on, and who would do it. (An asterisk (*) indicates a person who will advise on the make-up of the panel if other members are needed. Bold type indicates a member of NCAHF.)

Subject and Consensus Panels

DIAGNOSTIC TESTS

Subjects
Accupath 1000 (electro-diagnosis)
Arthur Amid Test
Bolen Test
Burton Test (protein fraction balance)
Burzynski Test (balance of peptides)
Darkfield Microscope
Hair Analysis
Hemacytology Index
Hubbard E-meter
Live Cell Analysis
Metabolic Typing
Navarro Test
Nutritional Analysis Tests

Consensus Panel:
William Jarvis, Ph.D.*
James Lowell, Ph.D.
Charles Moertel, M.D.
Lawrence Mulkerin, M.D.
John Renner, M.D.
Ben Wilson, M.D.

DIET, NUTRITION, DETOXIFICATION

Subjects:
Abscisic acid
Acidophillas
ADS tea
Aveloz
Blue Green manna
Chapparral Tea
Cell Salts
Chase Method
Coffee Enemas
Collodaurum
Colonic Irrigation
Comfrey

Enzymes
Gerson method
Gibson method
Glandular therapy
Intenzyme
Ipse Roxo
Iscador
Kelley Therapy
Liver Juice
Macrobiotic
Manner
Neiper
Pau d'Arco
Proteolytic
Retenzyme
Taheebo
Trace Elements
Vitamin A
Vitamin B-13
Vitamin B-15
Vitamin B-17
Vitamin C
Vitamin F
Vitamins, multi
Vitamin P
Wheatgrass
Wigmore
Winter Tea

Consensus Panel:
Edward R. Blonz, Ph.D.*
Victor Herbert, N.D., J.D.
James Lowell, Ph.D.
Jeanne B. Martin, Ph.D., R.D., L.D.
Guy Newell, M.D.
David V. Schalira, M.B., Ch.B, F.R.C.P.*

DRUGS, BIOLOGICALS, IMMUNE APPROACHES

Subjects:
Amygdalin
Antineoplastons
Autogenous vaccines
Auto-urine therapy

Live Cell
Beard method
Benzaldehyde
Burton therapy
Burzynski therapy
Brych Therapy
Carcalon
Carcin
Cell Therapy
CH-23
Coleys Mixed Toxins
Crofton Immunization Method
DBMG
DMSO
Ehrmer Therapy
Essiac
Glover Serum
Glyoxylide
Greek Cancer Cure
HCI
HCL
HLV
Hydrazine Sulfate
Hydrochloric acid
Hydrogen peroxide
Immunoaugmentative Therapy (IAT)
ISOO
Issels Combination
Keller Therapy
Koch Anti-Toxins
Lincoln Bacteriophages
Livingston
Laetrile
Lysozyme
Mercerene
Niehans
Purified Antigen
Reams
Rodaquin
Staphyloccus Phase Lysate
Thymosin
Urine

Consensus Panel:
Zal Arlin, M.D.
Neil Ellison, M.D.
H. Hugh Fudenberg, M.D.
Bridget Leventhal, M.D.
Peter Mansell, M.D.*
Charles Moertel, M.D.
David Schapira, M.D.

ETHNIC, FOLK, HERBAL, ROOT, AND BOTANICAL MEDICINES

Subject:
Botanicals
Escarotic pastes
Fasting
Folk medicine herbals
Hoxey
Iscador
Roots
Teas
Yellow and black salves

Consensus Panel:
Stephen Barrett, M.D.
Charlotte Gyllenhaal, Ph.D.*
Michael J. Huft
Lawrence Mulkerin, M.D.

PSYCHOLOGICAL, PSYCHONEUROIMMUNOLOGICAL APPROACHES

Subject:
Biofeedback
Imagery
Simonton
Visualization

Consensus Panel:
Barrie Cassileth, Ph.D.*
Michael Lerner, Ph.D.
Irv. Lerner, M.D.
Jim Lowell, Ph.D.

The list that the project worked from was not limited to just the ones named in the consensus panel studies. As a matter of fact, they included a chart, which follows:

Chart 2. *Major Questionable (Dubious) Remedies to Prevent or Treat AIDS*
Note: BTS [Barnett Technical Services] recognizes that there are some remedies on this list under investigation that are unproven but may be determined later to be productive, and that this list is not necessarily all inclusive. The project will be restricted to dubious therapy currently reporting.

Accupuncture [sic]
African Bio-Mineral Balance
AL-721
Allsafe Gel
Allsafe Liquid
Amino Acids
Anti—Microbial treatments
Autogenous vaccines
Auto-Immune system
Beta Carotene
BHT
Bone Marrow aspiration
Burton's protein fractions
Chinese herbal treatments
Conceptrol
Colustrum
DCNB
Deionized water
Detoxification programs
Diets
Electro-accupuncture [sic]
AIDS
Evening Primrose Oil
Germanium
Gingsen
Guided Imagery
Herbs
Homeopathy
Hydrogen peroxide
Immune stimulation methods
Immunoaugmentative therapy (see Burton serum protein
    fractions, supra.)

Ion Factors
Isoprinosine
Lentinin (polysacharride/shitake mushrooms)
Ligustrum lucidum
Living Foods Program
Livingston vaccines
Macrobiotic diet
Massage
Megavitamins
Metabolic typing (nutritional therapy)
Minerals
Neurolinguistic programming (NLP)
Nutrient Correction of Autoimmune system
Nutritional Immunology or Immunotherapy
Ozone therapy
Penicillin (40 mil. units daily)
Polarity therapy
Psycho/immunity
Purified Antigen
ReBella (douche)
Red Blood cell transfusions
Reflexology
Rejuvelac
Revice's lipid therapy
Sani-fone (protections from saliva)
Sellinium
Somarin (Chinese mushroom extract)
Sound wave healing tapes
Thermobaric treatment
Thymus extracts
Translinoleic acid
Unproven methods of cancer treatment; all major unproven
    and questionable methods of cancer treatment offered at
    Mexican, Caribbean and U.S. Clinics are now being
    offered at those same sites for AIDS patients.
Vitamin C (60-200 mg. daily)
Vitamin Therapy
Viralaid
Visualization
Wheat grass and algae
Yoga
ZPG-1 (non-prescription anti-AIDS pill)

This list was used in 1988-1989. More than likely more subjects were looked into, and there is no doubt that more items and lists have been used in this campaign.

An evaluation of these alternative methods in health care was made and, according to plan, the reports on these items were made available to government agencies involved in health fraud and insurance fraud and to private organizations involved in health and insurance fraud. Insurance companies would also have access to the data through "lease access to the data base and computer program to insurers for use in evaluating claims." They also planned to make the data available to both Medicare and Medicaid and for use in investigations of fraud and abuse.

That this group will make this data available to agencies involved in the investigations of fraud and abuse opens up an area of great concern. If the federal and state governments and the insurance industry rely on this data, then these tainted studies of alternative products, treatments, services, therapies, modalities, clinics, and practitioners could be used to generate actions against these targets simply because some "experts" said this was bad for the public.

Although it was stated at the beginning of the lists that they "recognize that here are some remedies on this list under investigation that are unproven but may be determined later to be productive," it is highly unlikely—considering which "experts" were on the Consensus Panels—that they would endorse any of the alternative treatments, therapies, modalities, services, or products they were investigating.

For instance, consider a development which was reported in the May 13, 1993, San Diego *Union-Tribune* under this headline: "Mislabeled Drugs are Target of U.S. Probe." The lead paragraph, datelined San Diego, said, "Federal and state investigators fanned out across seven states yesterday to seize evidence in a sweeping probe of a San Diego-based network suspected of marketing dangerously mislabeled prescription drugs."

According to an FDA Talk Paper dated May 12, 1993, obtained through the FDA, the FDA teamed up with agents from the following federal and state agencies in their crack-down on these "dangerously mislabeled prescription drugs":

U.S. FDA
U.S. Customs
U.S. Internal Revenue Service (IRS)
U.S. Attorney's Office

California Department of Justice
California Bureau of Narcotics and Enforcement
California Department of Health Services
Food and Drug Branch, Fraud Section
Florida Office of the State Prosecutor
Florida Department of Law Enforcement
Florida Department of Health and Rehabilitative Services

These agencies executed raids in California, Ohio, Michigan, Illinois, Texas, Florida, and Indiana on the same day, against such targets as supplement manufacturers, sales and distribution outlets, offices, residences, post office boxes, and health food stores. Included among the "dangerously mislabeled prescription drugs" seized were many items that were in fact targeted in the Emprise Grant study, including:

Coenzyme Q-10
DMSO
Essiac Tea Liquid
Germanium
Gerovital H3
Herpes Products
Hoxey Herbal Therapy
Hydrogen Peroxide
Laetrile
Selenium

One or more of the firms that were raided may very well have been involved with "dangerously mislabeled prescription drugs." If so, then the actions taken may very well have been justified, *but only for those products.*

Apparently the federal and state enforcement arm of this Health Fraud Task Force included other items which did not fall under the broad and sweeping description of "dangerously mislabeled prescription drugs," but which apparently came to their attention due to the fact that these products were on the target list of products to go after in this campaign against the alternatives.

It is highly unlikely that health food stores in Texas, Illinois, Michigan, and Ohio were selling illegal "dangerously mislabeled prescription drugs."

What appears to have happened is that other items that did not fit into the broad description were included in the raids and seizures. It looks like the "war against drugs" now includes alternative products one can buy in health food stores. Is this just an isolated case, or is it part of a much broader scheme which includes targeting alternative product manufacturers and distributors, as well as clinics and practitioners?

What is this Health Fraud Task Force? From what information are they operating? Who gave them this information? Are the current actions described above a part of the overall pharmaceutical/FDA Anti-Quackery Campaign? Is this sharing of information between private groups and the government just an informal health-care coalition? Is it something more sinister and chilling, such as a massive attempt to eliminate the *economic competitors* of the pharmaceutical companies which have been planning and financing this campaign?

The following chapter outlines the birth of a Big Brother computer tracking system that is being used against the alternatives through the insurance industry, medical boards, law enforcement, regulatory agencies, and local, state and federal agencies. It shows how they may be linked together, sharing information that is apparently being used to destroy the alternative health-care movement in the United States.

Chapter 6

Merchants of Misinformation

"Reporter: 'You believe that this case, the government's action against him, caused your husband eventually to take his own life?'
"Mrs. Diefenbach: 'I believe that to the core.'"
[ABC-TV "Prime Time" interview regarding Dr. Bill Diefenbach losing his Medicare provider status based on misinformation disseminated about him by the system.]

Where was this information on alternative practitioners, manufacturers, products, treatments, therapies, modalities and clinics distributed? Who was going to use this data? For what reason? Was this data accurate? Could it damage anyone's career, character, or life?

Some of these questions may be answered with the following information about Dr. Renner and his relationship with the FDA. A memo dated February 26, 1988, from the Food and Drug Administration Associate Commissioner for Consumer Affairs, Alexander Grant, included a copy of the Health Fraud Status Report. The memo and the Report were distributed to all FDA Regional FDA Directors, District Directors, Consumer Affairs Officers, and MCMI, WEAC, and the New York Regional Laboratory.

The Report indicated the following FDA activities in the course of its efforts to build "health-fraud" coalitions and share information:

• The FDA is working closely with many other groups to build national and local coalitions to combat health fraud.

• In September 1985, FDA, FTC, and USPS co-sponsored a national Health Fraud Conference in Washington, D.C.. This was the first national conference on health fraud since 1966. [The previous one, which was called a Congress on Quackery, was also co-sponsored by the FDA, the FTC, and the U.S.P.S. as well as the AMA.]

• As a follow-up to the National Conference, FDA held regional health fraud conferences during 1986 in cities all across the country.

• FDA efforts, including Agency-sponsored health-fraud conferences held across the country, led to the formation of coalitions to combat health fraud in the following areas:

Kentucky	Dallas/Fort Worth
Kansas City	Des Moines
Chicago	Los Angeles
San Juan	Kent (Ohio)
Minnesota	Michigan
Jacksonville (Fla)	Arizona
Oregon	Washington State

• To build on the success of the coalition efforts, in 1987 FDA announced that the Agency would sponsor another National Health Fraud Conference (St. Mary's Hospital of Kansas City, Missouri—March 13-15, 1988). [This is the hospital from which Dr. John Renner worked in 1988.]

• FDA placed a priority on the sharing of information among organizations. Sharing data helps to avoid duplication of effort and to encourage joint initiatives. ["Sharing" information can also serve to provide data on a subject or product that the recipient of that information might never have heard of prior to receiving it. Such a partnership in a "health-fraud coalition" could also serve as a means to spread false and misleading data and propaganda designed to be used against the entity being reported on.]

• Other organizations also have also initiated information exchange initiatives. Barrett Technical Services [along with Emprise] with funding from the NIH's Small Business Innovation Research Program, is developing a PDQ System that allows health professionals to access health fraud information via their computers.

• The Association of Food and Drug officials (AFDO) and FDA have jointly developed a plan for the establishment of Health Fraud Surveillance and Action Teams (HFSAT). [AFDO is an association of state government officials involved in Food and Drug enforcement, investigation, etc.]

• The HFSAT plan is intended to be used by state and regional officials to implement a program to control health fraud.

The FDA's Health Fraud Status Report also stated:

Reports from consumers, the media, and health professionals are also used to monitor promotions for suspected fraudulent health-related products. Reports of Suspected Health Fraud are completed by field offices to provide data to the district office where the manufacturer of the product is located for appropriate regulatory action and to the Health Fraud Office. . .

It was further learned, in March 1992, that the FDA had received information directly from Dr. John Renner. Gary Dean, former Director of Compliance, FDA District office, Kansas City, Missouri, stated the following:

1. That in 1988 Gary Dean was assigned the project by FDA headquarters of setting up a National Health Fraud Tracking System and a Health Fraud Unit for the FDA.

2. That Dr. John Renner provided a great deal of information to the FDA via Gary Dean. Dean stated that he worked closely with Dr. Renner during the initial setting up of the FDA's health-fraud data base. Dean revealed that he had contacted Dr. Renner to "seek advice, assistance and direction" from Dr. Renner on health fraud.

3. That Dr. Renner had provided him with information and leads for more than twenty investigations for follow-up by the FDA over an 18-month period. Dean did not reveal which specific entities Dr. Renner had provided him, but he did say that he did receive leads for investigation from Dr. Renner.

Apparently Dr. Renner is the custodian of the health fraud and quackery files of the National Council Against Health Fraud, or some other entity he was working with at that time. His Resource Center on Health Fraud is located in Kansas City, and this is apparently where he got the information to feed to the FDA, which formed the data base for this National Health Fraud Tracking System.

In addition, another FDA document further revealed how the computer system came about, what its purpose was, and how it was designed to work. An FDA Investigations Activities Report (For Official Use Only), dated February 10, 1992, from the Division of Field Investigation to all FDA Directors, Investigations Branch, revealed on Page 9:

RELOCATION OF THE NATIONAL HEALTH FRAUD UNIT

The National Health Fraud Unit has officially transferred from KAN-DO (Kansas City-District Office) to the Division of Federal/State Relations (DFSR) in headquarters. The Unit began operations in May 1988, charged with the responsibilities of:

(1) preparing quarterly reports summarizing Agency actions against health fraud;

(2) coordinating federal/state/local government and private sector exchange of health fraud information and complaints;

(3) working closely with other Agency components to facilitate communication with interested public health professionals and regulatory officials;

(4) providing a central repository for FDA health fraud information; and

(5) establishing a system to allow Agency-wide access to that information.

The report stated that the Health Fraud Unit and its data base had been transferred to headquarters to provide ". . .a more diversified interaction with federal/state/governments and local organizations combating health fraud."

Although the Investigations Activities Report did not name the specific local organizations and private sector groups with whom they planned to exchange "health fraud and complaints," there is little doubt who this might be.

Also, in points (4) and (5) the report does not elaborate on how it was that the FDA came upon the data base for its "central repository for FDA health fraud information" or how it established ". . .a system to allow Agency-wide access to that information." However, Gary Dean in his interview did elaborate on how he obtained that information.

In its Health Fraud Status Report of February 1988, the FDA described how it helped form coalitions in over a dozen cities to combat health fraud. Who makes up these coalitions? How do they

work together? What data base do they share? How do they keep
informed of each other's activities? What is the source of this information that is the basis of their operations and activities?

The February 26, 1988, memo revealed that the FDA was getting
leads for its investigations into "health fraud and quackery" from a
variety of different sources. The Associate Commission for Consumer Affairs described these as being:

> Consumer groups
> Health-care professionals
> Consumers
> Media

There can be little doubt which "consumer groups" were giving
them leads. This information was then apparently included into the
FDA's National Health Fraud Tracking System, which was already
being put together out of the FDA's Kansas City office of the
Director of Compliance.

This massive tracking system was planned years before it came
into being. It has been improved upon and expanded over the years.
Additionally, another entity involved in this campaign, the insurance
industry, has also put together its own data base on alternatives,
apparently using information similar to what the FDA was given.
This is covered in detail in the next chapter but is mentioned here
because they are interrelated and apparently are connected in some
way.

Each of the Health Fraud Computer Tracking Systems has apparently included in its data base information on the targets in the
PAC/FDA Anti-Quackery Campaign. Together these systems make
up the anti-competitive network that brings together the private
sector (Emprise, Barnett Technical Services), the National Council
Against Health Fraud, the National Health Care Anti-Fraud Association (hundreds of private and government insurance companies), and
state and federal enforcement and regulatory agencies, including
licensing boards.

The formation of the Health Fraud Task Force apparently came
out of the birth of the National Health Care Anti-Fraud Association.
Federal agencies involved in the NHCAA form the basic core of the
Task Force. The networking that is going on includes not just the
computers, but also conferences, training sessions, workshops, lectures, consulting, advising, and referrals. For example, the FDA's

Health Fraud Status Report of 1988 lists as sources of information on combating "health fraud" the following people:

William Jarvis, Ph.D., President, National Council Against Health Fraud, Loma Linda, California

Grace Powers Monaco, Esq., Chairman of the Board, Candlelighters Childhood Cancer Foundation, White, Fine, and Verville, Washington, D.C.

John Renner, M.D., Director of Community Health, Trinity Lutheran Hospital, Kansas City, Missouri

Marsha Goldberger, Council of Better Business Bureaus, Arlington, Virginia

Helen Sheehan, American Cancer Society, New York, New York

In still another example of this networking between the private sector and government, the FDA outlined how it makes use of its data base on the alternatives. In a section of the Health Fraud Status Report entitled FDA Enforcement Report, it revealed the creation of the Health Fraud Surveillance and Action Team (HFSAT). The stated purpose of the HFSAT was to help facilitate the sharing of information about health fraud and health fraud products. This information was to be shared among federal, state, and local officials and used to help "state and regional officials to implement a program to control health fraud."

This same FDA Report announced a pilot system for reporting on medical device products. (This would include alternative medical devices which the FDA has been after for years.) Entitled "A Notice to Deceptive Products and Misleading Claims," this newly formed report section of the FDA's Weekly "Enforcement Report" would include the names of targets who failed to respond to FDA's Notice of Adverse Findings letters.

The purpose of publishing the list of names of targets involved in medical devices was so that "state and local consumer units, Better Business Bureaus, and others who receive questions from potential purchasers" can use this data in their "health fraud" activities. The FDA further indicated that "such listings do not preclude legal or regulatory action by FDA." Judging by their actions, it would apparently be more appropriate to say that such listings *precede* legal or regulatory action by the FDA.

Of interest is that on February 26, 1988, the FDA disclosed that Dr. John Renner was "collecting stories from victims or friends or

relatives of victims" of "quackery." This announcement was apparently sent to all FDA offices and participants who were to attend
the March 13-15, 1988, Health Fraud Conference in Kansas City.
Then, just prior to the Health Fraud Conference, the Department
of Justice announced that it had raised its priority for health and
insurance fraud. On March 7, 1988, the Justice Department reported
that it had transferred one of its key FBI agents who worked on
health fraud and insurance fraud in its Detroit office to its FBI
headquarters in Washington, D.C. This move was the first of many
in the Justice Department's effort to beef up the FBI's fight against
"health and insurance fraud."

To date, this Task Force on Health Fraud has acted against
hundreds of alternative practitioners, products, treatments, services,
therapies, clinics, and manufacturers all across the country. The day
I was preparing this text, I received a FAX, headlined:

Update: Vitamins and Minerals Seized.
FDA Raids International Nutrition
In Las Vegas, Nevada

The news included the fact that a warrant was issued by the U.S.
Magistrate from the U.S. District Court for 24 products. The raid was
carried out by six FDA agents and an assistant U.S. Attorney. The
FAX stated that the building was surrounded by local police and staff
were being "rounded up." Apparently someone in the company had
managed to get to a phone and get the message out to Citizens For
Health, a consumer/industry activist group based in Tacoma,
Washington. The staff member was in a room away from the action,
and in a hushed tone passed on the report of what was happening
before also being rounded up by federal agents.

All 24 products listed in the raid and seizure fell into one or more
of the categories listed in the Grant Study of alternative products.
These included Pau D'Arco, selenium, minerals and vitamins (E-
magnesium, bromelain, potassium-magnesium, and calcium).

These same products are included in the FDA's Health Fraud
Tracking Computer System. According to a source inside regional
FDA headquarters, FDA officials considered this raid and seizure so
important that it sent down its Director of Compliance, Steve Kendall, and its Director of Public Affairs, Janet McDonald, to handle
any media flap that might ensue.

What we are looking at here is an unchecked network of federal,
state, and local government agencies working with private organiza-

tions and groups which are all linked together with the purpose of fighting "health fraud" and "quackery." Some insight into who these groups and organizations are and how they maintain communications among themselves and coordinate their activities came to light in an investigation of the FDA's Division of Federal/State Relations (DFSR).

The FDA's DFSR sends an information letter, entitled State Action Information Letter (SAIL) to a long list of federal/state government agencies, as well as some private organizations. On a state level, it is sent to:

> State Health Officers
> Directors of Agriculture
> State Laboratory officials
> State Cosmetic officials
> State Device officials
> State Dairy officials
> State Veterinarians
> State Weighs & Measures
> Boards of Pharmacy
> Food officials
> State Food Service officials
> State Drug officials
> State Radiation officials
> State Feed officials
> State Shellfish officials
> State Attorneys General

It was also sent to just about every Associate Commissioner within the FDA, the Office of Regulatory Affairs, and the Office of the Commissioner of the FDA.

The routing in the December 27, 1991, SAIL also included the following on an informational basis: Regional Food and Drug Directors; District Directors; Branch Chiefs; Consumer Affairs Officers; and Directors of State Cooperative Programs. It was also sent to several associations made up of government officials, including the National Association of State Departments of Agriculture (NASDA); Association of Food and Drug Officials (AFDO); and the National Association of Attorneys General (NAAG).

The network of state and federal agencies involved in this campaign is enormous. In addition to the Health Fraud Task Force, there is also a Task Force on AIDS Fraud. This Task Force differs from the Health Fraud Task Force in name only. The FDA houses all its information on Health Fraud and AIDS Fraud at its Federal/State Relations Division in Rockville, Maryland. This Division also houses the Health Fraud Tracking Computer and is where the Health Fraud Status Report is published. The same FDA State Action Information Letter of December 27, 1991, announced that members of the National Task Force on AIDS were receiving funding directly from the FDA for their activities. The SAIL stated:

> The National AIDS Fraud Task Force Project is entering its third year of operation with several state task forces meeting on a regular basis and the possibility of new task forces being established in other states. An AIDS Health Fraud Conference was held in Orlando, Florida, in October [1991], and discussions are underway concerning conferences in addition states. During the coming year [1992] the emphasis will be to: 1) provide the resources needed to support the operation of the task forces, 2) initiate collection of data from the task forces for dissemination to all state and FDA AIDS coordinators, and 3) conduct conferences in additional states.

> Under an agreement with the National AIDS Fraud Task Force Project, four operating state task forces have been provided funds to assist in meeting costs and data collection. The state task forces receiving these funds are California, Louisiana, Michigan, and Texas. In return for this support, the task forces have agreed to provide FDA with copies of minutes of task force meetings, quarterly reports of all their activities, and information obtained on suspected fraudulent AIDS drugs and therapies. Funding of these activities will run through September 30, 1992.

Of interest is that on April 9, 1992, Dr. John Renner appeared before the Subcommittee on Regulation, Business Opportunities and Energy's Committee on Small Business and the Subcommittee on Health and Long-Term Select Committee on Aging and stated the following in his published testimony:

> I am John H. Renner, M.D., a family physician, President of Consumer Health Information Research Institute (CHIRI) in Kansas City, Missouri. A nonprofit organization, CHIRI has as its goals the dissemination of accurate information and the identification of misinformation on quackery.

I am a member of the Board of Directors of the National Council Against Health Fraud. I am also a Clinical Professor of Family and Community Medicine at the University of Missouri, Kansas City, School of Medicine and an Adjunct Professor of Preventive Medicine at the University of Kansas School of Medicine. I have been a consultant to the Food and Drug Administration on AIDS quackery and have been deeply involved in studying and investigating quackery for ten years.

From all indications, the Task Force on Health Fraud began in 1988, with the birth of the National Health Care Anti-Fraud Association. At about the time it came into being, an article appeared in *Medical Economics* on March 7, 1988, entitled "Insurance Fraud Cops Have a Whole New Set of Teeth," by Mark Holoweiko. The article highlighted several federal laws which were now being applied against the "health fraud and insurance fraud" targets. These laws included:

The Racketeer Influenced and Corrupt Organizations Act (RICO). It stated that the federal courts now allow private insurers to use RICO to seek criminal and civil action against their targets. They need only show a "pattern of racketeering activity." This would also apply to the federal government using the RICO Act against targets in this campaign.

The Mail Fraud Act. A favorite of Assistant U.S. Attorney James Sheehan of Philadelphia (a Task Force member and on the Board of Governors of the NHCAA), who stated, "With it we can freeze a practitioner's assets, confiscate his records, demand an accounting of all his business revenue, and so on. It's limited only by the prosecutor's imagination."

The False Claims Act. This really applies only to those who use the insurance industry in their practices and clinics. However, under this law, Sheehan said, "The government can nail a provider for triple the amount falsely billed plus legal fees. . ." He also said that "thanks to the 1986 Bounty Hunter amendment to the law, insurers can earn a 15 to 30 percent share of the recovery by suing the culprit on the government's behalf."

The Civil Monetary Penalties Law. Even if a doctor has already been convicted or found civilly liable for false claims, Medicare and Medicaid cops can clobber him for the same offenses under this law. They only have to prove that he knew or should have known that the service was not provided as claimed.

The Medicare Protection Law. Eileen Boyd (a founding member of the NHCAA and member of the NHCAA Board of Governors), of the Department of Health and Human Services (DHHS) enforcement arm, said, "A new provision says that if the Inspector General (of the DHSS) has reason to believe a practitioner may be subject to the Civil Monetary Penalties Law (CMPL), he can get a federal court to enjoin the person from concealing, removing, encumbering, or disposing of assets. . .or seek other appropriate relief."

Task Force activity got into high gear in September 1991. On September 23, the Office of the Inspector General of the Department of Health and Human Services announced that the FDA was hiring and training 100 new criminal investigators for the health-fraud area.

On the same day, it announced the creation of the new office of Criminal Investigations (OCI), which it described as another "bureaucratic instrument in the war against health fraud." This was to be housed at the FDA headquarters. Under OCI would be six criminal investigation offices set up in Chicago, Kansas City, Miami, Newark, New York, and San Diego, assigned to deal with fraud and fraudulent products. Unlike other divisions of the FDA, the Offices of Criminal Investigations would report directly to central control at FDA headquarters.

On February 3, 1992, the FDA announced that its newly formed Criminal Investigations Unit was going to be headed up by ex-Secret Service man Terrill Vermillion. On this same day, the Attorney General of the United States released a report entitled "Report on Enhanced Health Care Fraud Initiative." This report announced the Department of Justice's re-assigning of 96 FBI agents to be devoted full-time to the health-fraud initiative. He said that the FBI had "reprogrammed an additional 50 agents from foreign counterintelligence and domestic counter-terrorism to the health care initiative." It announced that "Health Care Units would be established in 12 cities where we believe health-care fraud is most acute. These Units will attack priority cases and serve as regional training and expert resource centers for surrounding field offices. The cities include Baltimore, Charlotte, Chicago, Dallas, Las Vegas, Los Angeles, Miami, New York, Newark, New Orleans, and Philadelphia."

The Report also outlined other areas within the Justice Department that were being beefed up to attack health fraud. It can be clearly seen that this "beef-up" is costing the taxpayers millions of dollars each year. All in an apparent attempt to fulfill the goals of the pharmaceutically-financed Anti-Quackery Campaign. It stated that approximately 100 Assistant United States Attorneys had been "assigned to criminal and civil health care fraud matters by the U.S. Attorneys in those twelve districts receiving enhanced FBI resources"; that "ten additional attorney positions have been assigned by the Department's Executive office for United States Attorneys to reinforce the initiative"; that "six attorneys have been assigned to a newly formed Health Care Fraud Unit within the Fraud Section of the Criminal Division to help coordinate and support the initiative." In addition, "22 Civil Division Attorneys have and will continue to coordinate and litigate matters of national significance in this area."

In conclusion, the Report stated, "The primary objective of our enhanced [health-fraud] initiative will be to put health care cheats in prison and to forfeit their ill-gotten gains. Civil remedies will be used to obtain monetary penalties and restitution will be greatly enforced."

The Report also indicated which other agencies the DOJ was working with in their efforts to fight "health Fraud." These included:

FBI
DHHS Inspector General
Postal Inspection Service
FDA
Drug Enforcement Agency (DEA)
Labor Department Inspector General
State Medicaid Fraud Units
Insurance Industry Investigators

Then on February 10, 1992, Gary Dykstra, the FDA Associate Commissioner for Regulatory Affairs (directly over the Health Fraud Units, National Health Fraud Tracking Computer System, and the Task Forces on Health Fraud and AIDS Fraud), said that the FDA was now using "strategic enforcement" as a tool against health fraud. He explained that this strategic enforcement was a policy of "keeping the industry guessing" where the FDA would strike next. He also said that the FDA was a "paper tiger" before FDA Commissioner Kessler got there. Now, he said, the FDA is "flooding our General

Counsel's office and the Department of Justice with food and drug cases."

As we saw in some detail in Chapter 4, the Department of Health and Human Services (DHHS) had been operating from a quota system. The actual policy had been developed on June 5, 1987, out of the Office of Enforcement, Division of Compliance Policy, Associate Commissioner for Regulatory Affairs. This quota system also applied to the Office of the Inspector General of the DHHS. The policy stated:

In evaluating regulatory actions against indirect health hazard products, the following factors should be considered by districts and the centers:

The cost of the product, the economic impact of this cost on the target user group, as well as the profit (per sale) realized from the sale of the product;

The amount (dollar and volume) of product sold, and the geographical scope of its distribution.

One point of interest in the FDA's Policy on health fraud products is that it required the Office of Compliance in each center to "designate a contact and a back-up person for primary consultation on health fraud action."

Of course, the danger in using such a quota system is that it opens the door for government abuse, illegal acts, malicious prosecution, and selected enforcement actions against targets.

As Associate Commissioner Dykstra stated, the FDA was flooding both its General Counsel's Office and the DOJ with "food and drug cases." Whether these cases have any merit is another matter in light of the following information regarding this quota system.

In the summer of 1992, a major scandal rocked the Department of Health and Human Services when the Inspector General, Richard Kusserow, was forced to resign *as a direct result of having a quota system.* On July 31, 1992, Inspector General Kusserow was scheduled to leave his position in the DHHS and reportedly was going to join Strategic Management Associates, a management consulting firm in Washington, D.C. The events leading up to his resignation included a demand by the American Medical Association for his resignation for more than a year prior to his actually resigning. Apparently Kusserow's "Gestapo" had impacted AMA members as well as alternative practitioners. One of the functions of the Office of Inspector General of the DHHS is to investigate and prosecute Medicaid and Medicare fraud. Within the loop of this "anti-quackery" campaign, the standard assumption is that at least 10% of all claims for services in the Medicaid and Medicare programs are fraudulent.

It is important to note that this figure has never been documented, nor has the outrageous assertion that health fraud and quackery cost the American public either $10 billion or $25 billion a year (both figures have been thrown around). Many experts say that these figures are used exclusively in political circles and have no real merit in fact.

According to Boston attorney Donald Zerendow, head of the Massachusetts Medicaid Fraud Control Unit from 1978 to 1986, "the 10-percent fraud rate cited today by politicians was proposed—without proof or supportive documentation—in an article published by HHS Inspector General Richard Kusserow more than 10 years ago. And he has subsequently built his career by continuing to convince Congress that fraud is rampant."

In an article published in August 1992 in *Private Practice,* Howard Fishman, former senior editor of *The Psychiatric Times,* stated, "Kusserow's strong-arm tactics have resulted in the necessary statistical achievements. He has reported to Congress that his office brought in almost $29 billion in settlements, fines, restitutions, receivables and savings from 1985 to 1989." The year 1985 was one year after the FDA entered into an agreement to finance and support the Anti-Quackery Campaign with the pharmaceutical industry.

Fishman says in his article, "Inspector General initiated almost 5,800 successful prosecutions during that period. These accomplishments earned the DHHS an annual budget of $57.5 million for 1992 and it has requested $108 million for 1993." The article also pointed out that the National Association of Medicaid Fraud Control Units (which is also a member of the NHCAA) had accused Kusserow of "imposing conviction and recovery quotas on them. This is a fundamental violation of prosecutorial standards." Attorney Donald Zerendow added, "This whole process can only be described as legalized extortion and medical McCarthyism."

One practitioner who fought city hall on the issue of accusations that he had committed fraud said of his ordeal: "[It was] the most traumatic event of my life. I was faced with an awesome political machine that made me feel like a helpless victim. I knew what it would have been like to be a concentration camp inmate being led to the gas chamber by a group of thugs with guns trained on me." This doctor (a psychologist) was awarded $600,000 in damages after a jury found that he was a victim of malicious prosecution, according to the Fishman story.

The article went on to describe how the Federation of Physicians and Dentists issued a report which criticized the "Gestapo tactics" of the Medicaid Fraud Control Units. They stated that agents of the MFCU's had burst into offices with guns and were prosecuting physicians for small amounts of money for what "physicians claim were billing errors or misunderstandings on Medicaid regulations."

All of this is nothing new to those alternative practitioners who have been the victims of this campaign for the past ten years. As a matter of fact, one of the very first victims of the insurance industry's tracking computer was a chiropractor in Florida who, along with his wife and son, was arrested at his clinic in front of patients, by agents with drawn guns. They seized his patient records and the address files and even contacted patients and staff threatening them with indictments if they didn't "cooperate."

The report went on to state, "Other colleagues believe the fraud unit is being used for political purposes and is unwilling to consider administrative hearings to resolve conflicts because it must find fraud, even if none exists, to justify the federal funds it collects each year [from Kusserow's office]."

The Inspector General, in his annual evaluations, according to Fishman, insisted that "the units be ranked and evaluated based on their indictments, prosecution and monetary recovery records. In other words, he established conviction quotas." This would certainly seem to be the case in light of a $600,000 judgment awarded by a jury on this very point, because being a victim of a conviction quota amounts to malicious prosecution.

Even the National Association of Attorneys General (NAAG), according to the article, issued a series of formal resolutions and protest letters between 1988 and 1990 noting, "Such numerical output measurers would specifically contravene the American Bar Association Standards Relating to the Prosecution and Defense Function, which explicitly condemn prosecutorial decisions motivated by a desire to improve a prosecutor's conviction record."

The article went on to describe how Kusserow also initiated (and denied the existence of) an incentive system that provided merit pay raises for staff members based on specified numbers of prosecutions and recoveries. Even the medical establishment accused him of "creating a bounty system" regarding a case in California in 1988 brought against a local physician there.

Fishman conducted an interview with Kusserow during which he denied that he was rewarding his employees for imposing a sanction which "was found to be lacking in merit." But, as Fishman explains, in 1990 U.S. District Court Judge Robert E. Coyle ordered Kusserow to discontinue his merit pay/bounty system. In that case, a "smoking gun" was found in the performance appraisal of James Patton, director of the Division of Health Care Administrative Sanctions in the Office of the Inspector General. According to the record, to qualify for a pay increase, Patton was required to "assess 10 percent more sanctions than he had in the prior fiscal year" and, the article disclosed, "exceed by 10 percent the number of successful sanctions in dollar penalties."

Judge Coyle ruled in favor of the physician, noting that the merit pay/bounty system violated his Constitutional right to due process, according to the article.

Fishman reports that Kusserow had frequently criticized Medicare peer-review organizations for failing to produce sufficient sanctions and for not excluding a large number of physicians from the federally funded program. Peer Review Organizations (known as PROs) are made up of doctors who review claims sent into the federal government for Medicare and Medicaid cases, as well as for private insurance plans.

The article reports that in September 1990 ABC-TV reporter Chris Wallace interviewed Kusserow on several of these issues dealing with the merit pay/bounty system and quota system. Wallace asked Kusserow about a specific case involving Dr. William Diefenbach who, after a PRO review, was excluded from being a provider for Medicare patients. Kusserow stated, "There was evidence that in a number of cases, that he was an impaired physician—he was suffering from drug abuse—and that as a result of that, he was considered unwilling or unable to change his practice."

According to Fishman, Kusserow had later retracted his statements, but "while admitting that Diefenbach was not drug impaired, he persisted in contending that the physician should have been excluded because of inadequate performance." The ABC-TV segment concluded with the following dialogue:

Wallace: "But Bill Diefenbach gave up the fight to clear his name. His family says from the day he was excluded from Medicare he slowly sank into a deep depression from which he never recovered. Three months ago he shot and killed himself. Last month a memorial service was held on the grounds of the hospital where Dr. Diefenbach practiced for more than 20 years. . ."

Mrs. Diefenbach: "He was a healer, and he was a physician, and he was that first. And when you kick somebody in the heart, I think that's where his depression began. . ."

Wallace: "You believe that this case, the government's action against him, caused your husband eventually to take his own life?"

Mrs. Diefenbach: "I believe that to the core."

Some observers, according to the article, have suggested that Kusserow's most questionable "achievement" may be his distortion of the Civil Monetary Penalty Law process. Since 1985, two administrative law judges in his employ have been assigned responsibility for interpreting and applying CMPL provisions. A clear pattern has emerged in their rulings. Fishman explains, "Kusserow had the authority to impose sanctions on providers whose negligence resulted in erroneous billings. The prosecutor no longer had to show that the provider intentionally attempted to deceive the payer. Simple negligence is now grounds for a $2,000 *per-item* fine and exclusion from Medicaid and Medicare."

Probably the most important aspect of all of this is that, considering the insurance crisis in America today, Kusserow's quota system has diminished the ranks of the providers for Medicare and Medicaid. As a result of this campaign, the poor and elderly patients have been deprived of the necessary treatments they need to continue to live.

Are these Gestapo tactics being carried out against alternative and other health-care providers by design? Do we need a totalitarian-medical-police state to rid society and the health-care system of "undesirables" (those in the alternatives) while at the same time dictating to the public what is good and not good for them? Apparently some feel this way.

On April 9, 1992, during the Congressional Hearings on Recent Trends in Dubious and Quack Medical Devices, Dr. John Renner gave oral and written testimony which attacked every single major aspect of the alternative health-care system. The bottom line of his testimony was in his recommendation that "a unified approach is needed at the federal level by FDA, FBI, Postal Service, FTC, the Inspector General and state licensing boards."

There is certainly a "unified approach" at work in this campaign. The question remains—who is running this show? The government? Or outside interests?

One of the worst fears of those involved in the alternative movement is that actual deaths have already occurred as a result of this campaign closing down clinics and alternative offices. Of concern, as well, is the act of denying patients much-needed alternative products. It is feared that more people will die as a result of being denied what Constitutionally is their right to choose for themselves what health-care practitioner they want.

One of the most effective ways of cutting off the public's access to the alternatives is by omitting them from insurance coverage, whether that be Medicare, Medicaid, or private insurance plans.

The following chapter details more of how these outside interests have been influencing not just government agencies, but also the entire insurance industry. The results have been devastating to those involved in the alternative health-care movement. Cut off from insurance payments, patients are being denied access to life-saving therapies, treatments, or products that have helped them survive. These are just some of the ramifications of this "Public Service Anti-Quackery Campaign."

With the health-care system in the crisis it is currently in, millions of Americans are not able to afford health-care coverage under private insurance plans. Perhaps one of the answers to these problems lies in opening up the door to competition, not slamming it in the face of the alternatives.

The following chapter takes a detailed look into the insurance industry's role in this anti-competitive campaign and examines how this has affected alternative practitioners and clinics around the country.

Chapter 7

Big Brother and the Insurance Industry

"We are concerned about NHCAA operations in un-authorized states. Any information sharing outside the boundaries of the current guidelines presents liability issues. "
[Confidential memo, 8/8/90, to National Health Care Anti-Fraud Association Board]

Unholy "Medlock"

The term *unholy* means "immoral or undeserving of respect," and *medlock* comes from the term *wedlock* to denote, in this case, the alliance between medical vested interests and others in the government, in the pharmaceutical and insurance industries, and in the private sector. This alliance becomes "unholy" when its actions result in chilling effects on the alternative health-care marketplace. What makes this alliance unholy is the distinct possibility that there is something about it that is illegal and distinctly anti-competitive.

The Pharmaceutical Advertising Council (PAC) and the FDA kicked off their first National Health Fraud Conference in Washington, D.C., on September 11, 1985. The insurance industry conducted a similar conference a week later, also in Washington, D.C. A group of insurance companies that later became the National Health Care Anti-Fraud Association (NHCAA) met to discuss health/insurance fraud. This group was made up of health insurance companies from around the country.

Although the NHCAA formally incorporated on December 5, 1985, in Washington, D.C., the group actually started its anti-fraud activity in September of that year. The group was apparently brought together by Aetna Insurance company, which already had a "health fraud" team operational within its headquarters. According to its Certificate of Incorporation, the NHCAA articles included the following:

> To evaluate the feasibility of establishing a national health care anti-fraud organization, to formulate a general policy for

the promotion and control of health care fraud, to facilitate cooperation among health care organizations, law enforcement agencies and professional disciplinary bodies and to promote and develop anti-fraud activities among and between health care agencies and other organizations, and to act as an association.

Among the sixteen founding members of the NHCAA were officials representing the following agencies: U.S. Department of Health and Human Services—OIG (Eileen Boyd, Larry D. Morey); U.S. Department of Justice (Donald Foster); Florida Medicaid Fraud Control Unit (John G. Morris, Jr.); National Association of Medicaid Fraud Control Units (Barbara Zelner).

This was the early beginnings of what was to become known as the Task Force on Health Fraud. These government agencies (as well as many others which have since become members of the NHCAA) formed a working coalition to share information on targeted alternatives with the 350 members of the organization, including hundreds of insurance companies such as Aetna, Travelers, Metropolitan, CIGNA, The Guardian, Employees Health Insurance Company, Massachusetts Mutual Life Insurance, Mutual of Omaha, EQUICOR, and Blue Cross/Blue Shield of Ohio and of Michigan.

Today the membership in the NHCAA consists of the government agencies listed above and several more, including the Department of Justice's Federal Bureau of Investigation, as well as several hundred more insurance companies.

When the NHCAA began, government agencies accounted for about 25% of its Board of Governors. Its official First Annual Meeting took place in 1986, but the one in 1985 appears to have been the founding meeting. In 1987 the Second Annual Meeting was held in Hilton Head, South Carolina.

At its Third Annual Meeting in Phoenix, Arizona, some of the most outspoken critics of the alternative health-care movement were present as speakers. They held workshops headed by moderators with panels of "experts" on various subjects. Insurance executives were in attendance to learn about these subjects in order to become better equipped to do their jobs.

At this November 1988 meeting, Panel Nine, on Quackery, consisted of the following:

Moderator: Grace Powers Monaco, Esq., President, Emprise, Inc., Washington, D.C.

Panelists: Ronald Schwartz, Esq., White, Fine and Verville, Washington, D.C.

Peter W.A. Mansell, M.D., Houston, Texas
James A. Lowell, Ph.D., and Alison Lowell, Ph.D., Arizona
Council Against Health Fraud, Tucson, Arizona

Each of these people was directly involved in the National Institute of Health Grant Study reported on by Emprise (covered in the earlier chapters), with the exception of Ron Schwartz. He was one of the people listed in the original plan to study the alternatives—and was listed as working for a law firm in Washington, D.C., with which Grace Powers Monaco once was associated. While working for this law firm, one of Grace Monaco's chief clients reportedly was the American Cancer Society.

Dr. John Renner was also included in the 1988 membership list of the NHCAA. Here is another connection between the insurance industry and the spokesmen for the PAC/FDA Anti-Quackery Campaign.

It is a matter of record that the Emprise study of the alternatives stated that "commercial possibilities for the project" included:

Barnett Technical Services offering a consulting service utilizing the data base developed and the support of core working group professionals to review and evaluate insurance claims based on unproven and questionable cancer therapies from a legal and scientific basis.

The record shows that they had planned to test "the effectiveness of these products [included in the Consensus Panel reports] on a sample of potential users." (Page 2E-9 Item 6 of the Grant).

As part of this effort, there are three conferences each year at which Mrs. Monaco will be presenting papers on questionable and unproven therapies in 1987/1988. These conferences include the annual meetings of the American Society of Clinical Oncology, (New Orleans, La. May 22-24, 1988, and San Francisco, Ca., May 21-23, 1989), American Academy of Family Physicians (San Francisco, Ca., September 14-17, 1988, and New Orleans, La., October 3-6, 1989), Health Insurance Association of America (Toronto, CA., October 24-28, 1987) and National Council Against Health Fraud, Phoenix, Az., 1989).
. . .Ms. Monaco will also make presentations at conferences sponsored by the Florida Pediatric Oncology Committee, the Florida Cancer Council and the Food and Drug

Administration's Second Health Fraud Conference in March of 1988.

The information in the data base included everything mentioned in Chapter 5. Of interest as well was thr goal of "entering the rest of the reference libraries onto the computer."This appears to mean that the entirety of the libraries of the National Council Against Health Fraud, the Lehigh Valley Committee Against Health Fraud, and Dr. John Renner were entered into the computer data base.

According to the October Plan of 1986, this information was supposed to be fed to government agencies and to the insurance industry to use in making determinations on policy issues dealing with definitions, payments, and reimbursement.

The Grant report also proposed that the information developed be used by the insurance industry. Planned as well was the presentation of this propaganda at seminars and training workshops for professionals. With Grace Monaco, Jim Lowell, Peter Mansell, and John Renner all involved with NHCAA, there can be little doubt that the insurance executives would learn about "quackery, health fraud and insurance fraud," only from the limited perspective of these "experts."

The following headline and story appeared in *Insurance Advocate,* an insurance industry publication, on November 12, 1987:

First Computerized Network Designed to Combat Health Fraud is Unveiled.

The nation's first computerized network designed to combat health care fraud, said to be a $10 billion-a-year drain on the economy, was unveiled at the third annual NATIONAL HEALTH CARE ANTI-FRAUD SEMINAR in Washington.

The network, a central information system monitoring all health claims—both those submitted to MEDICARE and private insurers—begins operations this month in FLORIDA and will be implemented nationally next spring. Through this network, the insurance companies and the federal government will pool claims data on health care providers in all states.

Establishing the network has been a major thrust of the anti-fraud association. The association will now be able to provide physicians and hospitals with the names of physicians convicted of fraud or barred by the federal government from receiving Medicare or Medicaid benefits.

The insurance industry has lost billions of dollars over the years in payment of inflated health-care costs related to orthodox medicine and hospitals. This would especially include the unnecessary costs involved in over-testing, which is the hallmark of "defensive medicine," a term orthodox medicine uses to describe and justify batteries of tests that are performed on patients in order to defend against the possibility of malpractice lawsuits. There are some who feel that defensive medicine is just another means to further cover up medical incompetence in the operating room or hospital. Ultimately, it has been the insurance industry which has been burdened with the bill generated by these inflated medical costs.

It is, therefore, no surprise that the insurance industry would jump at the chance to save billions of dollars by joining in on this Anti-Quackery/Health Fraud campaign. It could be used as another means to cut corners on payout on insurance bills. Additionally, if "experts" describe the horrors of alternative medicine and show how to systematically cut alternative medicine out of insurance payments and reimbursement, this would further justify such cost-cutting activity in the name of consumer protection.

Under the guise of cost containment programs, peer review, utilization review, and outside "independent" insurance consultants (IME = Independent Medical Evaluators), the insurance industry simply incorporated new ways to increase profits. However, with the "experts" seizing this as a golden opportunity to further the cause of the "anti-quackery" campaign, it would appear that the insurance industry may have been directed against the alternatives and therefore used as pawns in an anti-competitive game. For that matter, this may also be true for the government agencies involved.

Any way one looks at this, the bottom line is economics. It is apparent that the economic competitors of the alternatives have simply taken advantage of the insurance industry's crisis by showing the insurance industry how to save money. Using this crisis, they have now apparently been able to help, direct, instruct, advise, consult, and otherwise adversely influence the insurance industry against the economic competitors of the medical/pharmaceutical industry. By simply identifying those entities in the alternatives as quackery, health fraud, or insurance fraud (in reports or other communications to insurance companies) they have apparently interfered with the business of the alternative practitioners, clinics, and manufacturers.

As an illustration of this point, consider the following example of how Emprise and their Consensus Panels' studies and reports impacted on one alternative target identified and persecuted via the insurance industry.

On June 29, 1990, a law suit was filed in the United States District Court for the Southern District of Texas, Houston Division, on behalf of Stanislaw R. Burzynski, M.D., and the Burzynski Research Institute (BRI) against Aetna Life Insurance Company, Emprise, Inc., Grace Powers Monaco, and a law firm. Among the actionable offenses (torts) were four counts of racketeering under the RICO Act.

The suit alleged that the action was brought against Emprise, Monaco, and the other defendants based on "defendants' multi-faceted fraudulent scheme" designed, among other things, "to interfere with and damage plaintiff's business in order to reduce Aetna's liability to pay for non-FDA approved cancer treatments, for which Aetna is obligated under law to pay. . ." [Point (i)] and ". . .to cause other insurance companies to reject payment for BRI's treatment for which the other insurance companies are obligated to pay. . ." [Point (iii)]

The suit further explained the Nature of the Action in Point (ii).It stated:

> The illegal conduct alleged herein is part of a nationwide scheme conceived and executed by defendants to defraud insured persons and their treating physicians by wrongfully denying health insurance benefits which Aetna and other insurers are lawfully obligated to provide.

> The goal of the scheme is to drastically reduce Aetna's and other insurers' claims exposure by eliminating a vulnerable part of its claims liability. Aetna's principle tactics to achieve this goal include harassment of doctors and other medical professionals to force them to forego their fees for Aetna-insured patients by instituting or threatening to institute frivolous claims against them.

The suit describes the nature of the alleged actions:

> . . .and most importantly providing false or incomplete information to law enforcement authorities to hector and goad government agencies into pursuing investigations of plaintiffs for the purposes of injuring plaintiffs in their business and gaining an advantage in its civil litigation with BRI.

. . .As part of their scheme to reduce its insurance liability and to drive plaintiffs and other similar clinics out of business, Aetna and the other defendants have also created a purportedly unbiased data-base reviewing Medical practitioners such as Dr. Burzynski who provide non-standard or alternative treatments to cancer.

To organize the data-base, defendants created a new entity, defendant Emprise, Inc. ("Emprise"). This entity ostensibly has no direct connection to Aetna or any other insurance company; however, the undisclosed purpose and agenda of Emprise is to publish negative reviews of alternative medical practitioners, which purport to be objective, but which are biased and are without objective basis, solely in order to justify and legitimize insurers' unlawful decision to deny payment for unconventional treatments otherwise reimbursable under the terms of many insurance contracts.

. . .Emprise obtained its initial funding from United States government grants, yet its grant applications failed to disclose its real purpose and the close working connection between its principals and Aetna and other insurance companies, the fact that defendant Monaco was a consultant or attorney in legal actions relating to one or more subjects of the data-base, or the fact that the research findings ostensibly being prepared for the benefit of taxpayers were being privately disseminated to insurers before publication of its results.

It was also discovered that Grace Powers Monaco had, as an attorney, represented one of the very alternative practitioners (Virginia Livingston) that Emprise was looking into during the grant study. The suit elaborated on this as follows:

The creation of the data-base also provided an opportunity for defendant Grace Monaco to pursue what amounted to a separate but related protection scheme. When it became known that Emprise was collecting information about the alternative practitioners, its principal Grace Monaco let it be known that as a practicing health care attorney, either alone or through her law firm she was available to be "retained" by alternative health care professionals for legal work. The implied message was that if she or her law firm was retained, Emprise might be more favorably disposed to the practitioner in its review. Thus, it appears that the defendants intended in part to finance part of their overall scheme with the funds of the very practitioners they sought to discredit.

At the time of the suit, two items related to Burzynski's alternative therapy were under study and evaluation by the "expert" consensus panels. Under DIAGNOSTIC TESTS was listed: Burzynski Test (balance of peptides). On the Consensus Panel evaluating his test were William Jarvis, Ph.D., James Lowell, Ph.D., and John Renner, M.D. Burzynski's attorney was apparently accurate about the study being biased and not objective in that regard. As far as the charges that the reports that Emprise disseminated included "false or incomplete information" is concerned, the suit stated:

. . .Aetna had been following BRI for years and by Aetna's own admission had a "large file" on BRI; that in 1980 Aetna's senior medical investigator had done a thorough investigation of Dr. Bryzynski which revealed several articles provided by him and concluded that his therapy while not FDA-approved had some "promise as a chemotherapeutic agent."

Developments in antineoplaston chemotherapy, as it is now known, have been the subject of numerous international conferences. The U.S. Department of Defense, via researchers at the Uniformed Services Research Hospital have commenced work with antineoplastons and their preliminary results offer validation that antineoplastons are effective and that Dr. Bryzynski's theory that antineoplastons reprogram cancer cells is well-founded.

The fact is that according to an Interoffice Communication dated October 14, 1980, from D.C. Kellsey, M.D., Medical Director, Medical Claims for Aetna to Russ Robertson, Senior Examiner, Group Claim, Aetna, their conclusion after reviewing materials about Burzynski's therapy was: "Antineoplaston A still remains an experimental drug albeit one with a suggestion of promise as a chemotherapeutic agent in the battle against cancer."

Apparently the Emprise study group did not include this information in the reports which, the suit charges, got into the hands of the insurance industry and law enforcement and other government agencies. In other words, the study group was selective in what they chose to report.

The National Health Care Anti-Fraud Association (NHCAA) must have greeted these "health fraud and quackery experts" with open arms. The goals and purposes of NHCAA are strikingly in tune with the National Council Against Health Fraud's activities on "quackery and health fraud":

To improve the prevention, detection and civil and criminal prosecution of health care fraud.
To assist law enforcement agencies to prosecute health care fraud.

With the anti-alternative "experts" advising the insurance industry on which alternatives *not* to pay, and otherwise influencing the insurance industry against alternatives, it is little wonder that many practitioners and treatments have (1) been cut out of coverage totally, (2) had payments withheld, or (3) faced insurance company policies of "low, slow, or no payment" to alternatives.

The Bryzynski lawsuit against Aetna outlined another tactic that the insurance industry apparently has used against alternative practitioners:

> Upon information and belief, Aetna together with other defendants devised a series of tactics and a fraudulent scheme to solve its liability problems. First, it decided that it would deny the claims submitted by alternative medical practitioners and put the burden on the patient to sue to collect benefits rightfully owing under insurance policies.
>
> Second, upon information and belief, based on the advice of defendant Monaco and others, Aetna decided that if a patient did sue, Aetna would initiate a third-party or other claim against the treating physician.
>
> Third, Aetna decided to encourage and support the creation of an on-line data base containing negative evaluations of alternative medical practitioners so that it could rationalize and legitimize its prior unlawful decision not to pay legitimate claims. Such a data base would permit it to refer to a purportedly objective body of research ostensibly prepared by unbiased taxpayer-funded investigators who were looking out for the public interest. Based on Aetna's support and at its behest and with its approval, defendant Monaco and as other as yet unknown defendants founded defendant Emprise.

The suit points out that Emprise had one of its Grant Applications denied:

> However, its application was denied after, *inter alia,* the granting authorities learned of the conflicts-of-interest and the close connection between the principals of Emprise and Aetna and other insurance companies.

With respect to the statement that Monaco and others founded Emprise allegedly with Aetna's support and "at its behest and with its approval," the following information (obtained during my 1986 investigation into Emprise and its predecessor, the Public Issues in Health Care Choices: a Project of the Ohio Council Against Health Fraud) is of interest.

In 1986, two years prior to Emprise incorporating in Washington, D.C., Grace Monaco and several people met to discuss the funding of this newly formed "project." According to one source present at this meeting, money was to come from several sources, including The American Cancer Society, the pharmaceutical industry, and the insurance industry. My informant did not specify which insurance company would be helping to fund this group at that time, but Aetna could very well have been one of the insurance industry funding sources back in 1986.

One thing is very clear. This campaign has been on-going for almost ten years and has consistently directed its attacks against those in the alternative movement who were in direct economic competition to the pharmaceutical industry, which has been involved in funding this campaign from the start. The pattern of the overall activity does in fact constitute a continuing group of persons associated together (whether they call themselves a coalition or a campaign) for a common purpose of engaging in a course of conduct which has been designed to injure those involved in the alternative health-care movement.

This has apparently been done by defaming and otherwise injuring those practitioners, manufacturers, and others in the alternative movement by devising a scheme to deprive them of payment from insurance companies, as well as denying patients and consumers the products that some of them depend on for good health. It is very possible that denying consumers some of these products, services, treatments, therapies, and modalities will result in death as a direct as a result of this "anti-quackery" campaign.

A national data bank on alternative practitioners has been assembled as part of the network that the insurance industry put together. Hundreds of insurance company members of the NHCAA share this information on the targeted practitioners. Take into account first that the members apparently have access to the Emprise study reports on the various treatments, services, products, and practitioners. Add to this the fact that the insurance industry is passing on names of "defrauders" to federal and state government agencies, as well as state licensing boards. It's no wonder that practitioners all over the country are coming under fire by the Medical Boards, in addition to having insurance claims denied and (in some cases) being placed under investigation by the Task Force on Health Fraud. It is, in many cases, a type of medical McCarthyism.

Each of the insurance company members of the NHCAA have, in this fashion, involved themselves in an industry-wide campaign directed against the alternatives. They have apparently allowed themselves to be adversely influenced by members of the anti-quackery campaign and those involved in it who have been advising, consulting, instructing, and otherwise adversely influencing the insurance industry against those targeted by this campaign.

What is occurring is that a massive "health-fraud coalition" has been formed, sharing information outside its structure as well as within it. The structure includes the insurance industry, federal and state governmental agencies, "anti-quackery" groups, medical boards, and others, all working with a common purpose to eliminate "health fraud and quackery" in the name of public interest. However, the actual effects are stunning when viewed against the existing laws on the books that detail violations of the Sherman Antitrust laws, RICO laws, civil rights laws, and conspiracy laws.

From all indications, the NHCAA computer is shared by its members. This includes Blue Cross/Blue Shield, which apparently has a massive computer tracking system at a facility just outside Harrisburg, Pennsylvania.

In a Confidential Memorandum dated August 8, 1990, Thomas Brunner, the attorney for the NHCAA (based in Washington, D.C.), wrote the NHCAA Board of Governors outlining his concerns about the massive computer network that had been set up. He stated to the Board members:

> As you know, The Pennsylvania Project has been carefully structured to minimize any threats of civil liability from information sharing. With this goal in mind, we have arranged a system where the disclosure of information is strictly limited, based on agreements by all participating companies on how information can be used.

> We are concerned about NHCAA operations in unauthorized states. Any information sharing outside the boundaries of the current guidelines presents potential liability issues.

Mr. Brunner's concerns are well founded, in that the U.S. federal antitrust laws clearly set the guidelines for such information sharing. The law clearly states that *it is illegal to share information when it is used for anti-competitive purposes.*

Timothy J. Muris, Director of the Bureau of Competition of the U.S. Federal Trade Commission (FTC) once referred to the FTC's position on this very issue when he stated, "Sharing information is lawful, unless it reduces competition."
With this in mind, it can be deduced that what is going on is in fact illegal. The economic competitors of the alternative health-care system have combined their efforts and have formed a network which has:

1. Identified treatments, modalities, services, products, therapies, practitioners, and manufacturers to attack in this "anti-quackery" campaign.

2. Conducted "independent studies" using "experts" on "quackery" who form consensus panels to sit in judgment of these alternative targets. Many of these so-called experts have made careers out of attacking the very same alternatives addressed by these "independent" studies.

3. Issued "reports" on the efficacy of those alternative targets.

4. Distributed these reports to insurance companies, federal and state enforcement and regulatory agencies, and licensing boards, as well as other health professionals and groups across the country.

5. Encouraged use of these reports as industry guidelines. (Insurance companies have been enlisted to act as gatekeepers within the insurance industry to keep alternatives out, and to report targeted physicians to state Medical Boards.)

6. Influenced the governmental agencies involved to use these reports to determine which targets to go after in the campaign against the alternatives.

7. Solicited and obtained the financial support of the pharmaceutical industry, which resulted in a joint agreement with the FDA.

8. Assisted the FDA in its work with other federal and state agencies to coordinate efforts against targets in the alternatives by forming coalitions and health fraud task forces around the country.

All of this makes for a very powerful coalition which has banded together to eliminate the economic competitors of the very industry that has been discovered to be funding this campaign.

We have the federal government involved in co-funding a campaign against alternatives with the very industry they should be policing—the pharmaceutical industry.

We have the federal government working with people who are avowed enemies of the alternative movement.

We see these spokespersons presenting training seminars and lectures at insurance industry conferences, joint government conferences, and health-care professional conferences, thus adversely influencing their audiences against the alternatives.

We see massive computer systems set up to link private groups with government and insurance industry outlets to spread their propaganda against the alternative movement.

We see practitioners, clinics, health food stores, multi-level sales companies, product manufacturers, and distributors all being targeted by this campaign. The result has been raids, seizures, embargoes, bad publicity, de-licensing, the destruction of businesses, and the disruption of lives—all in the name of "public service."

Is it really public service? Who is really being served here, the public or the vested interests?

In the Emprise Grant Progress Report it was proposed that Grace Monaco test the information developed during the project study by presenting some of this information to several conferences she planned to attend. One conference she listed was the FDA's National Health Fraud Conference for 1988. This conference was held March 13-15, 1988, in Kansas City, Missouri. It was cosponsored by the U.S. Food and Drug Administration, the Department of Health and Human Services, St. Mary's Hospital in Kansas City, and Trinity Lutheran Hospital in Kansas City.

The Program for the conference listed Linda Koller Strub as Conference Coordinator. Interestingly, she is one of Dr. John Renner's staff and has worked with him for years on the Anti-Quackery/Health Fraud Campaign.

One stated objective of this conference was to "assist local, state, and national agencies, plus consumer, health professionals, and industry organizations, in strengthening their health fraud programs." The conference held various workshops/seminars and had several lecturers on subjects related to the anti-health fraud issues. Some of the moderators and speakers at the workshops included: John Renner, M.D.; William Jarvis, Ph.D.; Stephen Barrett, M.D.; Victor

Herbert, M.D.; and Grace Powers Monaco, Esq. All of these people
are known members of the National Council Against Health Fraud,
or were on Consensus Panels in the Emprise study of alternatives, or
assisted in planning it. Two of the workshops that directly related to the insurance industry were listed as follows:

> WORKING WITH HEALTH INSURERS
> TO COMBAT HEALTH FRAUD
> (Panelists will discuss how to involve health insurers in
> anti-fraud activities, the type of information they can most
> effectively use, and ways to assist insurance companies in
> identifying fraudulent claims.)

> THE ROLE OF THE INSURANCE INDUSTRY
> IN COMBATING HEALTH FRAUD
> (A review of how insurance companies combat health
> fraud, the type of information they collect, and how they work
> with other organizations.)

Most of the speakers and panelists involved were from the FDA,
National Council Against Health Fraud, Council of Better Business
Bureaus, or representatives of some other state or federal agencies
that have been involved in this campaign from the start. The apparent
objective was to network on information that could be shared on
"health fraud and quackery." In fact, one of the stated objectives at
this conference was to "create effective networking links." Dr. John
H. Renner, M.D., as the Chairman of the Midwest Council Against
Health Fraud, headed the Welcome Session on the first day of the
conference, sharing the stage with John A. Norris, Deputy Commissioner, Food and Drug Administration.

The role of the various anti-health-fraud entities becomes clear
when one reviews the original October Plan, along with the National
Institute of Health's Grant Progress Report, the National Health Care
Anti-Fraud Association's activities, in concert with the Pharmaceutical Advertising Council/FDA's Public Service Anti-Quackery Campaign. This coalition's activity is a key factor in how the alternative
health-care system is being eliminated from the health-care
marketplace through propaganda.

Thus far we have examined what amounts to sometimes-confus-
ing pieces of a puzzle. Each piece by itself doesn't make a lot of

sense, but when it is all placed together the entire picture can begin to be seen as a whole.

No complete conclusion can be drawn without first examining the pharmaceutical industry itself. The drug companies that came forward to finance this "anti-quackery" campaign back in the beginning all had something in common. Their products were in direct economic competition with products within the alternative health-care movement. To examine and analyze these products would be a big part of understanding what the motivation has been behind this campaign. Which companies are involved? What products do they produce? Against which alternative products do they compete? What do these companies stand to lose if the alternatives are not eliminated and the public continues to have access to these competing products?

In light of what appears to be a growing acceptance and recognition by science as to the benefits of vitamins, supplements, herbs, and other alternative products in combating heart disease, cancer, and arthritis (among the many diseases for which alternatives are used) another question arises. Why are the pharmaceuticals, the FDA, the insurance industry, and "consumer experts" still pounding away with the propaganda campaign against these approaches?

It is believed by some that the acceptance and recognition of certain alternative products by established science would serve to support and reinforce the charges that are presented in this book. It may very well be that there is, in fact, a massive anti-competitive campaign going on against the alternatives and their related products, solely because these drug-less alternatives are *known to work*.

The following chapter on the drug industry serves to further define and detail the apparent motivation behind the pharmaceutical industry's relentless campaign against its competition in the alternative field. A possible answer to the riddle of why they are doing this may become obvious. It is probable that this data is a vital piece in completing the puzzle and is a piece which makes all the others fall quickly into place.

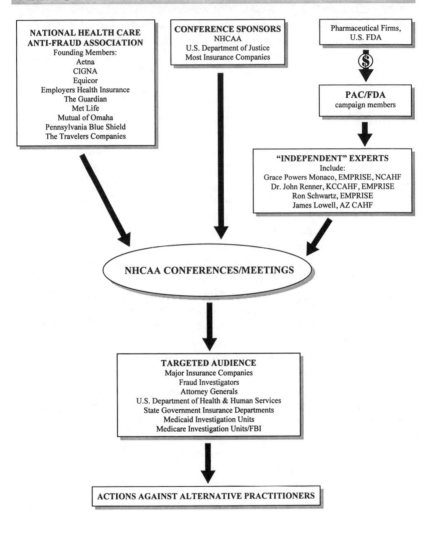

NATIONAL INSURANCE CAMPAIGN CHART

NATIONAL HEALTH CARE ANTI-FRAUD ASSOCIATION
Founding Members:
Aetna
CIGNA
Equicor
Employers Health Insurance
The Guardian
Met Life
Mutual of Omaha
Pennsylvania Blue Shield
The Travelers Companies

CONFERENCE SPONSORS
NHCAA
U.S. Department of Justice
Most Insurance Companies

Pharmaceutical Firms,
U.S. FDA

PAC/FDA
campaign members

"INDEPENDENT" EXPERTS
Include:
Grace Powers Monaco, EMPRISE, NCAHF
Dr. John Renner, KCCAHF, EMPRISE
Ron Schwartz, EMPRISE
James Lowell, AZ CAHF

NHCAA CONFERENCES/MEETINGS

TARGETED AUDIENCE
Major Insurance Companies
Fraud Investigators
Attorney Generals
U.S. Department of Health & Human Services
State Government Insurance Departments
Medicaid Investigation Units
Medicare Investigation Units/FBI

ACTIONS AGAINST ALTERNATIVE PRACTITIONERS

EMPRISE CAMPAIGN CHART

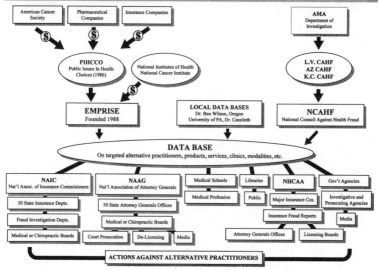

Chapter 8

The Business of Drugs

"The Task Force considered. . .what steps are necessary to ensure that the existence of dietary supplements on the market does not act as a disincentive for drug development."
[Gary Dykstra, FDA Associate Commissioner for Regulatory Affairs, as Chairman of the FDA Dietary Supplements Task Force, Final Report, May 1992.]

Chapter Four named three of the pharmaceutical companies that initially financed the Anti-Quackery Campaign: Syntex, Lederle, and Hoffman-LaRoche. On November 15, 1985, I received a letter (on *joint* Pharmaceutical Advertising Council and FDA letterhead) from Paul Chusid, Coordinator of the PAC/FDA Anti-Quackery Program and President of Grey Medical Advertising. He attached a list of all of the drug companies that helped finance the campaign up to that time, including the following. (* indicates client of Grey Advertising or one of its subsidiaries, including Grey Medical Advertising.)

Beecham Laboratories*
Bristol-Myers Company*
Burroughs Wellcome Co.
Carter Wallace, Inc.*
Gilbert Labs
Hoeschst-Roussel Pharmaceuticals*
Hoffman-LaRoche, Inc.*
Janssen Pharmaceutical
Jeffrey Martin, Inc.
Johnson & Johnson*
Knoll Pharmaceutical Co.
Lederle/American Cyanamid Company*
McNeil Consumer Products
Merck, Sharp & Dome
Organon, Inc.
Pennwalt Corporation
The Proprietary Assn.

A.H. Robbins
Rorer Group
Sandoz
Schering Corp.
Squibb*
Sterling Drug Inc.
Stuart Pharmaceuticals
Syntex Corp.
Warner Lambert Company

The targets selected in this Anti-Quackery Campaign were based on the survey mentioned in Chapter Four. Vitamins were on the top of the category list. Under this category are thousands of products and manufacturers. The drug products produced by these pharmaceutical companies are in direct economic competition to the vitamin/supplement industry against which the pharmaceutical campaign has been directed.

We have drug companies teaming up with the FDA to go after the economic competitors of the very drug companies that are financing this campaign. Working with government, they have sought to have the government investigate, indict, prosecute, and jail many of their competitors. When one has the government telling one what one can buy and cannot buy, one has a totalitarian/fascist state of affairs in the marketplace. What then exists is a market of government-endorsed products or services—a vital ingregient for creating a monopoly.

Economics is at the bottom of this campaign. But the specifics of the economic interest of these particular pharmaceutical houses are of interest as we attempt to better understand this campaign. In what part of the economic pie do these pharmaceutical companies have an interest? Do the areas in which they have market shares have competitors in the alternative health-care system? What specific products do the drug companies financing this campaign (hereafter referred to as the PAC firms) produce? The following gives some insight into these questions and thereby helps make more sense out of this attack.

Gary Dykstra's statement at the beginning of this chapter underlines the entire motivation behind the "vitamin/supplement wars" into which the drug industry and the FDA entered. How could a dietary supplement "act as a disincentive for drug development"? If certain vitamins in fact help to alleviate or cure diseases, the obvious result of their widespread use would be less demand for drugs produced by the pharmaceutical industry. Less demand would of course result in less motivation for the pharmaceutical companies to develop new drugs. The FDA is in essence saying that it will take "what steps are necessary to ensure" that the existence of the vitamin industry in the market does not interfere with the sale of drugs. There are billions of dollars at stake here.

To fully comprehend the enormous scope of the financial war that is being waged against vitamins, minerals, and supplements, one must first look at the overall health-care-spending picture in the United States.

In a 1992 *U.S.A. Today* article, spending on overall health-care and specifically for drugs in the years 1981-86 was calculated as follows:

Year	Billions	Spent on Drugs (Billions)
1981	$287.0	$20.7
1982	$323.6	$22.1
1983	$357.2	$24.5
1984	$391.1	$26.5
1985	$422.6	$28.7
1986	$458.7	$30.6

Figures for 1987-89 were unavailable, but the article put health-care costs at $666 billion for 1990 and at $817 billion for 1991. The figures for 1981-86 show a steady 7% of overall health-care costs being spent on drugs. If we project that percentage and estimate the amount spent in 1991-92, the chart continues as follows:

Year	Billions	Spent on Drugs (Billions)
1991	$666.0	$46.6
1992	$817.0	$56.7

According to figures released from the U.S. Office of Management and Budget (OMB), overall health-care spending by 1997 is projected to be $1 trillion, $475 billion dollars. That reads like this: $1,475,000,000,000. If we continue our assumption that 7% of that figure will be spent on drugs, we can project that Americans will spend *$103.25 billion ($103,250,000,000) on drugs* in 1997. The term "big business" does not adequately describe the stake the pharmaceutical manufacturers have in the future of drugs.

We have just seen how much American consumers spend on drugs. Another interesting set of figures shows how much the drug companies spend on advertising to generate the drug sales figures and to counteract the development of competition from alternative therapies. Keeping in mind that many of the drug advertising dollars go to the medical journals which the AMA publishes, the following figures are of interest:

Year	Spent on Drug Advertising (Millions)
1970	$ 38
1975	$ 50 (approximately)
1980	$ 79
1981	$ 84 (approximately)
1982	$ 89
1983	$105
1984	$135
1985	$148

The earliest recorded planning stages of the PAC Public Service Anti-Quackery Campaign took place in 1983. In that year, Paul Chusid sent letters out to hundreds of pharmaceutical companies to solicit their financial support for this campaign. By 1984 they had the television and radio media advertisements worked out and selected. By 1985 they were ready to launch the campaign, which they did in September in Washington, D.C.

Let's examine how the drug advertising figures correlate with the campaign's progress. Prior to the campaign, in 1981, $84 million was spent on drug advertisements. In 1982 there was an increase of $5 million. However, in 1983, the year that Chusid started up the drive to collect money from the drug companies, the amount spent on advertising jumped $16 million, and in 1984 it jumped another $30 million. By the time they put the campaign into full swing, in 1985, it had jumped to $148 million, an increase of $59 million from 1982. That is a 66% increase in drug advertising between 1982 to 1986. The figures from 1986 to 1992 were not available, but one can reasonably project that the amount has continued to increase comparably each year.

These figures are vital to an understanding of pharmaceutical companies' motivation in the war against alternative medicine in two ways. First, it's obvious that these figures represent an enormous investment in and of themselves; $148 million is not an amount to be written off lightly. Second, the size of that figure shows just how profitable drug sales must be, for the industry to spend that much to protect such sales.

Who are the big players in this drama? Who dominates the production of drug products, and what percentage of the products are produced by PAC members? The following figures show the strength of PAC members and therefore their interest in eliminating competition from alternative therapies. It's important, as we look at these star players, to remember that, from an initial list of targets, the PAC/FDA campaign against the alternatives eventually listed hundreds of products, treatments therapies, services, modalities, clinics, and manufacturers involved in alternative medicine. Each of these entities represents some form of a threat to the control over the marketplace by the drug companies financing the campaign. The Roper Survey (Chapter 4) named and identified the economic competition to the drug houses. This then served as a target list for the campaign. The original list targeted the following categories:

1. Vitamins for better health
2. Chiropractic for back pain
3. Psychological counseling for better mental health
4. Laetrile for cancer
5. DMSO for arthritis treatment
6. Pills for sobering up
7. Pills for a better sex life

Following the analysis of companies' investment in drug categories, when appropriate I have inserted the alternative therapy which threatens to compete with the products and is therefore targeted for elimination.

Who's Who of PAC Drug Peddlers

AIDS Products
Burroughs-Wellcome manufactures 100% of Retrovic (AZT).

Hoffman-LaRoche manufactures 100% of the experimental DDC.

Products for AIDS Related Complex (ARC)
Six companies manufacture products for the treatment of ARC. Three of the six are PAC members, and they produce 11 (78%) of the 14 available products. Roche, Burroughs-Wellcome, and Schering are the biggest PAC members who produce these products.

[Note: Dozens of products used in the alternative health-care community are popular with AIDS patients. See Chapters 5 and 9.]

Arthritis Drugs

Nine (39%) of 23 manufacturers of arthritis drugs are PAC members. They produce 35 (60%) of the 58 available products. Three manufacturers, all of whom are PAC members, produce gold compounds. They are Merck, Sharp & Dohme; Smith, Kline & Beecham; and Schering. They each produce 1 of the 3 available products. Five of the 10 manufacturers of steroids are PAC members. They produce 19 (70%) of 27 available products. Two companies— Merck, Sharp & Dohme and Syntex—produce 13 (48%) of the steroids available.

[Note: Syntex produces one particular product, Naprosyn, which had $366.5 million dollars in sales in 1985, the year PAC started its campaign in earnest. One of its chief economic competitors in the alternative field is an herb—APR—manufactured, distributed, and sold by the multi-level company Herbalife. It is little wonder, then, that Syntex was one of the first companies to help finance the Anti-Quackery Campaign; it is in direct competition with Herbalife. (See Chapter 10.) It is also no wonder that Herbalife was at the top of the target list put together for the PAC/FDA campaign (Chapter 4). DMSO and other alternatives also came under attack.]

Analgesics

Thirteen (30%) of 43 Manufacturers are PAC members. They produce 80 (46%) of 175 products. The producers of the largest numbers of analgesics are McNeil Consumer (13 products), Bristol-Myers (13 products), Knoll Pharmaceuticals (9 products), Janssen (6 products), and Smith, Kline & Beecham (6 products).

Of the 175 analgesic products, 88 are narcotic. They are produced by 25 manufacturers, 8 (32%) are PAC members. These 8 companies produce 28 (32%) of the 88 narcotic analgesics. Most of the products are produced by Knoll Pharmaceuticals (9), Sandoz (4), Roche (3), Janssen (6), and A.H. Robbins (2).

[Note: Chiropractic for the treatment of back pain has gained tremendously in popularity, and its success has caused it to be listed as the #2 target in the campaign.]

Biologicals

Two companies manufacture toxoids. One of them, Lederle, is a PAC member and manufactures 3 (60%) of the 5 toxoids available.

Biological response modifiers are manufactured by 7 companies, 3 (43%) of whom are PAC members. Those 3—Roche, Hoeschst-Roussel, and Schering Corporation—produce 3 (43%) of 7 available products.

Vaccines are produced by 11 manufacturers, 6 (55%) of whom are PAC members who produce 19 (66%) of the 29 available vaccines. Nine of the 29 vaccines (31%) are produced by one company, Merck, Sharp & Dohme.

[Note: Within the alternative health-care community there is a strong outcry against giving children vaccines because in many cases the vaccine itself causes more deaths than the disease it is supposed to be preventing. There are hundreds of cases of deaths and severe reactions recorded each year to vaccines.]

Antineoplastics for Cancer/Leukemia

Nine (33%) of the 27 manufacturers of products for cancer and leukemia are PAC members. They produce 44 (53%) of the 83 products available. Thirty-eight of the products are produced by 5 PAC members: Bristol-Myers (16), Roche (7), Schering (5), Lederle (5), and Burroughs-Wellcome (5).

[Note: Of all the types of drugs that are in competition with alternative products, this category probably brings in the most in dollar sales to the drug industry. This may well explain why the Emprise study targeted Burzynski's anti-neoplaston therapy, which resulted in him filing a RICO lawsuit against Emprise and Aetna insurance. (Chapter 7)]

Detoxifying Agents

One manufacturer—Bristol Myers, a PAC member—manufactures the only detoxifying agent on the market.

[Note: Chapter 5 noted that detoxification programs were targeted with other alternative methods used in fighting cancer and AIDS. These would include any detoxification program used in alcohol and drug rehabilitation which employs large doses of vitamins and minerals. Such programs have been used with great success in Agent Orange studies, in handling exposure to dangerous levels of industrial chemicals, and in detoxification from street drugs, around the world. Orthodox medicine has continually attacked these programs despite their successes.]

Fertility Agents
Two companies manufacture fertility agents. One—Sandoz—is a PAC member and produces 2 (33%) of 6 available products.
[Note: Pills for Sexual Rejuvenation were among the targeted products in the survey. Within the alternative products sold there are certain vitamins, and mostly certain herbs, which are used to enhance one's sexual drive.]

Gout Treatment
Two—Merck, Sharp & Dohme and Burroughs-Wellcome—of 5 manufacturers of gout treatments are PAC members. They produce 3 (60%) of 5 available products.
[Note: The alternative treatment of gout uses vitamin therapy and diet.]

Headaches/Migraines
Two (29%) of 7 manufacturers of remedies for headaches\migraines are PAC members, and they produce 5 (45%) of 11 available products. Sandoz produces 4, and Organan produces 1.
[Note: Some of the more common alternative treatments used for headaches/migraines include: vitamin therapy,chiropractic, acupuncture, acupressure, homeopathy, naturopathy, and electro-acupuncture/herbs.]

Preparations for Cardiovascular Problems
Fifteen (31%) of 48 manufacturers of drugs for treatment of heart problems are PAC members. They produce 97 (31%) of the 316 available products. Merck, Sharpe & Dohme produces 36 products, Bristol-Myers produces 8, Burroughs-Wellcome produces 8, and Schering produces 8.
[Note: Alternative health care's largest single treatment for heart problems is chelation therapy. Also used are vitamin therapy, supplements, and herbs to bring down blood pressure and to lower cholesterol to reduce the potential for heart disease. Acupuncture is also used.]

Psychotropics
Of 28 manufacturers of psychotropics, 9 (32%) are PAC members. They produce 64 (52%) of the 123 products available.
Smith, Kline & Beecham (who produces Thorazine) manufactures 23; Roche (who produces Valium and Librium) manufactures 15.

Anti-depressants are produced by 17 manufacturers, 9 (53%) of whom are PAC members. Of the 29 anti-depressants on the market, 4 are produced by Roche and 4 by Schering.

Of 7 manufacturers of hypnotics, 3 (43%) are PAC members. They produce 4 of the 12 available products. Roche produces 2, and Sandoz and Stuart each produce 1.

Of the 14 manufacturers of products for nausea/vomiting/vertigo, 5 (36%) are members of PAC. They produce 28 (57%) of 48 available products. Smith, Kline & Beecham manufactures 20 of the products.

[Note: Considering the billions of dollars spent on these narcotics in the name of "mental health" it is obvious why this was high on the PAC/FDA survey list in the campaign. It is also obvious why certain psychiatrists (who are the main distributors of these narcotics) would be whole-heartedly against such things as faith healing, spiritual healing, Christian Science, visualization, imagery, and all other forms of non-pharmaceutical religious practices. It is also of interest that the National Council Against Health Fraud has, in articles in its newsletter, criticized each of these religious entities. There are also vitamins and herbs used as substitutes for these often-dangerous drugs.]

Drugs for Treatment of Obesity and for Weight Reduction
Of 4 manufacturers of amphetamines, 1—Smith, Kline & Beecham (who makes Dexedrine)—is a PAC member and produces 3 (50%) of the 6 available products.

Of 9 manufacturers of appetite suppressants, 3 (33%) are PAC members. The 3—Sandoz, A.H. Robins, and Smith, Kline & Beecham—each produce 1 of the 10 products on the market.

[Note: The weight reduction/obesity alternative market represents billions of dollars in lost drug sales. During the FDA/PAC campaign, many weight reduction plans and companies were targeted and attacked. Included were Jenny Craig, Diet Centers, Herbalife, Shaklee, and others involved in weight reduction plans and products.]

Drugs for Sleeping Disorders
Three (43%) of the 7 manufacturers of preparations for the treatment of sleeping disorders are PAC members, and they produce 4 (33%) of the 12 available products. Roche manufactures 2 of them.

[*Note*: Acupuncture, vitamins, minerals, and herbs, used for sleeping disorders in alternative medicine, are competition for the big business of sleeping pills.]

Vitamins/Multi-vitamins

Of 32 pharmaceutical companies who manufacture vitamins, 7 (22%) are PAC members. They produce 25 products, among which are 9 produced by Roche and 6 produced by Lederle.

Both of the pharmaceutical companies—Burroughs-Wellcome and Lederle—who manufacture anti-folic acid are PAC members.

Of the 3 manufacturers of parenteral (injectable) vitamins, 2 are PAC members. Roche and Merck, Sharpe & Dohme each produce 1 of the 3 available products.

Nine manufacturers produce other vitamin products; 5 of these are PAC members, and they produce 8 of 12 available products.

[Note: The war over vitamins and supplements includes the fact that the pharmaceutical industry wants to take over the manufacturing of all vitamins. Lederle, for example, is currently running a million-dollar TV ad campaign for one of its vitamin products, promoting antioxidants (vitamins A, C, and E). These vitamins are now recognized as helping in the prevention of heart disease. Yet they have been targeted by the very same pharmaceutical firms who are themselves selling these vitamins and supplements. While the FDA is raiding and seizing vitamins from alternative manufacturers, the drug companies are diversifying into vitamins. We don't see the FDA raiding drug companies who make vitamins. On the contrary, the FDA has focused its attack against the alternative manufacturers of vitamins, supplements, and herbs, as well as health-food stores. Should it succeed in its relentless attack against these alternative targets, then we will see most vitamins manufactured and sold by the pharmaceutical companies. Thus there is a grand irony in this entire situation. Material which follows will defend the use of vitamins and supplements and our right to use them; yet how absurd that such a defense is needed against the pharmaceutical industry's claim that they are ineffective, when that industry is poised to take over the marketing of vitamins and supplements! But such is the ludicrousness of this battle.]

The preceding paragraphs identify the strong PAC-member players in the pharmaceutical drug market. What does their strength mean to the consumer?

Market share is the percentage of a total market of a product held by a company. A company—or a group of companies who cooperate and pool their resources, as do the PAC firms—with strong market shares gains *market power.* Market power which becomes a legal issue, under antitrust laws and anti-monopoly laws, is defined as follows:

> At some inexact point "market power" becomes "monopoly power" (that is the power to control prices and exclude competitors). Such power is marked by high (monopoly) profits over an extended period of time and the failure of other goods (the competition's goods) or services to respond as substitutes. ["Antitrust," *Gilbert Law Summaries*, Harcourt Brace Jovanovich Legal and Professional Publications, 1983-84.]

Now, this last phrase— *"the failure of other goods or services to respond as substitutes"*—is very important to an analysis of this campaign. This is the exact point that FDA Associate Commissioner Dykstra must have had in mind when he stated that the Task Force on Dietary Supplements considered ". . .what steps were necessary to ensure that the existence of dietary supplements on the market does not act as a disincentive for drug development." Here the FDA is seeing to it that vitamins do not prevent or discourage the sales or the development of drugs in the marketplace. This in effect is monopoly power at work. The drug companies are using the FDA to ensure that vitamins will fail as a substitute for drugs in the marketplace.

This is being done in several ways:

1. A campaign is being waged against vitamins and other supplements which alternative medicine uses as substitutes to drugs, in an attempt to identify them as "quack products" in the public's eye.

2. Once items are identified as "quack/health fraud products," the FDA then justifies their investigations, indictments, prosecutions, seizures, embargoes, and anti-competitive activity using the Task Force.

3. Congressional hearings are being held for the purpose of attacking the vitamin, supplement, and herb industries, thus making it easier to pass new laws which would make it

almost impossible for the public to continue to use vitamins, supplements, and herbs as substitutes for drugs.

For example, the Nutrition Labeling and Education Act (NLEA) could result in Vitamin C being available only in amounts equal to the RDA (Recommended Daily Allowance). Instead of consumers being able to purchase 100-tablet bottles of vitamin C in 1000 mgs, they might be able to legally purchase vitamin C only in 50-mg size. This makes the use of vitamins and supplements and herbs cost-prohibitive because one would have to buy 20 bottles to get the same potency of vitamin C that was available before.

It may also be possible that vitamins in larger potency dosages may have to be purchased through a medical doctor with a prescription. For example, when vitamin C is used to fight cancer, or the common cold, mega-doses are taken, up to 10,000 mgs per hour. With the new law in place, this dosage would be possible only by taking thousands of vitamin pills—to achieve the same result that one could previously achieve with just a handful of vitamins.

Such a law would most certainly restrict the consumption of vitamins/supplements/herbs. It would complete the "monopoly circle" by the drug industry, driving their number-one economic competitor out of the marketplace.

This three-step process appears to be the means through which the drug industry is attempting to capture the vitamin/supplement/herbs/alternative market. If laws such as the NLEA succeed, alternative treatments using vitamins/supplements and herbs will disappear from the marketplace as valid substitutes for pharmaceutical drugs. The FDA will have succeeded in its goal, as expressed by Associate FDA Commissioner Gary Dykstra, to *not let the existence of vitamins and dietary supplements to stand in the way of drug development in the marketplace.*

Acknowledging the Benefits of Vitamin Therapy

Many reports, studies, papers and articles—many more than we could address here—support the use of vitamins in treating certain diseases. Scientists from around the country, and the world, recognize the benefits of vitamins in the treatment of many diseases, including the following:

Cancer
Breast cancer
Cancerous tumors

Cervical cancer
Colon cancer
Esophagus cancer
Gastric cancer
Lung cancer
Mouth lesions
Pancreas cancer
Prostrate cancer
Stomach cancer
Weakened chromosomes and immune system

Heart Disease
Arteriosclerosis
High blood pressure
High cholesterol
Weak blood vessels
Conditions leading to heart attacks
Conditions leading to strokes
Weak capillary walls

Other Diseases
Birth Defects
Infections
Cuts
Gum ailments
Osteoporosis/Parkinson's

Over the years, the scientific community has begun to research the benefits of vitamins and supplements and is just now learning about their unique healing properties, knowledge that alternative medicine has had and used for more than 30 years. The following are just a few examples examples.

1. A recent study by Paul F. Jacques, Sc.D., of the U.S. Department of Agriculture, Nutrition Research Center on Aging, indicated that vitamin C may reduce the risk of high blood pressure (and therefore reduce the risk of heart disease). He said, "Higher levels of vitamin C were consistently associated with lower blood pressure."

2. Judith Hallfrisch, Ph.D., with the National Institute on Aging, while conducting a study of more than 550 men and

300 women, discovered that "people with the highest blood levels of vitamin C also had higher levels of HDL." (HDL is high-density lipoprotein, popularly referred to as "good cholesterol.")

3. In a July 1991 study, researchers reported that pregnant women who took folic acid supplements "had a much lower risk than women who did not take the supplement" and that "the women who did not take the supplement had a greater risk of their babies having neural-tube deformities such as spinal bifida, or open spine, and anencephaly, a deadly defect in which much of the brain is missing."

4. Dr. Gladys Block, formerly with the National Cancer Institute and now at the University of Berkeley, recently completed a comprehensive analysis of 15 epidemiological studies on cancer rates and the intake of vitamin C. She ranked individuals according to how much vitamin C they consumed, and she determined that people who were in the top one-fourth had only one-half or one-third the rate of cancer of the esophagus and stomach found in those in the lower quarter.

Other studies have shown a significantly reduced risk for tumors of the pancreas, cervix, lung, and breast when high amounts of vitamin C, vitamin E and beta carotene are eaten. Dr. Block said new evidence suggests that vitamins C and E work to prevent cancer.

5. Raymond B. Bridges, Ph.D., of the University of Kentucky, a leading researcher in the area of heart disease and cigarette smoking, said, "We found that cigarette smokers showed 25 to 30 percent reductions in blood levels of vitamin C when compared to non-smokers." He suggests, "If you smoke you should take in at least 100 to 200 milligrams of vitamin C daily to maintain adequate blood levels of the nutrient—that's about twice the amount nonsmokers need."

6. Studies by Dr. Joseph Witztum, of the University of California at San Diego, and Balz Frei, Ph.D., of Harvard's School of Public Health, indicate that vitamins C and E and beta carotene help to inhibit the destructive process that harmful

free-radicals do to the arterial walls, leading to arteriosclerosis.

7. A study in the British medical journal *Lancet* reports that foods rich in vitamins C and E may also protect against angina, the strangling chest pain caused by a build-up of fatty deposits in the arteries of the heart.

8. Beta carotene, which turns into vitamin A in the body as needed, was found to help patients with cardiac disease. Doctors at Harvard Medical School, who have been following 22,000 male physicians during a 10-year study, made a stunning discovery about beta carotene. They found that men with a history of cardiac disease who were given beta carotene supplements of 50 mg every day suffered half as many heart attacks, strokes, and deaths as those popping placebo pills. Beta carotene reportedly may be a powerful supplement in combating cancer. In Japan and Norway, where the diets are rich in beta carotene, the populations have a low incidence of lung, colon, prostrate, cervical, and breast cancers.

9. A study at the University of Arizona Cancer Center found that three to six months of daily beta carotene pills dramatically reduced precancerous mouth lesions in 70% of patients.

10. Vitamins C and E have been reported to reduce the risk of cataracts by at least 50% according to a Canadian study. Scientists at the National Eye Institute estimate that if cataract development could be delayed by 10 years, about half of cataract surgery could be eliminated.

Other studies have shown that:

• Vitamin C plays a vital role in forming and maintaining collagen, the substance that binds cells together.

• Vitamin C builds and repairs body tissues; heals cuts; combats infections and disease; minimizes bruising and hemorrhaging of blood vessels.

- Vitamin C helps promote the absorption of iron and calcium for healthy bones, joints, and teeth and helps regulate breathing.

- Vitamin C helps in regulating blood pressure and building strong capillary walls and healthy blood vessels.

- Folic acid reportedly counteracts cancer by strengthening the chromosomes and thus prevents dangerous viruses from infiltrating deep into cells and touching off a tumor.

- Vitamin E, taken in high doses by elderly patients, was discovered to have stimulated the growth of warrior white blood cells and fired up the production of immune signaling molecules.

- Vitamin K given to post-menopausal women inhibited the precipitous loss of calcium thought to prefigure osteoporosis.

- Vitamin E and ascorbic acid are reported to possibly help older people in the oxidation of the body tissues.

- Vitamin E has been reported to hold special promise for patients with Parkinson's disease. It has been also reported to delay the appearance of tumors, rigidity, and loss of balance.

- Vitamin E has reportedly helped to speed recovery in patients who have had coronary bypass surgery.

In an article entitled "Vitamin Revolution" (*Newsweek*, June 7, 1993), Dr. Walter Willett, a Harvard epidemiologist studying diet, supplements, and chronic diseases, was quoted as saying, "Until quite recently, it was taught that everyone in this country gets enough vitamins through their diet and that taking supplements just creates expensive urine. I think we have proof that this isn't true. I think the scientific community has realized this is a very important area for research." According to the article, what Dr. Willett says is an understatement. A *Newsweek* poll shows that seven out of ten Americans use vitamin supplements. And there are many experts who feel that although the Recommended Daily Allowance (RDA) has been updated periodically, they still reflect the old thinking and have begun to show their age.

In light of the studies and research going on and the findings pointing to vitamins and supplements as necessary for the prevention of disease, it would seem that any "expert" who denounces vitamins and supplements or says that we "get all the vitamins we need in our diet through the foods we eat" is simply behind the times. Either that, or they are propagandizing for the pharmaceutical industry, which has a lot at stake in seeing to it that its number-one economic competitor loses ground in the marketplace as a substitute for drugs.

According to the *Newsweek* article, the "big stars" of the vitamin "craze" are the so-called antioxidants: vitamins C and E and beta carotene. The dollar sales of these supplements have soared over the past five years. Since 1988, the United States market for beta carotene supplements has shot up from $7 million to $82 million a year, while sales of vitamin E have increased from $260 million a year to $338 million a year.

These figures are just for two supplements; there are hundreds on the market. These figures leave little need for any explanation as to why the pharmaceutical industry is pulling the FDA's puppet strings in Washington, D.C., to go after the vitamin/supplement industry.

In the summer of 1993, the FDA proposed new rules that call for full disclosure on labels of vitamins and minerals. At the same time the FDA announced it was going to take a *"serious look into herbals"* that are used *"as an alternative to pharmaceuticals"*—another statement consistent with Gary Dykstra's statement about how the FDA's Task Force on Supplements considered what steps they needed to take in order to prevent vitamins from acting as a "disincentive for drug development." The FDA also raised questions about the nutritional value and safety of amino acids (some of these products are aimed at body-builders and dieters). Such a move by the FDA could result in some supplements being pulled off store shelves and re-categorized as drugs which require a medical doctor's prescription.

FDA Commissioner David Kessler, in remarks regarding the FDA's Task Force Study, stated, "The Task Force acknowledged the strong desire of American consumers for access to dietary supplements." He added that "freedom of choice for these products *should be allowed as much as possible.*" [Emphasis added.] This is an incredible—and extremely offensive—statement; nowhere in the Constitution of the United States does it state that "freedom should be allowed as much as possible." Freedom is not something to be considered to *be allowed* in any sense, let alone *be allowed as much as possible.*

The Declaration of Independence states: "We hold these Truths to be self-evident, that all Men are created equal, that they are endowed by their Creator with certain unalienable Rights, that among these are Life, Liberty, and the Pursuit of Happiness." It further states that ". . .whenever any Form of Government becomes destructive of these Ends, it is the Right of the People to alter or to abolish it." This is not to suggest revolution. It is simply to point out that the people (consumers) have rights to life, liberty, and the pursuit of happiness which the campaign by the FDA and the pharmaceutical industry has been designed to erode. Having a government despot dictate that the American public's freedom to choose vitamins and supplements (which certainly qualifies as pursuing life, liberty, and happiness) should be *allowed as much as possible* is a classic example of totalitarianism.

The Declaration states that the people have the right *to alter* government; the situation addressed here demands that changes be made. These alterations could be something as simple as holding Congressional hearings on monopoly in order to change the current FDA relationship with the pharmaceutical industry. (Part Three addresses such changes in detail.)

What the FDA refers to as "questionable products" are in fact supplements that have been the subject of scientific studies which have proven their effectiveness in fighting certain diseases. Among these diseases are cancer and arthritis. Within these two diseases there are more than a dozen different alternative treatments and therapies that employ supplements of some sort. Despite the scientific evidence to the contrary, the FDA still insists that such alternative substitutes for drugs are "questionable products." The general public—and many scientists—know differently. As a matter of fact, *so does the FDA.* It is aware of the scientific studies as well as the public support for vitamins and supplements and for alternative treatments and therapies.

According to the FDA's own Health Fraud Status Report of February 1988, it commissioned a survey on alternative products and treatments for cancer and arthritis. The following is taken from that report. Regardless of its findings, the FDA persists in referring to these products and treatments as "health fraud" or "quackery."

EVALUATION

Although there have been several estimates of the costs of health fraud these calculations have not been based on hard data. Also, information about those people affected by health fraud is often conflicting. More systematic, statistically reliable surveys and research are needed in order to better focus and target public and private health fraud activities.

In order to obtain better information on the nature of the health fraud problem, FDA worked with Department's Office of Planning and Evaluation which contracted with Louis Harris and Associates to conduct a national health fraud survey in 1986. The survey screened respondents for the presence of two target diseases, cancer and arthritis. These areas were of special concern because of the potential adverse consequences resulting from the use of questionable arthritis and cancer products. For the rest of the respondents, the survey collected information on a representative list of fifteen treatment areas, e.g., disease prevention, stress reduction, promoting hair growth, etc.

Within the cancer, arthritis, and fifteen treatment areas, products and treatments were classified as scientifically acceptable (if there was a body of scientific evidence to support their effectiveness) or "questionable" (no body of scientific evidence, e.g., electrical stimulators to restore hair, body wraps to remove cellulite, or vitamins to relieve stress).

Some of the highlights are:

1. Of those who sought a treatment in one of the fifteen areas studied: 41% used only scientifically acceptable treatments; 34% used both acceptable and questionable treatments; 25% used only questionable treatments.

2. More than a quarter of the American public reports having used one or more questionable products in one of the fifteen treatment areas studied. Fifteen percent (15%) of the cancer suffers and thirty-six percent (36%) of the arthritis sufferers used a questionable treatment for the condition.

3. Sixty-five percent (65%) of questionable product users in the fifteen treatment areas believed that the treatment was very effective or somewhat effective. Thirty-three percent (33%) of those who used a questionable cancer treatment thought it

was very effective or somewhat effective. Forty-one percent of those who used a questionable arthritis treatment thought it was very effective or somewhat effective.

4. Word of mouth is the primary mechanism for the diffusion [the dissemination or spreading] of questionable products in the fifteen treatment areas.

5. There is some evidence that the poor and the sick are at special risk to the use of questionable products.

6. Those with the greatest trust in doctors and traditional medicine are least likely to use questionable treatments.

7. Doctors appear to be one of the most effective points of intervention for discussing the use of questionable products.

   [The highlight of this survey, and probably the piece of information most damaging piece to the FDA's credibility, is found in the last point:]

8. Most users of questionable products have never complained to anyone about their products. None of the survey respondents said that they had ever complained to a government agency, consumer group, or media source.

This was the survey that identified the Big Three targets for the PAC/FDA campaign.

If consumers are happy with the products, if they feel that the treatments are *either very effective or somewhat effective* (65% of the respondents did), and they are not complaining to any government agency or consumer group, then. . .someone else is obviously selecting and targeting products and treatments within the alternative community. This is not news in light of the information that has been presented in this book. However, the FDA's survey is proof by its own admission that the FDA isn't receiving complaints from the public users of these "questionable treatments and products." This certainly opens up a can of worms as to what is *really* behind the FDA's relentless attack against vitamins, supplements, herbs, treatments, and therapies used in alternative medicine.

The government agencies have been given direction from several sources. By their own account, they have received leads from consumer groups, other government agencies, health-care professionals, and media. What they have *not* listed in their public documents, or told Congress, is that they have also been receiving direction from the pharmaceutical industry.

The one source of a lot of help, assistance and direction for the government agencies has been the representatives of "consumer groups" involved in the "health fraud/quackery" issues. One such group has been the National Council Against Health Fraud, and one of the most active members associated with that group has been Dr. John Renner.

On April 9, 1992, the House Small Business Committee's Subcommittee on Regulation, Business Opportunities and Energy, chaired by Congressman Ron Wyden, conducted hearings in Washington, D.C., entitled Recent Trends in Dubious and Quack Medical Devices. Among the "experts" testifying was Dr. John Renner. In his testimony, he stated, "I am a member of the Board of Directors of the National Council Against Health Fraud. . .I have been a consultant to the Food and Drug Administration on AIDS quackery and have been deeply involved in studying and investigating quackery for ten years."

In his testimony, he submitted a long list of what he referred to as "dubious medical devices" and he stated the following about those "devices":

(1) Live Cell (whole blood) analysis, using a microscope, T.V. projector, T.V. monitor, and an instruction book that can supposedly diagnose almost any illness known to mankind. I have heard practitioners say they saw "diabetic cells," "arthritis cells," and even an AIDS virus. The first two do not exist, and it would take an electron microscope to see a virus. These people fabricate results. Ads run for these gadgets regularly in alternative medical magazines. This gadget generates $60,000 a year per practice. [Note: These is hearsay evidence, undocumented.]

(2) Electronic diagnostic gadgets, some with computer and bizarre instruction books, like Vega, Prophyle, Electronic Acupuncture voll (EAV), Interro, or Computronix. Some use a "disguised research project" to give the impression of legitimacy." [Note: These machines, by law, are allowed to be operated under a "research project" or if the operator informs the research subject (patient) that it is "experimen-

tal." By law there is nothing wrong with using these devices under those conditions.] The operators of these machines are M.D.s, D.O.s, homeopaths, naturopaths, chiropractors, and lay persons. These people generally find something wrong with the subject being tested, later requiring the subject to take herbs, food supplements, or large doses of vitamins. [Note: It is no surprise that a practitioner would "generally find something wrong with the subject being tested," given that the patient was seeking help for some illness or disease! Dr. Renner's implication is that there is something wrong with giving the "subjects" herbs, supplements or vitamins.]

(3) Phony Chronic Fatigue Syndrome laboratory tests, even though this can be a real illness. [Note: Dr. Renner failed to submit any supporting scientific evidence that such tests were "phony," yet he admits such an illness, which in fact does exist, "can be real."]

(4) Phony Osteoporosis measuring tests, using fingertip X-rays mailed in for analysis. [Note: Again, Dr. Renner failed to submit any supporting scientific evidence that such tests were phony.]

(5) Computerized nutritional questionnaires programmed to give only abnormal results, thereby "requiring" mega-nutritional supplements. [Note: The questionnaires are designed to find out where a subject is deficient in certain vitamins and minerals, so naturally the answers would show abnormal results. Again we see that Dr. Renner's emphasis is on "requiring" mega-vitamins.]

(6) Phony testing of the iris of the eye (iridology), using a camera and so-called geographic map of the iris, showing areas of the body that supposedly correspond to organs of the body and illnesses. One such quack was busing people to his office and diagnosing "Impending health problems" and then recommending herbs and nutritional supplements." [Note: Again, Dr. Renner fails to present any scientific evidence to support his allegations that there is something wrong here, and once again, the implication is that something is wrong with people having herbs and nutritional supplements recommended to them.]

(7) Activator gadget used by chiropractors to show where the spine or pelvis or temporal mandibular joint (TMJ) is out of place. Blue Cross/Blue Shield pays for this one. Workmen's Compensation Insurance also pays for this in some areas.

(8) Magnetic healing devices—small ones from $25 to $1,500—for a magnetic mattress so as to "align" all the cells in the body to a north/south pole. [Note: Even orthodox science is now coming to the realization that high-voltage wires are linked to altering the electro-magnetic fields of the body, resulting in such things as tumors and cancer.]

(9) Hair analysis—using head or pubic hair to diagnose and treat a variety of illness, thereby recommending nutritional supplements to treat the "identified" illness. [Note: The analysis does show if one is lacking in certain vitamins or minerals. It does not show illness or disease. However, if one is deficient in certain vitamins/minerals, it is possible to develop a related illness or disease. Even orthodox medicine and science support this. Once again Dr. Renner implies that something is wrong with getting supplements.]

(10) Devices used to diagnose or treat illness, depending on the imagination and/or ethics of the practitioners.
   a. Urine amino acid tests
   b. Nutritional kinesiology (muscle testing)
   c. Pendulum testing
   d. Water purification devices
   e. Yeast sensitivity diagnosis
   f. Ozone therapy
   g. Pyramid power
   h. Saliva analysis
   i. Handwriting analysis
   j. Thermography
   k. Toftness device
   1. Mercury amalgam testing devices
   m. Urine probability test
   n. Dried blood crystal test
   o. Infrared test
   p. Weird allergy testing

[*Note*: Most of these are used in alternative medicine but not by all practitioners. However, with all due respect to Dr. Renner in his efforts to point out to the Congress what he feels are "dubious medical devices," he does not submit anything to support his allegations.]

The bottom line of Dr. Renner's testimony came when he remarked about what should be done about all of this.

License to practice a healing profession is governed by state governments. Devices are regulated by federal government. State licensing boards rarely communicate with the Food and Drug Administration. Only a few state attorneys general offices have large enough staff to investigate adequately consumer health fraud. FDA and some states' attorneys general offices have recently teamed up to go after multi-state quackery activity. *A unified approach is needed at the federal level by the FDA, FBI, Postal Service, FTC, the Inspector General and state licensure boards. [Emphasis added.]*

[*Note*: Dr. Renner suggested here something that was already going on to some extent. The federal government already had a Task Force on Health Fraud and a Task Force on AIDS Fraud in place. Each of the federal agencies he listed was already involved in these task forces. The Justice Department had already released its report on the Health Fraud Initiative one month prior to this hearing. The only thing new was having the state licensing boards connect with these federal agencies. From all indications this looks to be happening now. They may even be sharing the same alternative priority lists.]

Dr. Renner's testimony makes it apparent that recommending nutritional supplements, vitamins, mega-nutritional supplements, or mega-vitamins is in some way a very bad thing to do. This message is repeated over and over in the testimony. What is also very clear is that he does not lend any support to his presentation. He does not bring to the table any hard documentation or scientific evidence to support his implications that recommending vitamins/supplements is not good for people. Much of his testimony appears to be opinion, based on his credentials as an "expert" on "health fraud and quackery," and it ignores the fact that much of what he implies regarding vitamins and supplements is countered by recent scientific reports, articles, and papers on vitamins, minerals, herbs, and supplements.

Dr. Renner submitted a list/chart entitled "Estimated Annual Costs of Quackery Devices and Quack Products." One common denominator of these entries is that most of the alternative practitioners or entities listed (as quacks) use multi-vitamins, mega-nutritional supplements, or herbs in their practices or business. It is unknown how Dr. Renner arrived at these figures, but here they are:

Practitioner	Total	Quacks or dubious practitioners	Dollars generated using device/ quackery	Total costs
M.D.s	630,000	1% or 6,300	$200,000	$1,260,000,000
D.O.s (osteopathic doctors)	50,000	10% or 5,000	$200,000	$1,000,000,000
D.C.s (chiropractors)	40,000	60% or 24,000	$200,000	$4,800,000,000
Nurses (R.N. & L.P.N.)	1,500,000	1% or 15,000	$ 25,000	$375,000,000
Dentists	141,000	1% or 1,410	$200,000	$282,000,000
Veterinarians (treating humans)	300	100% or 300	$125,000	$37,500,000
Pharmacists & Chain drug stores	100,000	1% or 1,000	$150,000	$ 150,000,000
Dietitians	60,000	0.2% or 120	$100,000	$12,000,000
Non-licensed Psychological practitioner	11,200	90% or 10,080	$100,000	$1,108,000,000

Health Food Stores	7,300	80% or 5,840	$350,000	$2,044,000,000
Homeopaths	500	98% or 495	$200,000	$ 99,000,000
Health mail order Gadgets & pills	50	90% or 45	$500,000	$ 22,500,000
"Herbalists"	1,000	80% or 800	$25,000	$20,000,000
Acupuncturists	1,500	90% or 1,350	$200,000	$270,000,000
Multi-level sales of nutritional products, herbs, weight loss products	500,000	80% or 400,000	$ 50,000	$20,000,000
Grand Total Estimates				$31,448,000,000

Once again it must be emphasized that nowhere in any of Dr. Renner's testimony does he enter into public record any documentation, evidence, studies, statistical analysis, or data to support these figures. Whether such information exists or not, it simply was not presented to support the doctor's figures and his charts. Being an "expert" does have its privileges—apparently including the right to throw out figures as fact without presenting supporting data.

In the past, the so-called experts on health fraud and quackery have thrown around such figures as $1 billion, $10 billion, $25 billion, and now $31.448 billion, being spent on "quack products." The fact is that a lot of money *is* being spent on alternative medicine, treatments, products, services, modalities, vitamins, supplements, and herbs; and the fact is that these products and services are in direct economic competition to the pharmaceutical industry and the medical establishment.

It is also a fact that the pharmaceutical industry would like to get rid of the alternatives and it is doing something to bring this about. It is a fact that the FDA, FBI, IRS, FTC, U.S. Postal Service, Department of Justice, and others are doing the dirty work for the vested interests in the drug industry. A nationwide computer network, linking government agencies, the insurance industry, and private "consumer groups," allows them to share information on alternative targets. They are highly organized and are working toward a common goal. A powerful combination.

This is what the alternative community and consumers are up against. Using laws designated to attack the Mafia, this network's campaign is destroying lives, ruining businesses, and breaking up families.

There is an irony in all of this. At the very first National Health Fraud Conference in Washington, D.C., on September 11, 1985, one of the key spokesmen for the "consumer groups" involved in the health fraud/quackery issue described the alternative health-care movement as "a highly organized, nationwide, computer-operated conspiracy."

To paraphrase Shakespeare, they protest too much. Having been inside both camps, I can honestly say that the alternative movement is, in fact, the absolute opposite of a highly organized, nationwide, computer-operated conspiracy. That seems to be one of its main problems. The members are not these things. If they were they could easily defeat the opposition that has been bent on destroying them for the past ten years. What *is* a highly organized, nationwide, computer-operated entity is the National Health Fraud/Anti-Quackery Campaign.

The following quotes will serve to sum up the arrogance of this anti-competitive movement. These are taken from the first National Health Fraud Conference. Speakers were heard to say the following:

1. On strategy in fighting against the "quacks":

   "Divide and conquer by specialization."

2. Of people who use alternative treatments and products:

   "You really can't protect people from themselves."

   "I hope someday we can license patients."

The following chapters present several case histories of private practitioners, medical doctors, homeopaths, naturopaths, chelation therapists, chiropractors, vitamin and supplement manufacturers, and sales and distribution companies all involved in alternative medicine. Documentation and evidence gathered in these cases all point to the fact that those singled out in the case studies were victims of a planned campaign against them.

It will become very clear that all the information presented in Part One can be seen at work in each case outlined in Part Two. Exposing what has been behind these attacks opens the door to hope for the future. Once the truth is known, then something can be done about it. You can help, and you should. Your own personal freedom of choice is at stake.

Part Two

Case Histories

Chapter 9

The Nutri-Cology Case

"Check with potential informant about getting inside firm [Nutri-Cology] let FDA know outcome and cost."
[Notes by Jim Eddington, California State Food and Drug, Fraud Section at joint investigation meeting with FDA, August 1988.]

Background and Political Atmosphere

Nutri-Cology is a small company located in the California Bay Area city of San Leandro. Headed by Stephen Levine and his wife Susan, it started out in 1980 as a small business but quickly grew because its products were in high demand within the alternative health-care community. Practitioners throughout the United States and even some from foreign countries were ordering their products. The business started to bloom, and their products were being marketed on a broad scale geographically prior to any campaign being launched by the pharmaceutical industry and U.S. FDA.

Nutri-Cology came on the scene at a time when California state agencies, such as the California State Food and Drug Branch (FDB), were under fire by the state legislature. The State FDB was specifically singled out for criticism by the legislature in Sacramento for its methods of investigation and enforcement, especially its tactics and methods applied in the investigations regarding laetrile, chelation therapy, and retail health food store.

An example of the tactics which caused such criticism was a joint raid that the U.S. FDA and the California State FDB conducted on a small health food store in the Watts area of Los Angeles some years prior to this reprimand from the legislature. After conducting an undercover investigation, the agents determined that the proprietor of the store had a six-shooter revolver in his desk in the back room of the store. That he had a permit for the weapon apparently made no difference to the agents. This was cause enough to enter the store at 7 A.M. Guns drawn, a dozen agents stormed the targeted store with network television cameras and press in pursuit. I asked Grant Leake, the supervisor of the California FDB, what the crime was and he responded, "They were selling a Chinese herbal tea for earaches." This was just one example of hundreds of instances of overkill on the part of the Food and Drug Fraud agents.

At this time, there was a pro-alternative-health-care atmosphere in California and a lot of consumer lobbying in favor of legalizing laetrile and chelation therapy. Two bills were introduced in 1977 in support of these alternative treatments, as well as a bill which would have exempted "giving nutritional advice" from the definition of *the practice of medicine*.

California, being the hub of "alternative anything," came under extensive government scrutiny throughout the 1970s. That decade also saw an increase in investigative/enforcement activity directed against "quackery" targets from the California Attorney General, county prosecutors, California FDB, U.S. FDA, and the AMA. For years prior to Nutri-Cology coming under fire, these agencies had worked closely together in pursuing the "quackery" targets fed them by medical vested interests, including the AMA, the California Medical Association (CMA), the American Cancer Society and its California affiliate, the American Heart Association, the Arthritis Foundation, and others. Also on the scene in the 1970s was the California Council Against Health Fraud, later to become the National Council Against Health Fraud.

During this same decade, John Miner, the Deputy District Attorney for Medico-Legal Affairs, introduced legislation which made it a felony under the California Business and Professional Codes to practice medicine without a license. He worked closely with the AMA's Department of Investigation during the time it took to get this bill passed into law, and he received the full support of the CMA getting it pushed through. Miner was very active in working with the medical vested interests on a state-wide and national scale in fighting such things as laetrile and alternative cancer treatments. Strict cancer laws were also passed, designed to further restrict the use of alternative medicine in that area.

Doyl Taylor of the AMA's Department of Investigation thought so much of John Miner that he had him featured at one of the AMA sponsored Congresses on Quackery. Taylor often referred to the law as Miner's Law and felt it was a perfect model for all states to use to "strike a blow against quackery." Miner's Law was specifically written to address the use of "quack products and treatments" such as laetrile in the treatment of cancer and other alternative treatments for other diseases. The alternative health-care movement posed a very large threat to organized medicine's little monopoly in California, because the alternatives were stronger and more popular in California than in any other state in the country during this time. It was only natural that the opposition to alternatives would be the strongest in that state. If they could defeat "quackery" in California they could defeat it anywhere.

In July 1978, priorities were set for the Food and Drug Branch (FDB), Fraud Section. These were outlined in its Operations Manual (used in fraud investigations), which was a guideline on how to investigate "quackery," who to work with, what to look for, and so on. The manual was the Bible for all fraud investigators. This was and is the *only* operations manual the FDB people operate from in their work on health fraud cases. Although it was written in 1978, it has been added to over the years and is still used today.

In the Operations Manual under "Liaison Activities," the FDB instructed its investigators to "conduct a concerted effort toward contacting several health oriented groups and associations." The manual explained that the reason for this was so that the Food and Drug Branch, Fraud Section could "solicit their help in defining the problems" related to quackery and fraud in California.

This directive translated into the following process:

1. The FDB would liaise with private outside health-oriented groups and associations in order to determine what targets these groups and associations felt the FDB should attack. They called this soliciting "help in defining the problem."

2. They approached groups such as the American Cancer Society, the Arthritis Foundation, the American Medical Association, and the California Council Against Health Fraud (later to become the National Council Against Health Fraud).

3. It would appear from all indications that a large part of what the FDB did was based on what direction ("help") it received from these private groups and associations.

This pattern and mode of operation, consistent through the years, apparently still exists today.

In its work plan, the FDB had its priorities set. Under the targeted area of fraud investigations, the manual was divided into sub-categories and each was then defined. The Operations Manual described the types of fraud and set them into priorities. The following quotes are taken from the section "Priority Two (2)—Food Supplement Frauds":

> Most of the fraudulent products that fall within the food/supplement food additive category. . .can represent a serious economic rip-off to consumers in that these products generally do not and cannot deliver what they promise.
>
> [Health fraud products in this category include B-15, B-13, ginseng, rose hips, vitamin C, GH-3 and others.]
>
> We will attempt to control the manufacture and distribution in California at their source, wherever possible. Our enforcement activities in this area will be focused at the wholesaler/distributor level of the chain of commerce. . .
>
> Our objective in this area of fraud control will be to stop the distribution of misbranded and adulterated products with a minimum amount of time and manpower.

At the time this work plan was introduced to the Operations Manual, the very existence of the Fraud Section of the FDB was in question. Proposition 13 had just been passed into law, making government agencies more accountable to the public and the legislature and requiring them to account for all expenditures. The head of the FDB even stated that his branch was faced with the question, "Is there a need for a Health Fraud component within the Food and Drug Section as a separate unit?"

The Unit's existence was therefore treatened. It had to produce in order to justify to the legislature the money required to run the Health Fraud component. It had to *increase the number of investigations, prosecutions, and enforcement actions* in order to justify to the legislature its continued operation as a unit. All of this was on top of the pressure and criticism it had received for its investigative and enforcement tactics.

A decision was made to increase the number of investigations and enforcement actions, as well as prosecutions. A quota system was devised which dictated the production numbers in order to guarantee that there would be a "need for a Health Fraud Unit within the Food and Drug Branch as a separate unit." This quota system is still in use today. The quota under which Nutri-Cology fell was as follows:

Priority Two —Food Supplement Frauds:
8 trials, 24 lab test samples, 2100 man-hours statewide.

[This was to be directed at manufacturers/wholesalers and distributors of food supplements, vitamins, minerals etc.]

Other Priorities included:

Priority One—Economic Fraud:
30 food samples, 30 cases statewide.

Priority Three—Herb Fraud:
3 Trials, 1200 Man-hours statewide.

Priority Four—Cancer Fraud:
6 Trials, 600 man-hours (undercover work), 30 cases statewide.

In total they set a quota of 8.25 man-years in 3 regions in the state for the four priority categories.

The Operating Manual outlined and defined the various types of fraud they were to investigate:

Direct Health Hazard. Products that have a reasonable potential for causing direct serious effects to the user or the patient when used as directed. [This definition would later be used against Nutri-Cology for two of their products—L-tryptophan and Germanium.]

Indirect Health Hazard. An indirect health hazard is a product that will have a significant adverse impact on a patient's health due to:

(1) The promotion of the product for a use which is not effective.
(2) The delay or denial of proper medical treatment which results in the reliance on the product.
[This category of "fraud" has been applied to the Nutri-Cology products over the years.]

Major Economic Frauds. This category includes products distributed on a national or statewide basis. The consumers may be expected to purchase them for bodily improvements or for the benefit of their general health. [Nutri-Cology products came under attack under this definition also.]

Minor Economic Frauds. There are generally two types of products within this category. They are labeled or promoted by minor unsupported nutritional, health, or cosmetic claims in addition to their labeling—vitamins fall into this category as well as Major Economic Frauds.

The Operations Manual also gave the following instructions:

Cooperation With Other Agencies: . . .before undertaking an investigation, consultation should be done with other agencies. . .to be able to work with us for a more effective investigation at a lesser cost.

Sources of Complaints: Contact voluntary health agencies. . .to be better able to define the problems of quackery and health fraud.

One month after the FDB adopted its Operations Manual with its accompanying quotas, the Council Against Health Fraud came out with its first press story. The August 1978 article appeared in the *Los Angeles Times* and quoted William Jarvis, the president of the Council, as proclaiming that vitamins, minerals, and especially "megadoses" of vitamins are the "biggest health fraud in dollar volume."

In the same article, Mr. Jarvis attacked the proposed legislation to legalize laetrile. Both of these issues, vitamins and laetrile, happened to be on the FDB targeted priorities. This leaves a question. Did the FDB solicit the Council's "help in defining the problems" and thereby determine these two items to be targeted priorities? Did it "conduct a concerted effort towards contacting" voluntary and private health-oriented groups and associations? Is this how vitamins and laetrile became priority targets, as outlined in their operations manual?

Regardless of how the FDB arrived at its decision to go after vitamins and laetrile, the fact remains that it did. Its decision to do so has adversely affected many independent vitamin and supplement manufacturers.

Nutri-Cology: Targeted for Elimination

This, then, was the political setting. Eighteen months after Nutri-Cology started in business, it came under attack by the U.S. Food and Drug Administration. Agents conducted an inspection of the Nutri-Cology facility in Concord, California, and followed it with another inspection in March 1982. The FDA sent then Steve Levine a Notice of Adverse Findings letter. The head of the Office of Compliance of the FDA's San Francisco office outlined several points needing correction related to products and labeling, based on the FDA's inspection. The U.S. FDA turned over a copy of this letter to the California State Food and Drug Branch, Fraud Division, to get them involved.

Not taking this warning from the FDA lightly, Steve Levine responded quickly. He sent the FDA a letter expressing his puzzlement about why the FDA was concerned about tryptophan. He stated to the FDA that he did not feel that it was the same as a drug.

By now the California FDB, Fraud Division, had opened a file on Nutri-Cology. Its files indicate that its first contact with Nutri-Cology was in May 1983, when it conducted an inspection of Nutri-Cology. This was conducted under a General Inspection category and not classified as a fraud investigation, but this was to change.

It is important to note here that by now the Pharmaceutical Advertising Council (PAC) and the FDA had their Anti-Quackery campaign underway. Between 1983 and 1984 the PAC/FDA campaign had:

1. Received funding from the drug companies to conduct their campaign.
2. Received funding from the FDA.
3. Named Vitamins for Improved Health as its number-one target in the campaign.
4. Developed a list of priority targets to go after which included vitamins, supplements, and companies. This list was expanded upon over the years and directly impacted the Nutri-Cology case.

On July 11, 1983, Warren Crawford, head of the FDB, placed an article from the American Council on Science and Health's newsletter into the Fraud Division's Operations Manual as a guideline and reference for investigation into "health food stores promoting fraudulent foods and drugs." The article attacked various supplements, including vitamins and spirulina. Both of these were on the PAC/FDA list of priorities for their campaign. The article also included quotes from Dr. Victor Herbert on spirulina, bee pollen, RNA, and B-12. In the same newsletter, articles appeared attacking naturopathy and nutritionists. Quoted were both Dr. Victor Herbert and Dr. Stephen Barrett. These men were involved in the PAC/FDA campaign early on, as spokesmen for the campaign as well as Board members of the National Council Against Health Fraud. It appeared that these articles were a direct result of the PAC/FDA Anti-Quackery Campaign on the specific targets mentioned in the articles.

Three days later, on July 14, 1983, Sally Osterhout of the FDB filed a report on Nutri-Cology under the Fraud Program. This was based on her general inspection on May 12, 1983. In her report, she recommended that "legal action be referred to the District Attorney." She stated that the people at Nutri-Cology "refused to release information on product labels, manufacturers of products, storage of products and testing of products." This refusal, she reported, was based on the advice of the Nutri-Cology attorney. She also recommended a Regulatory Letter to address the "unlawful behavior in refusal of the aforementioned information."

On July 19, 1983, Jim Eddington, FDB Supervisor, called Steve Levine regarding these reported refusals. Levine stated that he would cooperate in every way, but he wanted the FDB to contact his attorney, Scott Bass. Eddington called Bass and was assured full cooperation by Nutri-Cology. Bass asked for a letter outlining all the points that the FDB felt needed to be addressed.

On July 21, 1983, Eddington sent Bass such a letter. His letter asked for (1) labels for all products, (2) all promotional materials, (3) locations of other manufacturers, distributors or warehousing facilities, (4) names of all manufacturers of firms products, (6) scientific evidence of the use of the term "hypo-allergenic."

Nothing official took place against Nutri-Cology between July 1983 and December 1984. However, several events took place during this time that directly and indirectly impacted on Nutri-Cology.

On May 23, 1984, a meeting took place in California which was to change and influence several government agencies' actions directed against alternative targets in that state. Harold Loffler, a member of the National Council Against Health Fraud, met with representatives of the following government agencies:

U.S. Food and Drug Administration
California Food and Drug Branch

U.S. Postal Inspectors
Federal Trade Commission
California State Board of Medical Quality Assurance

This meeting was apparently held in total alignment with the guidelines in the Operations Manual of the FDB concerning Cooperation With Other Agencies and Sources of Complaints.

According to interviews with several people who attended this meeting, the National Council Against Health Fraud representative directed the government agencies present against several targets. These also happen to have been on the PAC/FDA priority list. These targets included Herbalife, chiropractic, and vitamins and health promoters. According to one highly placed source at the meeting from the California FDB, Mr. Loffler's role was that of directing the government agencies as to their priorities for investigation and regulatory actions.

Again, this was all in accordance with the guidelines and quota system delineated in the Operations Manual on Food Supplement and Herb Fraud. The result of this meeting was that the government agencies involved now had specific targets to pursue. Or, as the Food and Drug puts it, they were now better equipped to "define the problem." They stated:

> We will attempt to control the manufacture and distribution in California of such fraudulent products by stopping them at their source, wherever possible.

> Our enforcement activities in this area will be focused at the wholesaler/distributor level of the chain of commerce.

This May 23, 1984, meeting is absolute evidence that the FDB, as well as the FDA and the others present, were assigned priorities by outside interests, apparently as part of the campaign that was being run and financed by the pharmaceutical industry. These priorities did in fact become government targets for prosecution.

Some of the people who were directly involved in the investigations and enforcement activities directed against Nutri-Cology were in attendance at this meeting. One of the categories that the National Council Against Health Fraud apparently directed the agencies to pursue, vitamins and health promoters, applied to Nutri-Cology. The following people attended this meeting and then worked on the Nutri-Cology case:

Dale A. Kenner—FDA San Francisco

Hal Keener—Supervisor, Special Investigations of the California State Board of Medical Quality Assurance. He attempted to tie Nutri-Cology into an undercover intelligence investigation that was directed against a practitioner who used Nutri-Cology products.

Mike Bogumill—FDB, Fraud Division. As head of the Fraud Division he supervised the investigation into Nutri-Cology. He was directly over Jim Eddington and Sally Osterhout.

Chambers Bryson—FDB Sacramento. He was directly over Bogumill and Eddington.

Jim Waddell—FDB San Diego. His Fraud Branch sent data to FDB Berkeley on Nutri-Cology.

Ralph Lowensbury—FDB Los Angeles. His office also sent data into the Nutri-Cology file in Berkeley.

Five months after this meeting, in October 1984, the PAC/FDA Anti-Quackery Campaign completed its survey of the alternative targets. (However, as early as 1983 it had a published list of intended targets which included specific manufacturers of vitamin, minerals and supplements.) A month later, in November 1984 (apparently as a part of the stepped-up Anti-Quackery Campaign against nutritional targets, vitamins, and health promoters), the U.S. FDA and California FDB went after General Nutrition Corporation (GNC) for its sale and distribution of primrose oil.

The FDB's Operation Manual for Fraud Investigations lists as one of the sources of complaints "anonymous calls or letters." Sadly, it is common knowledge that investigative and enforcement branches within government agencies have been known to either have allies outside of government send or call in complaints anonymously or send letters to themselves in order to justify opening up case files on those they want to investigate or prosecute. There have even been cases in which government investigative agency personnel have *manufactured* non-existent informers, then turned in information allegedly obtained from these informants, submitted vouchers allegedly to pay off these informers and then pocketed the cash designated for the informants! This type of activity is another argument against the quota system, as well as reason not to automatically accept anonymous tips.

In the case of Nutri-Cology, an anonymous letter was sent to the FDB in December 1984. It was attached to thirteen pages of Nutri-Cology promotional literature on their products and stated, "These are drug claims and protocols distributed directly to the public. *You want work. . .here look at this.*"

Almost immediately after receiving this anonymous letter, Jim Eddington sent a "pretense letter" under the name of Dr. J. Jacobson to Nutri-Cology. His December 4, 1984, letter stated, "Please forward your protocols as offered in Bestways magazine 12/84 issue." A Post Office box was given as a return address.

The file does not contain a reply to Eddington's covert query, but the absence of one did not prevent the FDB from acting on its anonymous tip. On December 12, 1984, the FDB conducted an inspection based on the premise that Nutri-Cology was making "drug claims" in its promotional materials for its products. The FDB's efforts to uncover some blatant violation of the law must have been fruitless because no action was taken as a result of this particular inspection. They found nothing wrong. However, the bureaucratic machine moved forward in an effort to justify its existence.

Eddington put Nutri-Cology under physical surveillance on January 10, 1985. In his report, Eddington noted that the investigator was to "do a surveillance check of subject firm location. Attempt to determine status of the location." What that meant is still a mystery.

On January 14, 1985, a "surveillance" of the Nutri-Cology firm's location was conducted. The surveillance amounted to one FDB investigator going over to the Nutri-Cology plant and offices and hanging around outside the facility at "the coffee vending truck outside the building" during a coffee break. The totality of this undercover investigator's astute surveillance activity was to strike up a conversation with a female employee of Nutri-Cology who had come out of the building for a break at the vending truck. The result was that the investigator recommended a follow-up inspection of Nutri-Cology.

On January 30, 1985, Jim Eddington instructed Sally Osterhout Lum to "conduct inspection of firm. . .and check label claims closely." He ordered her to "pick up labels of approximately 10 most popular products for label review at office if indicated."

Sally Lum attempted to conduct an inspection of Nutri-Cology on February 8, 1985. In her report of the inspection, she stated that she was "refused" entry to do her inspection of Nutri-Cology. She called Jim Eddington to report that the refusal was due to the fact that no one in authority was present at the time she wanted to inspect.

Any employee interested in keeping a job would make such a reasonable protest. It is a logical request to have the president of the firm present during an inspection, but it was not reported this way by the inspector. Eddington, having received Sally Lum's phone call, called Steve Levine at home and noted that there was no answer there when he called.

Eddington's notes about Lum's telephoned report about the February 8 attempt to inspect Nutri-Cology show the following notations:

> Any day next week
> Not let in. . .
> We will seek forced entry. . .
> Jim will check with D.A.
> Running out back door. . .
> Willing to set rat traps at back door. . .
> Scenarios—
> Stake out to and from. . .watch leaving of personnel,
>   will be. . .
> Search all places. . .
> Got to be opened. . .
> Wash out. . .
> We have to get full access to everything. . .
> Locked doors. . .
> Regroup and meet with D.A.
> Try to talk boss to get refusal of entry from him
> Indirect Health Hazard

Steve and Susan Levine, however, in Nutri-Cology's dealings with the FDA and the FDB, had cooperated all along. Their stated intentions had always been to fully disclose anything either agency ever demanded from them. At no time did any employee or official from Nutri-Cology ever prevent either the U.S. FDA or FDB from doing their jobs. Nutri-Cology officials asked only to have Steve Levine present or to have their attorney notified as to what the inspectors wanted from them. In every case where this reasonable request was granted, Steve Levine or Nutri-Cology's attorney provided these agencies with what they demanded. At no time did they use deceit, pretense or under-handed means to prevent the government from doing its job.

On the other hand, at no time did either the FDB or the FDA notify Steve Levine, his attorney, or any employee of Nutri-Cology that these so-called inspections were in fact *investigations* being conducted as a result of Nutri-Cology being targeted for fraud investigation. This information was deliberately withheld from them during every single contact by the government with the firm, its officials, and its attorney. Clearly the government demonstrated both bad faith and deceit.

The FDB Operations Manual instructs its Fraud Investigators that one of the functions of a fraud investigation is to ". . .prepare an investigation report containing, among other things. . .proof of bad faith knowledge of participants. . ." It further defines the three types of investigations in the fraud area as (1) the front door approach, (2) undercover actions, and (3) surveillance activities.

Its investigation into Nutri-Cology employed all these approaches, but the one used most was type two, undercover action. The manual's guidelines stated clearly that undercover operations may be required:

1. To observe fraudulent operations.
2. To obtain evidence of the involvement of others or higher-ups in a company or scheme.
3. To give a suspect or firm the opportunity to act unlawfully while under surveillance without "entrapping" him or them.

In the legal world, *entrapment* excuses a defendant from criminal liability for crimes induced by certain governmental persuasion and trickery. This simply means that the predisposition of the defendant to commit the offense must be balanced against the police (or investigative or enforcement agency) conduct to determine whether the enforcement/investigative officers can be said to have caused the crime to begin with. In other words, did the enforcement officer persuade the ordinary law-abiding citizen into committing a crime?

The last comment in Jim Eddington's handwritten notes about Lum's phone report of what occurred at the February 8, 1985, attempt to inspect was "try to talk with boss to get his refusal of entry from him." This amounts to entrapment.

Contrary to the Operations Manual's instructions to give an *opportunity* for an individual to act unlawfully, the FDB directive was essentially an order to entrap Stephen Levine. They had no reason to assume Levine would refuse their entry if he were present; in fact, the notes from the meeting clearly indicated Levine's willingness to allow entry "any day next week." Why, then, was the directive not to "try to talk with boss to obtain entry"? The FDB's purpose in talking with Stephen Levine was not to determine if he was a law-abiding citizen who was willing to cooperate; it was to use trickery and deceit to entrap him into violating the law—for the sole purpose of creating a case against Nutri-Cology in its attempt to fill the quota.

Sally Lum's report that she was denied and refused entry to Nutri-Cology on February 8, 1985, although groundless or a matter of interpretation (depending on who is telling the story), was to come up later against Nutri-Cology in the government's case against them.

The FDB did in fact conduct an inspection on February 15, 1985. During this inspection, Sally Lum, in compliance with her boss's order of January 30, and in order to take actions in alignment to the quota system, seized 100 thyroid capsules. She also seized the labels and literature for the product, for FDB use. She report, "Labels for products are relatively free of drug claims."

Immediately following this inspection, Levine sent a letter to Lum stating that the thyroid product she had seized was sold only to physicians and not to the general public. Scott Bass sent a letter on April 15, 1985, to Jim Eddington, addressing and answering all the points the FDB made about the products and labels seized.

Even though Nutri-Cology complied with the FDB's request, and despite the fact that its own investigator found no fault with their labels, Eddington called the U.S. FDA in San Francisco and spoke to Compliance Branch Director Ron Fischer. According to Eddington's notes of that phone conversation, he told the FDA man that the FDB would hold FDB follow-up in abeyance, pending the outcome of the FDA's Regulatory Letter sent to Nutri-Cology and the firm's response. Apparently the FDA's Regulatory Letter was based on information and data received from the FDB on Nutri-Cology and the FDB's inspection.

In spite of the fact that Nutri-Cology had demonstrated full cooperation, compliance, and good faith, the machine of injustice moved forward. The FDB had been working behind the scenes, feeding the U.S. FDA the findings of the FDB's inspections as well as the data on Nutri-Cology products and labels.

On the very day the FDB received a compliance letter from Nutri-Cology's attorney, Scott Bass, meeting the points of the FDB's demands on labels and products, Eddington called up the FDA and they in turn sent out a Regulatory Letter to Nutri-Cology. Eddington never bothered to inform the FDA that Scott Bass had sent him a compliance letter in response to the FDB's demands.

The FDA's Regulatory Letter of April 15, 1985, stated that several products were considered (1) drugs or new drugs, (2) misbranded, (3) falsely labeled. Among the products cited were Immuno-Gland-Plex, Sodium Selentite, and Aller-Aid (hypoallergenic product). All these products were part of the FDB's inspection follow-up of February 15, 1985, and were addressed in their letter to Scott Bass. The U.S. FDA's Regulatory Letter used the fruits of the FDB's inspection on the very day that Scott Bass and Nutri-Cology demonstrated full cooperation and compliance to the FDB. Yet this information was withheld from the FDA by Jim Eddington.

According to the records contained in the FDB's Fraud Investigation files on Nutri-Cology, neither the FDB or the FDA took any actions against Nutri-Cology between April 15, 1985, and January 1986. However, one major external event took place which affected Nutri-Cology and would serve as a never-ending source of attack against the firm and Mr. Levine.

On September 11, 1985, the Pharmaceutical Advertising Council and the U.S. FDA launched their Public Service Anti-Quackery Campaign in Washington, D.C. This was the first public announcement of this campaign, although it had been planned and had been actively impacting such firms as Nutri-Cology, Herbalife, GNC, and others since May 1984.

The Anti-Quackery Campaign was covered in great detail in Chapters 4 and 6 in this book, but is mentioned here in that this served as a catalyst for the FDA's quota system, and a justification for its increased activities in the area of alternative health care investigations, indictments, and prosecutions.

Immediately following the kickoff of the PAC/FDA campaign in Washington, D.C., the FDA began to collect data from around the United States on Nutri-Cology and its products. The FDA had each of its district/field offices around the country send any complaints or data that they had on the firm. They did have some minor complaints from a couple of customers. In each case the customers had contacted Steve Levine directly, and he had resolved the problems to their satisfaction. Also, in each case where there was a complaint to field offices of the FDA, the FDA personnel had contacted Levine to make him aware of these complaints. He had swiftly taken care of them. An example of the most serious of the complaints was a woman who had ingested too many supplements, resulting in a reaction which amounted to some stomach cramps. Levine spoke to the woman and instructed her simply to cut back on the amount of the supplement she was taking which would cure the problem. Small problem—simple solution.

However, such complaints (there were about five of them) amounted to making a federal case against Nutri-Cology. Among the complaints the FDA had assembled was a report from an informant, who most likely was a creation of the FDA's San Francisco office. On February 6, 1986, the FDA received a phone tip from this informant, whom it described as a former employee at the Nutri-Cology facility. The report stated that Nutri-Cology was:

(1) Illegally selling Germanium, that is used for cancer.
(2) Ordering employees to "hide products, literature, as well as the firm's dog, when FDA inspectors showed up for inspections."

Following this phone tip, an FDA investigator debriefed this informant at FDA offices in San Francisco on February 18, 1986. The informant also told the FDA man that the firm was also "avoiding Customs inspections" (although it was not indicated just how this was being done, if at all).

Keep in mind that both the FDB and the FDA already had catalogs and literature from Nutri-Cology wherein it is no secret what products they were selling, including Germanium. Also recall that the FDB's investigation in February 1985 had found no fault with the labels at Nutri-Cology, which would have included labels for Germanium. The FDA's pursuit of Nutri-Cology can be explained only by two motivating forces: (1) the Anti-Quackery Campaign and (2) the quota system to make cases against alternative targets.

Following the interview (debriefing) by the FDA with the informant, the informant called the FDB on February 20, 1986, and gave them the same information that the FDA had received. On May 12, 1986, as part of a follow-up to the tip from the FDA's informant, FDB inspector D. Moore sent a pretense letter to Stephen Levine, saying, "My friend had given me some literature on this subject and said it might help with cancer. My grandmother has cancer and is not doing well. Please send information especially on the subject of cancer."Another attempt by the Food and Drug people to entrap Steve Levine and Nutri-Cology into violating the law (in this case prescribing supplements for cancer) by using trickery and deceit? Steve Levine, law-abiding citizen, did not forward any data that the letter asked for regarding cancer. Not because he knew this letter was from the FDB, but because he knew it was wrong to do so.

In a continuing show of cooperation and compliance in an effort to meet the FDB's and FDA's demands, Levine had his labels and literature changed on July 3, 1986, in compliance with the FDA's

Regulatory Letter. He did so even though the FDA and the FDB had found very little wrong with them.

Despite the obvious cooperation and compliance, and as further evidence of selected enforcement and malicious prosecution against Nutri-Cology and Steve Levine, the FDA and FDB still came after him. As part of the ongoing campaign against alternative products and manufacturers, and in keeping with their quota system, the FDA and FDB joined together in a major effort to close down Nutri-Cology.

On August 7, 1986, the FDA and FDB entered into still another a joint fraud investigation against Nutri-Cology. The joint investigation was given a Priority One status as part of the stepped-up campaign against alternatives. Both agencies entered the Nutri-Cology facility under the pretense of doing a routine inspection. When they arrived, they were temporarily detained by lower level employees of the firm. The reason for this delay (and it was not a deliberate attempt to prevent the government from doing their jobs) was that the owner, Steve Levine, was not present.

Anxious to move forward with their joint investigation, and in an attempt to bypass this temporary inconvenience, Jim Eddington, FDB Investigation Supervisor, used intimidation and threats in order to gain entry without Steve Levine present. He threatened to write a citation on one of the employees for not letting them into the facility. He took out a citation and his pen and began to write, but he did not issue it. This is a clear instance of intimidation and threats on the part of the government in order to force entry into the Nutri-Cology facility without Steve Levine present.

The official report of this joint investigation showed once again that the government interpreted their delay as a refused entry into Nutri-Cology's facility. The report stated that:

1. They were refused entry on several other occasions. (The facts are, however, that they were *never* refused entry on any occasion at the Nutri-Cology facility and were always afforded full cooperation with Steve Levine on the scene to assist the inspectors.)
2. They were not allowed into a room where promotional materials were stored. This was an example of refused entry. (The fact of the matter was that the only person with a key to the promotional room had already left for the day. This was specifically told to the inspectors during their visit.)

3. Although Scott Bass had informed the FDA in writing that they had made changes in their labels and product literature after the last inspection, the FDA reported that the firm was still making claims in violation of FDA laws.

Thse claims were made despite the fact that the report stated:

(a) They found no violations, or minor ones.

(b) The firm changed its labels and sent FDA copies of its revised labels and product brochures on 7/3/86.

(c) The revised labels do not appear to be making drug claims. [They never really did.]

(d) The inspection found that some of the promotional literature still appears to be making drug claims, but the claims have been toned down.

Then on September 23, 1986, Dale Kenner, from FDA San Francisco Investigation Supervision wrote to Jim Eddington regarding the fruits of their joint investigation. Kenner's letter revealed that the FDA didn't really feel it had anything against Nutri-Cology: "We are reviewing the labels, but I doubt our Agency will do anything more as the firm has made some corrections."

Had the FDA and FDB read Scott Bass's letter in July 1986 and reviewed the labels and product literature he sent them at that time, they could have saved the taxpayers a lot of money that was spent for nothing.

One can see a definite pattern by the government against Nutri-Cology. Inspection, regulatory letter, and compliance by Nutri-Cology, followed by more inspections, letters, and more compliance, resulting in more inspections. It appears that the more law-abiding Steve Levine became the more the government became interested in pursuing him as a target. It didn't stop in September 1986.

Between September 1986 and May 1988, there was a lull in the government's direct attack against Nutri-Cology. However, it was to pick up again after several events which apparently had a great deal of influence on the FDA's decision to go after the company.

One such event took place in October 1986. The infamous October Plan, described in detail in Chapter 5, was planned and apparently implemented when Emprise actively pursued an NIH (National Institutes of Health) Grant to study the alternatives. The Grant Study's list of products—which were also targeted by the FDA's priority list—included Nutri-Cology's products as well as treatments and therapies that used products sold by Nutri-Cology. Some of these products were:

Amino acids
Thymus extracts
Vitamin C (60-200 mg daily)
Immune stimulation methods
Enzymes
Germanium
Liver juice
Living Foods Program
Pau d' Arco
Mega-vitamins
Trace elements
Minerals
Evening primrose oil
Nutrient correction of auto-immune system
Beta carotene
Glandular therapy
Nutritional immunology
Vitamin therapy
Selenium

In June 1987, the FDA issued an "expanded policy on health fraud." Under Chapter 50, Guide 7150.10, "Health Fraud Factors in Considering Regulatory Actions," the new FDA policy laid out the guidelines which were to directly effect Nutri-Cology and others identified as targets:

1. Priorities are to be set on targeted health fraud products, treatments, services, modalities, and manufacturers.
2. Criteria for regulatory actions are to be based solely on the economic impact of products.
3. The size of the industry, the cost of the product, the profit of the product, the dollar amount of volume of product sales, and the geographical scope of the distribution are to be regarded as "key factors in considering taking action against a target product firm."
4. A Notice of Adverse Findings Letter is to be sent to promoters of new health fraud products with undetermined economic impact and limited health significance.

5. When it appears there is a growing national or substantial regional market for products of limited health significance, regulatory action is to be considered.

The measurement of the FDA's success in its Anti-Health Fraud Campaign, by its own statements and policy, is strictly based on the dollar amount of volume of a targeted firm's product sales and distribution. The smaller, less significant firms receive a simple Notice of Adverse Findings Letter. The larger firms receive FDA's Regulatory Actions directed against them, as was the case with Nutri-Cology. In 1982, when it was small and didn't have such an economic impact, it received an FDA Notice of Adverse Findings Letter. As it grew and developed a larger economic impact on the marketplace nationally and regionally, it became more of a target for the FDA and others.

Thus Nutri-Cology became a victim of the quota system set up by the government against health fraud products and manufacturers. Additionally, the government was using the alternative product priority targets fed to them by outside interests to determine its next victims.

On December 24, 1987, the FDA sent a Regulatory Letter related to several products manufactured and/or distributed by another California firm by the name of Natrol. The link between Natrol and Nutri-Cology was simply that both companies had been involved in the sales and distribution of some of the same products, and they were ones that had made the FDA's priority target list.

In the summer of 1988, in Kansas City, Missouri, the FDA was fed lists of products, practitioners, and manufacturers to start up its data base for the FDA's National Health Fraud Tracking System computer, as well as targets for the FDA. (See Chapter 6.) The FDA's alternative targets apparently came right out of the Emprise Grant study. This was all predicted in the 1986 October Plan described in Chapter 5.

The products Nutri-Cology produced, sold, and distributed were all non-pharmaceutical products. They fell into the broader plan to go after alternatives as described in the October Plan. These products were then specifically identified in the Emprise Grant study and ended up in the FDA's priority target list in their computer. This laid the groundwork and background for what was to happen to Nutri-Cology next.

In March 1988, the Federal Task Force on Health Fraud (which had been created within the structure of the National Health Care

Anti-Fraud Association) announced its stepped-up campaign against health and insurance fraud. It stated that its campaign would now employ several laws which would give them more clout, including the RICO Laws and the Mail Fraud Act. The government could use the Mail Fraud Act to: "(1) freeze assets, (2) confiscate records, (3) demand an accounting of all business revenues, etc." This law was used later against Nutri-Cology.

It was also discovered that the FDB had sent an undercover agent from their Santa Ana office to the 1988 Natural Foods Convention. He collected literature and materials on Nutri-Cology products, and this information was sent to the FDA. Additionally, the FDB collected over 50 pages of product promotional literature and Nutri-Cology catalogs between May 5 and 24, 1988; this data then ended up with the FDA.

From May through June 1988, the FDB worked on another joint investigation against Nutri-Cology. This time they worked with the California State Board of Medical Quality Assurance (BMQA). The purpose of this joint investigation, according to the investigative reports in the Nutri-Cology files, was to "obtain evidence of violation activities linking Nutri-Cology [with Rosalie Tarpening]." Rosalie Tarpening was a practitioner who used Nutri-Cology products. She was under investigation for practicing medicine without a license, a situation in which Nutri-Cology had no responsibility or involvement.

The Board reported to Dan Walsh (FDB) that Allergy Research Group (Steve Levine's company) was "doing coffee colonics and selling G-OXY-132 as a general cancer cure. They are selling Germanium Sequioxed. . .sold as a cancer cure." In a May 3, 1988, report, Walsh was specifically quoted as saying that "the owner has a felony conviction with BMQA."

This report was not true. It was full of falsehoods and misleading data. It would have led anyone not knowing the situation to believe that Steve Levine, Allergy Research Group, and Nutri-Cology were practicing medicine without a license (which was not the case). It falsely asserted that Steve Levine was a felon (which was not the case). Whether by design or stupidity, the FDB investigator had collapsed the BMQA's case on Tarpening onto the case of Nutri-Cology.

Two days after the FDB started up its joint investigation with BMQA, the FDA sent out a Notice of Adverse Findings Letter to Nutri-Cology. The FDA's Letter addressed products, literature, promotional catalogs, and materials, all of which were related to the FDB/BMQA joint investigation. They included:

Nutri-Pe9+ (Egg Lecithin-used by AIDS Buyers Clubs)
Nutri-Ge-132/GE OXY-132 (Germanium)
Oxysport/PO 2- (Germanium, Coenzyme Q 10, Carnitine, etc.)
Organic Flax Seed Oil

The FDA's letter was sent from the FDA Compliance Office in San Francisco by Steve Kendall. He requested a meeting in his office to discuss the points in his letter; the meeting was arranged for May 14, 1988, and later postponed until June. At the June 16, 1988, meeting, the FDA accused Nutri-Cology of selling drugs and new drugs and threatened further enforcement actions. These further actions came on June 29, 1988. Heinz Wilms, Director of Federal/State Relations, FDA Office of Regulatory Affairs, Rockville, Maryland (home of the FDA's Fraud Unit and National Health Fraud Tracking Computer), issued an Import Alert on the following products:

Germanium Sequioxide
Organic Germanium
GE-132
GE-OXY-132

Wilms stated in his Import Alert:

These products have been repackaged as health foods or as OTC drugs with claims for use in such severe medical conditions as AIDS or cancer. Advertising literature has been identified which promotes germanium products for use in treating or preventing serious disease conditions under the following names:

Germanium
GE OXY-132
Organic Germanium
Vitamin O
Bio-Oxygen
Nutrigel 132
Immune Multiple
Germax

This Alert came directly from the FDA's Clearinghouse Health Fraud Computer and the routing on the Alert included the California FDB.

Note that this Import Alert came at the exact time that the FDA was being fed information—targets to go after—for the Health Fraud Computer in Kansas City. It is known that Dr. John Renner monitored alternative journals, magazines, and publications and extracted information on manufacturers, products, and conferences for his use. He testified to Congress that he attended such meetings for years. It is even possible that the FDA had only become aware of the Natural Foods Conference in April 1988 (where it collected data on Nutri-Cology's products) as a result of Dr. Renner.

Almost all the products listed on the Import Alert were from Nutri-Cology. Two weeks after the Alert was issued, Steve Kendall called a meeting with the FDB to again join forces against Nutri-Cology. At the request of FDA San Francisco agents Janet Coder and Katherine Macropol, the meeting took place on August 2, 1988, at the FDA's office.

Once again the FDA and FDB teamed up to go after Nutri-Cology. Jim Eddington, representing the FDB, attended this meeting, and the following is taken from his notes:

FDA To Do:
1. Equip Honolulu Rep (FDA resident post) with phone and answering machine.
2. Solicit product information.
3. Buy products or use Las Vegas RP (Resident Post)/Tucson RP instead of Honolulu.
4. Find/create D.C or M.D.—solicit product and patient leaflets.
5. Monitor current ads.
6. Joint inspection—last event.

FDB To Do:
1. Interview Colleen Morton (Nutri-Cology employee).
2. Interview Mary Garcia (Nutri-Cology employee).
3. Check to see if Employment Data (unemployment insurance data) are available, and if so, interview recently discharged employees.
4. Check with potential informant about getting inside firm— let FDA know outcome and cost.
5. Joint Inspection—last event.

By law in California it is improper to access employment records of the unemployment agency without a court order. Also, it is unlawful to conduct electronic surveillance without first having a court order. There is no indication in the files that such a court order was obtained in this case. It is therefore possible that the government conducted illegal electronic surveillance, which would not be a first with government investigations into the alternatives.

Under Point 4, for the "FDB To Do," they planned the use of an informant for getting inside the firm. This raises the question of illegal entry using a former or current employee of Nutri-Cology to get a key, or someone to somehow get government agents inside the firm. This would amount to illegal entry or breaking and entry. It is not clear whether this was done or not; it is unlikely that the files would indicate this if they did.

In May 1990, the FDB received a tip from an informant that Nutri-Cology employees never wore "hair restraints, gloves, lab coats or masks" in the room where they prepared products for packaging. This tip resulted in another inspection by the FDB on June 13, 1990. FDB inspector Sally Lum spent one hour at the firm and reported that Nutri-Cology had failed to register as a food storage and repackaging facility.

The next day, Steve Levine called the FDB requesting the proper forms so that he could correct this oversight by registering as such a facility. It didn't appear to be too serious an oversight to the government because on June 18, 1990, they sent him the forms so that he could register the company per the inspector's request. Once again, Nutri-Cology demonstrated its good faith in cooperating and complying with the laws, yet the government still pursued him.

Following the June 1990 visit by the FDB, the FDA conducted a covert undercover operation against Nutri-Cology and Steve Levine. Beginning in June 1990 and continuing through May 1991, the FDA employed undercover agents posing as doctors, health professionals, or physicians in order to obtain samples of products and literature from Nutri-Cology. Now the question arises. . .why would the FDA stoop to covert undercover activities? All they ever had to do was to inspect the firm and seize products, labels, and literature. They had been doing so all along. Why would the FDA recruit health professionals, or pose as such, to obtain the very same information they could get themselves?

After at least two major joint investigations, as well as the FDB's investigations and inspections and after seizures, Import Alerts, and several Regulatory Letters, the FDA persisted in going after Nutri-

Cology. All of this despite the fact that they never really found anything wrong to begin with. The persecution of Nutri-Cology was relentless.

Even its own investigators reported the firm had no—or very few—violations. Those were only minor, and were corrected by the firm. Its own officials stated that the FDA didn't really want to pursue Nutri-Cology because they were either in compliance or had made changes in their product labels. Repeatedly over the years Nutri-Cology, Steve Levine, and their attorneys corrected any minor violations, complied with both the FDB and FDA's demands for change, and provided these government agencies with whatever information or products they demanded. Nowhere in the government files did any report show or state that they were in violation of a law. Minor oversights were always addressed within 24 hours of notification, corrected in each case completely and to the government's satisfaction.

Yet the government persisted, coming back in 1986, 1988, and 1990. In each instance, from the beginning and continuing today, a pattern or sequence of events could be seen as the motivation for the government's attacks—the pharmaceutical campaign against the alternatives was the common denominator behind the attacks. Why have they persisted from 1984 to the present?

The Alternative Hit List

It doesn't just happen that the government regulatory and enforcement agencies go after certain targets. It doesn't just happen that more than a thousand practitioners involved in the alternative health care movement are attacked by medical and dental boards. "Stuff" doesn't just happen. . .it is created.

Evidence has existed for years pointing to a priority list of targets, sometimes referred to as the *alternative hit list*. This list has been the subject of great concern by those in the alternatives. This hit list has been said to include the names of practitioners, clinics (both in the U.S. and in Mexico and the Caribbean), products, and product manufacturers, to name a few. Reminiscent of the insidious communist blacklist and the hysteria of the McCarthy era, this hit list has been carefully guarded by the opposition. Some of the information about this list and the practices surrounding it has come to light as a result of determined investigation, and some has been released to attorneys under Freedom of Information petitions. Still more has been collected from Anti-Quackery Campaign workers who thought they were giving information to others "on their side."

I first became aware of the probable existence of this list years ago. In looking into the Nutri-Cology case I came across information that would further validate the idea that such a hit list does in fact exist. During 1990-1991, additional evidence surfaced; this time I was made aware of it by an anonymous source inside the "opposition camp." I learned the following about this hit list:

1. There is more than one list.

2. List One, as it is called, was created by a Board member of a West Coast-based anti-fraud "consumer" organization. It is reportedly on letterhead of the group and is about ten pages long. This list contains the names of practitioners, clinics, and manufacturers who are to be given the highest priority. This is the short list and was apparently made up in August 1989.

3. List Two is the longer list. This list was generated by computer and is reportedly over 100 pages long, filled with names of practitioners, manufacturers, clinics, and others who are targeted. This list includes writers and authors, including me. This second list was created around December 1990. It is reportedly the creation of a Midwest-based anti-quackery consumer group.

4. These lists reportedly have been distributed to:
   Federal Government Regulatory Agencies
   Federal Government Enforcement/Investigation Agencies
   State Agencies/California State Food and Drug Branch
   Medical Boards
   Dental Boards
   Osteopathic Boards
   Private Insurance Companies
   Government Insurance Programs

5. There are at least two main custodians of these lists, the two group members who originated the lists. In addition, others have seen the lists or portions of them. The central repository is suspected to be located in the Midwest. The other location is said to be in Southern California.

According to my information, the California Food and Drug Branch, Fraud Division, has a copy of this list and has been working off it in pursuit of designated targets in California who manufacture vitamins, minerals, and supplements. According to all indications, the FDA also has a copy of this list and part or all of it may very well have been entered into its Health Fraud Tracking Computer.

It must be said the existence of these lists is not the cause of a person or product or service being targeted. Names that appear on this list have been the subject of attack for years prior to these lists being officially or unofficially published. In fact, in many cases they were put on the list as a result of having been targeted earlier. This has been the case with Nutri-Cology.

The following are just a few of the names that appear on one or both of the hit lists. These targets have come under attack by the FDA, U.S. Customs, the Task Force on Health Fraud, insurance companies, or medical, dental and/or osteopathic boards of examiners. It is very important to note that as a result of being on these lists those who have been individually targeted have been the victims of a planned campaign of selected enforcement actions and selected prosecution/malicious prosecution.

> Steve Levine/Nutri-Cology
> Dr. Dan Clark, Florida
> Century Clinic, Reno, Nevada
> Dr. Katrina Tang, Reno, Nevada
> Dr. Yiwen Tang, Reno, Nevada
> Fuller Royal, Las Vegas, Nevada
> Dr. Bob Doell, Denver, Colorado
> Dr. Warren Levin, New York
> Dr. Jonathan Wright, Washington
> Dr. Kurt Donsbach, California
> Dr. Julian Whitaker, California
> International Nutrition, Nevada
> AO Supply Co., Ohio
> Zerbo's Health Food Store, Michigan
> Neiper Products, Germany

Following the FDA's covert investigation of Nutri-Cology from June 1990 through May 1991, the government brought a case against them. The charges included violations of the U.S. Mail Fraud Act, as well as FDA laws.

The U.S. Mail Fraud Act was one of the favorite tools of the U.S. prosecutors. It gives the government the power to seize property, assets, company records, customer and patient files, and so on, of the targeted victim. This is what they planned to do with Nutri-Cology. The U.S. Attorney's office recommended seizure of assets, property and so on, in their motions to the court when they brought their case against the firm. This action against Nutri-Cology originated from the office of Stuart Gerson, Assistant Attorney General, Civil Division, Department of Justice, with the help of Susan Strawn, Office of Consumer Litigation, Washington, D.C.

Of interest is that Stuart Gerson, like Dr. John Renner, is connected to the Task Force on Health Fraud and the National Health Care Anti-Fraud Association. Perhaps then it is no coincidence that Nutri-Cology was targeted by the FDA and the U.S. Justice Department. It seems that it is no coincidence that its products were listed in the Emprise Grant study. It may be no coincidence that the government repeatedly came back to investigate and inspect Nutri-Cology year after year, even though it was in compliance to the FDA and FDB and showed full cooperation each time. It certainly doesn't appear to be mere coincidence.

On May 23, 1991, Judge Lowell Jensen denied the government's motion for a preliminary injunction against Nutri-Cology. However, the government's case didn't end there. They continued to push forward with their fraud case. During the time that the Nutri-Cology case continued (1991-1993), there were more activities taking place within the federal government which impacted Nutri-Cology and others involved as targets in this campaign.

September 23, 1991. Richard Kusserow announced that the FDA was hiring and training 100 new criminal investigators to be placed into the health fraud area. He also announced the creation of a new office within the FDA called the Office of Criminal Investigation (OCI), to be housed and headquartered at FDA offices in Rockville, Maryland. It was to deal solely with fraud and fraudulent products. Within OCI would be six criminal investigation offices located in Chicago, Kansas City, Miami, Newark, New York, and San Diego. Unlike all the other divisions and sections of the FDA, the OCI would report *directly* to central control at FDA headquarters.

December 27, 1991. Heinz Wilms, Director of the FDA's Federal/State Relations division sent out a State Action Information Letter (SAIL) to all State and Federal Task Force Coordinators, including the California Health Department (Food and Drug) and the California Attorney General's Office. He announced that all state AIDS Health Fraud Task Forces that receive funds from the FDA (California, Michigan, Texas and Louisiana) must report directly to the FDA. The reports must include the minutes of all Task Force meetings, quarterly reports, reports of all activities, and information obtained on suspected fraudulent AIDS drugs and therapies. Funding for the AIDS Health Fraud Task Forces was to "run through September 30, 1992."

February 3, 1992. The Attorney General of the United States released the Report on Enhanced Health Care Fraud Initiative. The Report announced the re-assignment of 95 FBI agents from the counter-intelligence and the counter-terrorism divisions to work exclusively on health fraud in 12 cities around the U.S. An additional 100 Assistant U.S. Attorneys were assigned to criminal and civil health fraud cases. Another 10 attorney positions were created by the Department of Justice to re-enforce the Health Fraud Initiative plan. Another six attorneys were assigned to the newly formed Health Care Fraud Unit within the Fraud Section of the Justice Department's Criminal Division. Another 22 attorneys were assigned to prosecute Health Fraud cases. Health Fraud was moved up as one of the top three Justice Department priorities.

The Justice Department also announced that it was working with several other agencies in bringing cases of health fraud. These agencies included the FBI, the U.S. Postal Service, DHHS-OIG, Postal Inspectors, the FDA, and state agencies. The Office of Consumer Litigation was reported to be working in conjunction with the U.S. Attorney's office in criminal investigations. (Note that these two agencies were both working to prosecute Nutri-Cology.)

February 10, 1992. Gary Dykstra, FDA Associate Commissioner for Regulatory Affairs (directly over the Health Fraud Units, National Health Fraud Tracking System computer, the Federal/State Relations Division and the Task Force on Health Fraud and AIDS Fraud), said that the FDA was now using what he described as strategic enforcement as a tool against health fraud. He explained that this included a policy of "keeping the industry guessing" where the FDA would "strike next."

He said that the FDA was a "paper tiger" before FDA Commissioner David Kessler got there. Now, he said, the FDA "is flooding our General Counsel's office and the Department of Justice with food and drug cases." The increase in the number of health fraud cases parallels the quota system set up by the DHHS-OIG for Investigations office.

Also in February 1992 the Field Investigations Division of the FDA issued an Investigation Activities Report (Official Use Only) which stated that the National Health Fraud Unit was now officially transferred from the Kansas City District office, headed by Gary Dean, to the FDA headquarters. The unit was charged with (1) preparing quarterly reports on FDA actions from around the country on health fraud, and (2) coordinating federal/state/local government and private sector exchange of health fraud information and complaints. [This was covered in earlier chapters.]

The Report also revealed that plans were underway by the FDA to conduct a series of inspections of AIDS Buyers Clubs in order to "more fully determine the nature and scope of their activities." AIDS Buyers Clubs are a network of AIDS victims who formed together for the purpose of purchasing various products, drugs, and treatments for AIDS. The Buyers Clubs have been allowed by the FDA to use experimental drugs that were manufactured by pharmaceutical companies with FDA approval. However, the Buyers Clubs have also been involved with alternative treatments and products for AIDS, which the FDA does not allow or condone. The FDA has used this friendly connection into the AIDS community as a means to covertly collect information about alternative practitioners and products, who in turn have come under fire from the FDA. Many Nutri-Cology products have been used by AIDS victims and practitioners treating AIDS victims, and the FDA attacked Nutri-Cology for those products.

April 9, 1992. Congressional hearings were held on Recent Trends in Dubious and Quack Medical Devices. Dr. John Renner spoke before the Congressional hearing committee and recommended that: "A unified approach is needed at the federal level by FDA, FBI, Postal Service, FTC, the Inspector General and state license boards" to go after health fraud. As we have noted, this "need" was already being met through the Task Force on Health Fraud, the Task Force on AIDS Fraud, and the National Health Care Anti-Fraud Association, to name a few.

May 7, 1992. More hearings were held on health fraud. Stuart Gerson and Larry Morey, Deputy Inspector General for Investigations of the Department of Health and Human Services spoke before the committee. Morey is on the Board of Governors of the National Health Care Anti-Fraud Association and testified before the Subcommittee on Human Resources and Intergovernmental Relations regarding the recommendation by the General Accounting Office (GAO) to form a National Commission on Health Fraud. Gerson stated he was against such a commission because this function was already an ongoing activity of the federal Task Force on Health Fraud.

More than two and a half years in the courts. One million dollars in legal fees. Bad press, lost business, and a tarnished image and reputation. This is the price that Steve and Susan Levine and Nutri-Cology have had to pay to keep their doors open and to continue their service to the alternative community. What have the U.S. government's relentless attacks produced? When the smoke cleared, the results were:

1. In the last week of September 1993, Judge Lowell Jensen of the Federal District Court in San Francisco ruled in favor of Nutri-Cology and granted it a Summary Judgment against the government. The Judge ruled basically that the FDA's and U.S. Attorney's charges of fraud were unfounded, and he threw out the fraud charges against Nutri-Cology.

2. The government continued to pursue its charges that the product claims made by Nutri-Cology were drug claims and that therefore the Court should order it to be closed down.

3. The Judge ruled that the claims were *not* for drugs or new drugs and therefore dismissed those charges as unfounded as well. The Judge stated that the government was overreaching in attempting to get restitution, and that the charges of fraud were also overreaching. He also stated that the government's evaluation of the Nutri-Cology products as being drugs was also overreaching.

That is the way this skirmish ended. However, one battle won does not mean that the war is over. Steve Levine stated in May 1994 that the government is still attempting to push forward on some other issues with Nutri-Cology. As of the time of writing, the fight continues.

Its actions in 1994 indicate that the government apparently has no intention of voluntarily stopping its pursuit of the alternatives. It has too much time and money invested at this point. The agencies involved would have a lot to explain to Congress and the people if they were to suddenly throw up their hands in defeat. As the saying goes, it would take an act of Congress at this point to force these agencies to cease their anti-competitive activities.

Those involved also have another power to answer to—the vested interests in the pharmaceutical industry who started this whole campaign. The government's alliance with the drug industry, and the government's attacks against the economic competitors of the drug industry, have always forwarded the pharmaceutical industry's purpose, which is to disallow competitors from interfering with the sales of drugs and to prevent them from freely competing.

Again, we need to emphasize the words of Gary Dykstra of the FDA in May 1992: "The Task Force considered. . .what steps are necessary to ensure that the existence of dietary supplements on the market does not act as a disincentive for drug development."

Furthermore, we need to re-emphasize that the FDA has cosponsored and jointly financed (with the pharmaceutical industry) a campaign designed to destroy the economic competitors of the drug industry within the alternative health care products community. All in the name of "protecting the public against health fraud."

The Nutri-Cology case suggests that there is a different type of fraud being committed. The victims of this fraud are the Congress, the media, and the people. The fraud is, from all appearances, this entire anti-health fraud campaign.

The Nutri-Cology case thus far serves as evidence that the majority of alternative product manufacturers are not guilty of health fraud, mail fraud, or any kind of fraud. The ones who apparently *are* guilty of fraud, and of many other violations of federal laws, are those who have perpetrated this massive hoax to begin with. They have apparently hoaxed Congress, the media, and the public. Government agencies have been duped into spending millions of taxpayer dollars in the pursuit of a campaign that serves no purpose other than to eliminate the public's freedom to choose its own brand of medicine. This forwards the pharmaceutical industry's plans to dominate the marketplace with their products.

Thousands of practitioners, companies and clinics simply do not have the financial resources to fight this battle in the courts. It would be to their benefit to rally behind the Nutri-Cology victory and to offer support. If Nutri-Cology can defeat Big Brother in the courts, there is hope for those who do not have the resources to do so themselves. How you, the reader, can help is covered in Part Three.

Chapter 10

The Herbalife Story

"April 26, 1984. Sacramento FDB. Walsh [FDB inves-
tigator] *recorded covert telephone conversations with a
Sacramento area Herbalife distributor. Several more
telephone conversations with this distributor were recorded
through 06/14/84. "*
[FDB Chronology of Herbalife Case, 02/26/85]

*"Health Fraud Products—Herbalife. . .Number One
Priority PAC/FDA Target List—1984 "*
[PAC/FDA Public Service Anti-Quackery Program 1983-
1984]

The Herbalife story is a classic example of how the PAC/FDA
Public Service Anti-Quackery Campaign attempted to destroy a
young company using the media, the FDA, and assorted dirty tricks.
As in the Nutri-Cology case, the California Food and Drug Branch,
Fraud Section, worked with the FDA and others in the campaign
against Herbalife.

It began in earnest in 1983-1984 when the Pharmaceutical Advertising Council joined with the Food and Drug Administration to
eliminate the chief economic competitors of the drug industry. Herbalife, who made herbal products that were used for a variety of
wellness purposes, was on the top of the target priority list in the
campaign. Some of the products addressed weight loss, while others
were used by customers for such health-related problems as arthritis.

One product for which the FDA came after Herbalife dealt with
arthritis, APR (Arthritis Pain Reliever). One of the first pharmaceutical companies to help finance the PAC/FDA Campaign was Syntex.
One of their best-selling drugs was Naprosyn, which was in direct
economic competition with Herbalife products used for arthritis. The
sales for Naprosyn when the campaign began were $366.5 million
for just one year. If Herbalife's products were taken off the market
and the FDA attacks could create bad press for Herbalife products,
Syntex sales would likely increase. It is, therefore, no revelation that

Herbalife was at the top of the priority target list, especially considering that Syntex was helping to finance the campaign.

According to the Herbalife case files of the California State Food and Drug Branch, Fraud Section, the very first complaint the FDB received on Herbalife was a minor one. A consumer wrote to the U.S. FDA, alleging nausea and constipation while taking the product NRG. The FDA sent this complaint to the State FDB for attention and investigation. The FDB Santa Ana District Office received the complaint. The Los Angeles District Office got one bottle of the NRG product and sent it to the Berkeley Microbiological Laboratory for salmonella analysis. On May 19, 1981, it was determined that the product was free of any salmonella. Herbalife officials explained that someone could get constipated and nauseous by taking too much of this herb product, and that the solution to the problem was very simple—cut back on the amount of the product taken.

Almost a year later, on May 13, 1982, the San Jose FDB office received a consumer complaint alleging dizziness, blackouts, insomnia, and hyperactivity symptoms as a result of taking an Herbalife product. Again, nothing came of this complaint. Again, it was determined that if one took too much, one could possibly experience such symptoms as were reported. Again, the simple solution, according to Herbalife officials, was to cut back on the amounts taken and the symptoms would disappear.

Following this complaint, however, FDB Regional Administrator Warren Crawford ordered his San Jose District to infiltrate an Herbalife group. His operative did so by becoming a distributor for Herbalife. From that point, and over the next year and a half, there were only two consumer complaints. Each was addressed by the Herbalife company officials directly, and the company refunded the money paid for the product, to the satisfaction of the consumer.

There were no significant complaints that would have justified federal and state government agencies taking the actions they did against Herbalife. Notwithstanding, these agencies spent taxpayer dollars to pursue an insignificant situation.

Interestingly, one of the complaints which apparently served as the catalyst that propelled the FDB and the FDA into a higher level of involvement in their investigation of Herbalife, was filed by the Arthritis Foundation. On January 15, 1983, James Waddell of the FDB San Diego office received a complaint about from Herbalife's product APR (Arthritis Pain Reliever), from the Foundation in San Diego. This complaint was then forwarded to the FDB headquarters in Sacramento. In turn, it was referred to the FDB's Los Angeles office for follow-up.

It was at this time that the Pharmaceutical Advertising Council and the FDA listed Herbalife as a number-one priority target in their Anti-Quackery Campaign, and so the complaint resulted in the FDB conducting a visit to Herbalife. They obtained several products for sampling regarding the labeling and literature of products, including APR. This action was followed up by an inspection of the Herbalife facility in Culver City, California, on July 22, 1983. Nothing really came out of this except a series of letters back and forth between the FDB and the attorney for Herbalife, Kirkpatrick Dilling.

While all of this correspondence was taking place, the FDB continued to collect data on Herbalife. Ray Wilson, FDB official in Sacramento, evaluated the Herbalife career book for claims on various products. Keep in mind that these products are herbs, not drugs. Attorney Dilling sent a letter to the FDB regarding the Wilson report on the Herbalife career book and the Regulatory Letter sent to Herbalife.

This volleying continued until 1984, when the FDB decided to send an undercover plant into Herbalife to become a distributor in the Sacramento area. Mike Bogumill, FDB Fraud Section Program Director, had received a consumer complaint about an Herbalife distributor in the Sacramento area. The files do not reveal any serious problems caused by any Herbalife products. This "consumer" complaint could have just as easily have come from one of the "anti-health-fraud" consumer groups in California. In April 1984, FDB official Dan Walsh of the Sacramento District office began to collect information on the company. He got data from the Attorney General's Office of Kentucky, the local Stockton newspaper, the Assistant District Attorney in Santa Cruz, medical expert witnesses, and U.S. Postal Inspectors, and then moved forward with his covert investigation.

On April 26, 1984, Walsh contacted the Herbalife Sacramento area distributor by phone. Unbeknownst to the distributor, Walsh recorded the conversation. The distributor, a man by the name of Clint Jones, was just one of the many people who made up the mass of Herbalife distributors around the globe. He obviously believed in the products and talked freely with Walsh several times. Walsh covertly recorded all his conversations with Clint Jones from April 26 through June 14, 1984.

No evidence in the files of this case indicate that Walsh or anyone at FDB had obtained a court order to conduct this type of electronic surveillance of the Herbalife distributor. It is in violation of federal laws to conduct electronic surveillance of a private citizen without a court order; even with a court order there are a number of restrictions. There is an exception—when a law enforcement agency is *directed* to do such surveillance by a prosecuting agency of government. However, there was no indication in the files that Walsh was acting under the directions, orders, or request—written or otherwise—from any prosecuting agency of government.

Instead of following the proper sequence of conducting an initial investigation based on inspections and other sources of data, then submitting a report to a prosecuting authority requesting authority for electronic surveillance, Walsh submitted his outline report *after* he had already started the questionable, and very possibly illegal, electronic surveillance. It wasn't until *after* he conducted his covert phone recordings that the FDB implemented a state-wide plan against Herbalife. It was only *after* he did this that he submitted his report to a prosecutor. This plan, developed by Walsh and approved by FDB Chief Chambers Bryson in Sacramento, was approved on May 16, 1984, right in the middle of his covert phone-recording investigation, which continued for another month.

On the day Walsh got approval for his state-wide investigation, FDB District offices around the state participated in a conference call regarding the investigation of Herbalife. The call involved Mike Bogumill, Dan Walsh, Vivianne Oates, Jeff Lineberry, Chris Wogee, Ralph Lounsbury, and Ozzie Schmidt. They discussed their strategy for the investigation.

On May 21 and 22, 1984, Dan Walsh went to Los Angeles to meet with the FDA and review its files on Herbalife. He copied their files with special attention to any complaints about the consumer fraud aspects of Herbalife. The following day, May 23, 1984, the multi-agency strategy meeting mentioned in earlier chapters was held regarding Herbalife and other issues dealing with "health fraud." A dozen people from the FDB attended. In addition, several federal agencies were represented, including FDA Los Angeles, FDA San Francisco, the FTC, and the L.A., Sacramento, and San Francisco offices of the Postal Inspector. The California Board of Medical Quality Assurance was also in attendance, as was the National Council Against Health Fraud's representative, Harold Loeffler, Ph.D. Loeffler, according to Dan Walsh, more or less directed the government agencies present at this meeting as to what his organization's priorities were, including Herbalife.

At this meeting, Dan Walsh was given, probably by Loeffler, a publication entitled "Let's Grow Younger," written by Richard D. Marconi of D&F Industries (which manufactured Herbalife products, as well as 30 other supplement company products). This promotional material dealt with a product called Schizandra Plus.

Following this meeting, the investigation of Herbalife intensified nationwide, involving all of the government agencies represented at the meeting.

There is a doctrine in law known as the Fruit of the Poisonous Tree Doctrine. Under this doctrine, any evidence gathered that is the direct result or immediate product of illegal conduct on the part of an official is inadmissible against the victim of this illegal conduct. This all comes under the principle of due process, as outlined in the Fourteenth Amendment of the Constitution. (This rule, by the way, does not apply to evidence resulting from such conduct on the part of a private citizen, unless there has been some complicity on the part of the government.) The doctrine draws its name from the concept that once a tree is poisoned (that is, the primary evidence is illegally obtained), then the fruit of that tree (any secondary evidence) is likewise poisoned or tainted and may not be used. This doctrine is applied in criminal cases, and may very well be applicable in the Herbalife situation and investigation conducted by Dan Walsh. It wasn't until *after* Walsh conducted covert electronic surveillance of Sacramento Herbalife distributor Clint Jones that Walsh began his investigation plan for a statewide action against Herbalife. His plan was based upon the fruits of his covert electronic surveillance, as well as his infiltration of Herbalife meetings and betrayal of distributor Clint Jones. In itself this raises the question of a violation of Jones' civil rights, as well.

In the twilight world of gum shoes (private investigators) and government undercover snoops, one tool used to obtain information on a target is either contact with an ex-spouse of the target or digging through divorce papers in the courts. Such tactics are considered standard practices in gathering information about a person's background. The logic at play here is to contact someone who may hate the targeted subject of the investigation in order to extract as much "dirt" as possible about that subject. It isn't considered unethical, or immoral, but it can be considered a "tabloid" tactic. Such tactics were not beyond the scope of Walsh's bag of dirty tricks in his pursuit of Herbalife. A week after the multi-agency meeting with the National Council Against Health Fraud, on June 6, 1984, Walsh received from Los Angeles FDB copies of a civil divorce suit filed in Los Angeles County Superior Court against Mark R. Hughes, the head of Herbalife. Apparently Walsh didn't gain much from the material. But whether there was embarrassing information or not, personal material is absolutely irrelevant to a company's business. Walsh's investigation also went through the trouble of checking the backgrounds of both Richard Marconi and Fred Siegel, who were doing business as D&F Industries, the company that manufactured the Herbalife product line. All that the Walsh file chronology reflected in this regard was that both of these businessmen "are closely linked to the Herbalife operation in Culver City." If that statement isn't an attempt to make something out of nothing, then nothing is. Since there is nothing unsavory or suspicious about having close business ties with a company, what we have here is a deliberate use of words with inflammatory undercurrents: "closely linked to" and "operation." The goal is apparently to insinuate some sort of wrong-doing. Had the sentence read, accurately, that D&F Industries had a business relationship with Herbalife, the report would have been more professional.

By the time the government had completed its investigation of Herbalife and had created a case against them in the press and in the courts, the company had experienced a huge economic loss. As an apparent extension of the PAC/FDA Anti-Quackery Campaign, television exposés on the company were airing in Kansas City. Newspaper accounts of the government's case against the firm were spread across the United States. There is no question that Herbalife was assaulted by one of the most organized and ruthless propaganda campaigns ever directed against any company of its kind. The attack was waged on all fronts. There was the FDA's federal case, the civil suits filed in California, criminal prosecutions in Canada, and the media blitz.

It all hit in March and April 1985. The company was experiencing its best quarterly sales in its five-year history. Rumors were that they were on target for a billion-dollar year in sales world-wide. Its first-quarter total sales of that year exceeded anything the company had done in the past. Many distributors were making over $15,000 a month in commissions and sales. The multi-level marketing plan designed by its founder was working.

By December 5, 1984, however, the end was near. U.S. Food and Drug Administration Compliance officer Debbie Grelle (who had attended the May 23, 1984, strategy session) contacted FDB's Jeff Lineberry (also at the May 23rd meeting) with a request for an ad hoc committee meeting. The request recommended to the U.S. FDA headquarters staff in Rockville, Maryland, "seizure of Herbalife products that are in apparent violation of the Federal Food, Drug and Cosmetic Act."

On January 31, 1985, the FDB people met with officials of the Attorney General's office in Sacramento to map out the case they planned to bring against the company. Five days later, on February 5, 1985, an article against Herbalife appeared in the Los Angeles *Times*. On the same day, it was noted in Walsh's file on his investigation that consumer advocate and reporter David Horowitz appeared nationally on the NBC "Today" television program with an "exposé" of Herbalife.

Nine days later, on February 14, 1985, according to Walsh's notes on the case, Don Gartner, Peter DeMauro, and Al Sheldon (representing the People, the Department, and the State, respectively) met in San Francisco with Herbalife attorneys Kickpatrick Dilling and Perry Turner, to discuss the issues raised in Gartner's letter of January 24, 1985, and to attempt to "reach a stipulated settlement in the case." The government's requests were so extensive and irrational that no agreement could be reached.

The result of this meeting was that the government filed its case against Herbalife in March 1985. The cards were stacked against Herbalife from the start. Whether the lawyers knew it or not, Herbalife was in fact targeted as a direct result of being on the PAC/FDA's Anti-Quackery Campaign priority target list. Whether or not their attorneys knew that this was part of a planned campaign is not known. What is known is that the company suffered substantial financial losses as a direct result of this campaign.

There were Congressional hearings which involved Herbalife. There was a blizzard of bad press. There were layoffs, and there was a resultant drop in sales world-wide. If ever a company could show a direct cause-and-effect relationship of financial losses and the campaign directed against it, Herbalife could.

It spent five years in the courts. Overwhelmed by the media onslaught, Herbalife distributors were subjected to a constant and relentless barrage of suspicion and ridicule. All this resulted in the loss of an estimated $5 billion over the five-year period.

The government also tried to link Herbalife to five deaths of clients who were on Herbalife products when they passed away. But even the government's own medical expert refused to make a direct connection between the deaths and Herbalife's products.

In vivid contrast to the few consumer complaints against Herbalife, we saw a severe response amounting to overkill by the government against Herbalife. On the surface there was no basis or foundation for what occurred. Where there were any complaints the company addressed and handled these customers in a timely fashion.

It evidently wasn't really a question of the public being harmed by Herbalife products so much as it was that Herbalife's chief economic competitors had mounted a campaign against them, using the FDA to close them down. This appears to be a classic case of a restraint of trade, or collusion and conspiracy to do so. It should be obvious that this was not just a coincidence that this happened to Herbalife. It wasn't just a parallel independent business justification that brought together more than two dozen pharmaceutical companies which then financed a campaign designed by a medical advertising firm and jointly carried out by the drug interests and the FDA.

It wasn't by chance that the pharmaceutical industry helped design, name, and then approve an agreement between them and the FDA to eliminate alternative products and manufacturers. It didn't "just happen" that the targets chosen were in direct economic competition with those financing the campaign. It wasn't just some fluke that those involved in the study of alternatives happened to pick the very people known to be diametrically opposed to alternatives to sit in judgment of these very same alternatives and to write reports about the safety and usefulness of these alternatives for distribution to the insurance industry and state and federal government agencies.

The agreement signed between the Pharmaceutical Advertising Council and the FDA in March 1984 should most certainly fall under a Supreme Court decision (*Standard Oil v. United States*, 1911) wherein the Court held "that certain types of business agreements among competitors would be held unreasonable as a matter of law— i.e., illegal per se." No fewer than 26 drug firms entered into the campaign by financing it, and as a result of the agreement, the parties involved named specific products and companies to go after in their campaign. In so doing they have apparently violated federal laws designed to protect the free marketplace from such conspiracies. The measurement of whether or not they succeeded can be seen in the fact that as a result of the campaign the targeted competitors lost ground in the marketplace and the drug firms benefitted. It's just that simple.

It is my considered opinion—and this is only my opinion—that in the case of Herbalife, the only ones who gained from this fight were the attorneys. The legal fees were astronomical, soaring into the millions of dollars over the years spent waging this battle against the government. Other observers of this situation are of the opinion that the company would have been much better off taking the offensive. It should have considered suing the government and the pharmaceutical industry and their allies in this campaign, for conspiracy. Some alternative lawyers who are familiar with this case feel very strongly that violations of the federal RICO laws are clear and evident on the part of the government and its allies in this campaign, particularly with regard to Herbalife.

The FDA and state agencies involved in the attack did so with the zeal of fanatics. They used every trick in the book to bring Herbalife down, and they did so apparently with the express agreement and financial aid of the pharmaceutical industry over a long period of time. The same goes for Nutri-Cology and other alternative product manufacturers who have become victims of this campaign.

In contrast to the Herbalife story, the following is presented as a clear-cut example of favored treatment of a product considered by many to be truly dangerous.

Would you consume a product which caused you headaches, migraines, neurological disorders, seizures, suicidal depression, impaired vision, menstrual and reproductive disorders, and even lesions of the brain? If you knew that scientists reported that such a product may cause damage to a fetus, including reduction of I.Q. in newborn infants, possible cancerous tumors, and possible addiction, would you want to consume such a product?

Such a product is on the market, and it is estimated that more than 100 million consumers are using it. It is a product known as aspartame (marketed under the names of Equal and NutraSweet). For years it was kept off the market by the FDA because of the potential danger to consumers. In 1977 the FDA even brought a grand jury investigation against the company that manufactured it (G.D. Searle & Company) for submitting falsified scientific data on the effects of aspartame. For some reason, the grand jury investigation was suddenly called off, but the product was still not allowed on the market.

The FDA's Public Board of Inquiry noted that more studies were needed to see if aspartame contributed to brain cancers. However, this all changed after the Reagan Administration installed Arthur Hayes, Jr., as the FDA Commissioner. Once in office, he reversed the FDA's decision and the FDA approved NutraSweet for foods in 1981. Then in 1983 this approval was extended to the lucrative diet soda market.

Shouldn't the FDA be more cautious with regard to a product that has reportedly caused such series maladies in humans? Of course it should! However, the FDA probably won't do anything until down the road, years from now, someone decides another product is better. The FDA might then declare NutraSweet dangerous and ban it from the market. This happened with cyclamates in 1970 after being linked to cancer and mutations. Next, saccharin was shown to increase the risk of bladder cancer (but remained on the market anyway). Then along came NutraSweet. The NutraSweet story, which is on-going, is intriguing.

One of the principle opponents to NutraSweet is Washington, D.C., attorney Jim Turner, of the law firm Swankin & Turner. Jim fought for years to keep NutraSweet off the market because he was convinced that there were serious health problems caused by the product. He handled several law suits against the company by consumers who felt they were harmed by aspartame. One such case involved a young boy five years old who was experiencing debilitating headaches. Jim described this horror story to me in detail. He said that when the boy first had these awful headaches he would throw his body on the floor and uncontrollably roll around screaming for his mother to help stop the pain. Turner also told me about scientific experiments with lab animals wherein lab monkeys exposed to aspartame had developed lesions in their brains. He said that the FDA had known about this study and others which pointed to the existence of dangerous and adverse effects of aspartame. He said that although the FDA knew of these studies, it relied on studies sponsored and financed by the industry, showing aspartame safe for human consumption.

In marked contrast to the Herbalife attack, based on what amounts to minor complaints, the aspartame (NutraSweet) situation was apparently a case of no-action by the government based on the power of the vested interests involved.

Herbalife had only a few consumer complaints against its products. NutraSweet had *thousands* of complaints, and some involved effects as serious as seizures. For example:

1. Dr. Richard Wurtman, Director of the Clinical Research Center and Professor at Massachusetts Institute of Technology, in April 1988 urged the FDA to issue warnings to physicians that aspartame may be associated with a syndrome including severe headaches, and in some cases,

grand mal seizures. Wurtman had received over 1,000 complaints at M.I.T. directly into his department.

2. FDA had received complaints as early as 1983. It reported having received 592 complaints from July 1983 through April 1984 from Searle Labs.

3. In November 1984 the FDA had another 85 complaints of seizures which it reportedly studied.

4. In 1985 the FDA became aware of another 1,000 cases from Searle of adverse reactions to the product.

5. In April 1986 Senator Metzenbaum sent the FDA 360 reports of alleged adverse reactions to aspartame.

6. In 1988 the FDA studied 35 seizure cases it had received as complaints from Dr. Wurtman.

7. In the March 7, 1988, issue of *Food Chemical News,* the FDA reported receiving 60 cases which raised the issue of eye damage from aspartame. The FDA reported at that time that these cases were among 152 they had already received.

The many complaints received from private sources outside government included:

8. Dr. Woodrow Monte of Arizona State University received about 200 complaints about the product's adverse reactions.

9. The Aspartame Victims and Friends, a consumer group in Ocala, Florida, had received another 450 complaints.

10. The Arizona Consumer Council in Phoenix, Arizona, had received 100 complaints about the side-effects of Nutra Sweet.

These complaints all came to the FDA's attention. There were *thousands* of them. Yet the FDA did nothing to take this apparently dangerous product off the market. In contrast, the FDA took rather heavy-handed and drastic actions against Herbalife for *fewer than six* complaints, according to the California Food and Drug files.

In the case of Herbalife, the FDA went for overkill. In contrast, the FDA worked out a special arrangement with Searle Labs for complaints about NutraSweet. On February 11, 1986, FDA Commissioner Dr. Frank E. Young, in response to a series of letters from Senator Metzenbaum regarding complaints about NutraSweet, wrote a letter to the Senator stating, "...we have an agreement with Searle that they file their complaint reports on a monthly basis." Young further noted that the FDA had "established a formal post-marketing surveillance system for improved evaluation of consumer complaints..." Young said that this system would allow the FDA's Center for Food Safety and Applied Nutrition scientists to analyze complaints to determine whether there were associations between adverse reaction and food products. He added that if an association is *suspected* then the FDA would "initiate an appropriate investigation."

The letter acknowledged the 360 cases that the Senator had reported to the FDA and said, "The 360 reports will be processed in the same manner as all other consumer complaints of adverse reactions to foods and food and color additives that come to the attention of the FDA." (That's government talk for "this is not a priority.") Young then explained how the FDA was going to step-by-step look into these complaints. He ended with stating that he would provide the Senator with a report on the 360 cases "and compare them with the much larger number of cases describing adverse reactions allegedly due to aspartame already in our system."

It was discovered that, in what seems to be a bizarre move on the part of the FDA, the FDA Commissioner had knowledge of almost 600 complaints that Searle wanted to turn in to the FDA between July 1983, and April 1984, but the FDA *did not accept them.* Young stated, "It would not be correct to state that Searle held on to these reports for over a year. . .The firm offered to submit additional reports but. . .the agency [FDA] decided to focus on an intensive evaluation of the larger number of complaints already received."

As it turned out, the FDA did an evaluation of 592 complaints it received from Searle, designing a 13-page questionnaire for use by the Center for Disease Control to conduct a "thorough investigation" of the complaints, which resulted in the following statistics:

67% of the 517 complaints were of headaches, dizziness, and mood alterations.
24% were of upset stomachs, diarrhea and other gastrointestinal problems.

15% were of rashes and other allergic reactions.
6% were of changes in usual menstrual patterns.
9% were of various other symptoms.

The FDA Commissioner also acknowledged that there were consumers in this study who had to seek medical attention as a direct
result of consuming aspartame.

Metzenbaum asked Young for a report on all Searle research on
aspartame, and Young replied that "the vast majority of academic
research being conducted on aspartame is either under the National
Institutes of Health sponsorship or well known to G.D. Searle." He
sent the Senator a list of research being sponsored by NIH plus a list
of studies provided by Searle. He noted that Searle was sponsoring
"several different studies at Yale University and Mt. Sinai Hospital
related to potential seizure effects of aspartame." He added that he
understood that Institutional Review Boards (which approve
academic research protocols) had approved the protocols for these
two studies, but the protocols for the studies were "intended to
challenge individuals who have reported seizure activity subsequent
to aspartame exposure."

The controversy surrounding aspartame continued when Dr.
Richard Wurtman attempted to involve the FDA in a joint research
project with MIT on aspartame and seizures. On April 21, 1986,
Wurtman met with officials of the FDA in an attempt "to urge them
to cooperate with him in a study to begin shortly at MIT on 10
subjects, five of whom are epileptics." Wurtman insisted that the
study would be a pilot for other larger, more meaningful experiments, but the FDA rejected his offer of cooperation, claiming "little
would be gained."

Wurtman tried for over a year to get support for his research, to
no avail. He said, "The present system, in which the companies that
sell our synthetic foods—like NutraSweet—fund virtually all of the
studies, FDA-mandated or not. . .is too vulnerable to misuse. . .when
outside investigators propose studies that might yield the 'wrong'
answer, a large bag of 'dirty tricks' is available for derailing those
studies."

In his presentation to the FDA, Wurtman also asserted that no
pregnant woman "should ever consume aspartame in any amount."
He also attacked Searle's own studies related to how much aspartame average Americans now consume. Wurtman called
NutraSweet's estimates of current use "spurious," asserting:

They show, among other things, that people consume less aspartame in the summer than in other months, a finding which violates good sense and reason. (This probably reflects the fact—affirmed in our laboratories at MIT—that people have much more difficulty accurately remembering snack than meal intakes. . .and most of the aspartame in the American diet comes via cold beverages and other snack foods.)

Wurtman also emphasized that animal studies have supplied enough evidence to suggest the link between aspartame and seizures, pointing out that what remains is to conduct a study in the only experimental animal in which the question can be realistically addressed, an individual who has suffered such a seizure.

In an article in *Food Chemical News* (April 28, 1986), Searle Vice President for Public Affairs stated that they were "funding studies and have ongoing studies for the purpose of evaluating the effect of aspartame on seizure activity." The same article reported that in responding to Wurtman's report on seizures, an FDA spokesman "acknowledged that FDA evaluated 85 cases of reported seizures since November 1984. About 17 could conceivably have been associated with aspartame use. . .[but] five of the persons had a history of epilepsy."

Here you have the FDA admitting that it found 17 of 85 reported seizure cases that could "conceivably be associated with aspartame use." Yet the FDA goes on to *justify* these cases and make less of the reported seizures by stating that "five of the persons had a history of epilepsy."

That being the case, the least the FDA could have done was to warn the public that anyone with epilepsy should not use any product with aspartame in it. At most the FDA should have issued a broad public statement in the press announcing that its scientists had found enough scientific evidence to point to the conclusion that there is a conceivable link between seizures and aspartame use. It did not do this and the product continued to cause seizures and other health problems.

Dr. Wurtman is not the only scientist who has evaluated the adverse effects of aspartame on humans, and he is not the only scientist who is critical of aspartame. Dr. Woodrow Monte, head of the Science and Nutrition Laboratory at Arizona State University, studied hundreds of cases dealing with the adverse effects of aspartame, including seizures. His scientific opinion of aspartame is summed up in his statement: "If you *tried* real hard to design a food additive that could cause health problems, you'd have to try *real hard* to design one as bad as aspartame."

Another scientist, Dr. William N. Pardridge of the University of California at Los Angeles, stated that liberal intake of aspartame may be harmful and toxic for human consumption.

Jim Turner reported that he knew of an internal U.S. Air Force memo, authored by an Air Force doctor, which warned Air Force personnel, especially pilots, about NutraSweet and seizures. This may have been based on another report which told of a pilot who had seizures after consuming a soft drink containing NutraSweet.

What is aspartame anyway? What exactly does it do once it enters the body? If it does harm people, how does it do this?

Aspartame came on the market touted as the ultimate in artificial sweeteners. This additive—200 times sweeter than sugar but with only one-tenth the calories—is now in a wide variety of foods, including diet sodas, breakfast cereals, chewing gum, lemonade mixes, dry foods, jello, and many other products we now consume.

Made by G.D. Searle & Co., a division of Monsanto chemical company, it is a synthetic compound of two amino acids— phenylalanine and aspartic acid. It is marketed by Searle as a "safe and natural product, a low-caloric sugar substitute" that they say is "an amazing discovery. . .which sounds a little too good to be true." Unfortunately, it *is* a little too good to be true.

A look at the three chemical components of aspartame provides a possible explanation for the discrepancies between the promising claims and the warnings of dangers by its critics in the scientific world as well as in the consumer-protection area.

Phenylalanine. This composes 40% of aspartame's weight and has received the most attention. It is undisputed that this chemical can be extremely dangerous to people afflicted with the rare genetic disease phenylketonuria (PKU), which is the inability to metabolize this amino acid. This rare disease often strikes small children and can be lethal if they ingest aspartame. People with PKU are at special risk from consuming NutraSweet, and warning labels have been prescribed by the FDA for products with the substance (although foods served in restaurants are exempt). Babies with PKU who ingest aspartame can suffer mental retardation if they consume NutraSweet. Logically, pregnant women shouldn't consume it either.

According to one consumer group, the Coalition for Alternatives in Nutrition and Healthcare (CANAH), aspartame in hard candy and cough drops is especially dangerous to young children with PKU. The FDA stated, "CANAH feels that the inclusion of aspartame in hard candies, and in particular those which are individually wrapped, will present a non-easily recognized hazard to some unsuspecting PKU patients, children in particular. On this basis alone, we feel there is enough concern to disallow the use of aspartame as a sweetener in hard candies in particular." (*Food Chemical News,* March 7, 1988.)

However, even those without PKU can be affected by phenylalanine. According to Dr. Richard Wurtman, studies performed at MIT would suggest that the buildup of the chemical in the brain could interfere with important brain chemicals when it is consumed with carbohydrates.The FDA refutes Dr. Wurtman's contention that there is a problem here, stating that it is "unlikely" that people would ever combine carbohydrates and phenylalanine. Maybe not in a test tube in some FDA laboratory, but it is *very* likely that someone would drink a diet soda while eating a hamburger or sandwich. The FDA's objection to Wurtman's study is not a very astute observation on the part of FDA scientists.

Aspartic Acid. Half of the weight of aspartame is aspartic acid, which has been proven to cause glandular disorders in mammals and to affect hormones that regulate the menstrual cycle in rats. Proponents of aspartame often point out that amino acids are essential parts of the diet. However, when absorbed in foods, amino acids are broken down a little at a time. With aspartame, the amino acids are quickly absorbed into the blood, and there may not be enough time to regulate them. Dr. Monte has stated that absorption of amino acids from NutraSweet is like "the difference between a time release capsule and main-lining."

Methyl Alcohol. This is the final part of aspartame, a poison better known as wood alcohol. (The alcohol in your booze is ethyl alcohol.) Symptoms of methyl alcohol poisoning include headaches, dizziness, weakness, and blurred vision. It is well known that 95% of methyl alcohol breaks down in the body into formaldehyde, which is a cancer-causing agent. Furthermore, aspartame is unstable at warm temperatures and breaks down in heat as low as 86 degrees, increasing the amount of methyl alcohol. For this reason, aspartame is not supposed to be added to products which must be cooked. Apparently this danger was overlooked in approving NutriSweet in gelatin desserts which require the use of boiling water. It is also worthy to note here that considering the danger that this product poses to children, it should be questioned why it is allowed in children's vitamins (manufactured by drug companies).

Jim Turner describes the FDA approval of aspartame as a "shoddy process riddled with conflict of interest that relied on scientific data which was mainly in excess of 10 years old by the time they approved it for diet soda."

During the Reagan Administration, the product made it to the market. According to Jim Turner, one of the most important aspects of how this product finally made it to the market was the fact that a former FDA official had left the FDA and went to work in public relations for G.D. Searle & Co. It was from that position that the former FDA man reportedly called in some favors. G.D. Searle & Co. began to push the FDA for approval, which they did receive.

Bill Vaughan, spokesman for G.D. Searle & Co., was asked in an interview about the large number of complaints that had been received about NutraSweet. He stated that he wasn't aware of a large number of complaints. Specific numbers were then given to him related to over 2,500 complaints. Being given these numbers must have jogged his memory, because he did admit to recalling about 1,500 of these complaints about the product. He downplayed these complaints and their significance by stating, "That's not bad, considering there are 100 million people using the product."

The Herbalife story is a bitter pill to swallow in light of the facts about NutraSweet. (By the way, Herbalife also produced a *natural* sweetener made from a South American herb which is reportedly much safer than NutraSweet, and tasted better too.)

Here we see a five-year-old company, making its way in the marketplace with products that are harmless, especially compared to something like NutraSweet. We then see it being targeted by its economic competitors in the pharmaceutical industry for economic destruction. The pharmaceutical industry, teaming up with the FDA, then financed this campaign and helped name the targets. The FDA proceeded upon a task of removing Herbalife as a threat to the drug companies which are in competition with Herbalife products.

There appears to be definite imbalances in the FDA's actions. The FDA brings out all its guns against Herbalife based on a handful of complaints. At the same time, the FDA works out an agreement for Searle to send monthly reports on their complaints. No action is taken against the company or its product, NutraSweet. The FDA turned a deaf ear to the thousands of complaints against NutraSweet, yet pursued Herbalife with a vengeance.

One can suppose that what is going on can best be explained by Gary Dykstra's statement that the FDA's Task Force considered it an important mission to ensure that dietary supplements would not stand in the way of drug development. . .and sales.

Regrettably, they seem to have succeeded in Herbalife's case. Is there any justice?

Chapter 11

The Conspiracy Against Chiropractic

"Since Chiropractors are here to stay, an adjunctive alternative, revolutionary in concept, is to establish a membership category within the structure of [the AMA] for those chiropractors who are ethical. . .

"Thus any campaign against chiropractic by the medical profession could not be interpreted as an effort to 'corner the market' in health-care delivery as often has been the case in chiropractic strategy. "

[Report on Chiropractic, Ad Hoc Committee on Liaison with the Health Related Professions, June 25, 1980]

The American Medical Association has a long history of combating chiropractors. From its beginnings in 1895, chiropractic as a profession was in direct opposition to orthodox medicine by the very nature of its philosophy and its approach to the cause and effects of diseases. According to modern dictionaries, the word *chiropractic* comes from the Latin word *chiro,* meaning "hand," and the Greek word *praktikos,* which means "effective or practical." It is described as a system of therapy in which disease is considered the result of neural (nerve) malfunction. Manipulation of the spinal column and other structures is the preferred method of treatment.

The key word here is *preferred,* because chiropractors do not use drugs, radiation, or surgery and therefore like to feel that they are giving the consumer a choice. The AMA from the start was violently opposed to chiropractic. During the first part of this century, the AMA considered chiropractic, along with other alternative schools such as homeopathy, naturopathy, and eclectics, as quackery. *The AMA and U.S. Health Policy,* by Frank D. Campion, a staff official with the AMA's Communication Department, described chiropractic as follows:

Chiropractors believed that diseases could be cured by the adjustment of the vertebrae. Chiropractic started in 1895, so the legend goes, when Daniel David Palmer, a Davenport,

Iowa, grocer, adjusted the spinal column of a local janitor and supposedly cured him of deafness.

This statement is typical of the AMA's cynical and sometimes bitter mockery of chiropractic. The AMA's Principles of Medical Ethics stated under Principle 3 that it was unethical for a physician to associate with an "unscientific practitioner." In 1966, the AMA's House of Delegates passed a resolution calling chiropractic an unscientific cult.

To complete the circle, in 1967 the AMA's Judicial Council issued an opinion under Principle 3 holding that it was unethical for a physician to associate professionally with chiropractors. The AMA's opposition included both "associating" with chiropractors, which would include a game of golf, and "associating professionally," which would include referring patients to a chiropractor or accepting referrals from a chiropractor.

As described in Chapter 2, the AMA had a long history of opposition to chiropractic, all of which is well documented. On January 4, 1971, the AMA's Committee on Quackery sent a memorandum to the AMA's Board of Trustees. The memo stated:

Since the AMA Board of Trustees' decision at its meeting of November 2-3, 1963, to establish a Committee on Quackery, your Committee has considered its prime mission to be, first, the containment of chiropractic and, ultimately, the elimination of chiropractic.

The memo went on to chart what progress the Committee on Quackery felt it was making along these lines: "Your Committee believes it is well along in its first mission and is, at the same time, moving toward the ultimate goal."

For more than a dozen years the AMA's Committee on Quackery and the AMA-directed Coordinating Conference on Health Information (CCHI) worked on the front lines—and behind the lines—to attack chiropractic. They worked to exclude chiropractic from coverage under Medicare (both Title 18 and 19) as early as 1967, and at the same time worked to exclude chiropractic from Workmen's Compensation laws. They also tried to adversely influence private insurance plans and chiropractic coverage and tried to discredit chiropractic education by pushing the U.S. Office of Education to refuse accreditation to chiropractic colleges .

To go into any great detail about the campaigns that the AMA ran against chiropractic between 1963 and 1975, when the Committee on

Quackery was dissolved, is a book in itself. [I have, in fact, compiled such a book: *Are You a Target For Elimination* (International Institute of Natural Health Sciences, Inc., 1985).] One memo in particular serves as a prime example of how the AMA used its allies in and out of government to "fix things" against chiropractic. In a memorandum to H. Doyl Taylor dated September 21, 1967, Robert A. Youngerman of the Department of Investigation reviewed the Committee on Quackery's Meeting of September 15, 1967. Youngerman reported:

> Basically, the Committee's short-range objectives for containing the cult of chiropractic and any additional recognition it might achieve revolves around four points:
> (1) Doing everything within our power to see that chiropractic coverage under Title 18 of the Medicare Law is not obtained.
> (2) Doing everything within our power to see that recognition or listing by the U.S. Office of Education of a chiropractic accrediting agency is not achieved.
> (3) To encourage continued separation of the two national chiropractic associations.
> (4) To encourage state medical societies to take the initiative in their state legislatures in regard to legislation that might affect the practice of chiropractic.

In his memo, Youngerman revealed a conspiracy between the AMA, Stanford Research Institute, and the U.S. Public Health Service directed against chiropractic inclusion under Medicare:

> If section 141 [of House Resolution 12080, which provided for a study to determine the feasibility of inclusion of certain services under Part B of Title 18 of the Social Security Act] is implemented, staff and Committee already have commenced investigating the possibilities of Stanford Research Institute of Menlo Park, California, being given the assignment by HEW to conduct such a study, or at least to conduct that part of the study that would include various aspects of the current status of chiropractic practice in the United States.
> We have been reliably informed the outcome of such a study would not recommend chiropractic services be included under the act, and might very well go so far as to call it a health hazard.

Steps have been taken with officials of both the United States Public Health Service and the Stanford Research Institute to have such a study made regardless of whether Section 141 is enacted.

Once this survey has been completed, and assuming it would be negative to chiropractic (and we have every reason to believe this is the case), it would almost strike the final blow to the future of chiropractic. State medical societies then could have their hands strengthened to such an extent that there is little doubt but state legislatures would seriously consider rescinding state chiropractic licensing laws.

This is but one example of the AMA working behind the scenes to "contain and eliminate" chiropractic as a profession. Just about every document that the AMA ever wrote about chiropractic in the years 1963-1975, and its plans to destroy that profession, have been made public. The documents in question found their way into the hands of the chiropractors, and eventually into the state and federal courts.

After bringing their conspiracy case to the courts, the chiropractors were opposed by the AMA every inch of the way along a 12-year road that cost millions of dollars. In the end the court ruled that, indeed, the AMA was found to have conspired against chiropractic as a profession and had worked to boycott them in medicine. The court finally ruled on September 25, 1987. Judge Susan Getzendanner, U.S. District Court for the Northern District of Illinois Eastern Division, published her opinion on the case. She stated:

> The AMA's Boycott and Conspiracy—In the early 1960s, the AMA decided to contain and eliminate chiropractic as a profession. In 1963 the AMA's Committee on Quackery was formed. The committee worked aggressively—both overtly and covertly—to eliminate chiropractic.

Her opinion went on to describe one of the principal means used by the AMA to achieve its goal: to disallow any AMA doctors from associating with chiropractors, as outlined and detailed in its Principles of Medical Ethics. She made several other points as to how the AMA carried out this conspiracy; however, this was her main point. There was nothing in the order addressing how the AMA conspired with other private health groups and with government agencies to further contain chiropractic through the Coordinating Conference on

Health Information (CCHI). Nor did she address how the AMA worked to destroy chiropractic by way of the insurance industry, Medicare, Blue Cross/Blue Shield, and the many other avenues they pursued behind the scenes.

She did state that under the Sherman Act, every combination or conspiracy in restraint of trade is illegal. She stated that the conduct of the AMA and its members constituted a conspiracy in restraint of trade, thus violating the Sherman Act, based on the following facts of the case:

1. The purpose of the boycott was to eliminate chiropractic.
2. Chiropractors are in competition with some medical physicians.
3. The boycott had substantial anti-competitive effects.
4. There was no pro-competitive effects of the boycott.
5. The Plaintiffs were injured as a result of the conduct.

The AMA's defense in the suit involved a "patient care defense"; the AMA explained that what it did against chiropractic was in the defense of good scientific patient-care—that, in essence, the AMA was protecting patients from the unscientific approach by chiropractic to disease. However, the Court did not buy this defense and struck it down.

The judge found that throughout this boycott (1966-1980), the AMA failed "to establish this concern was objectively reasonable." Finally, the court ruled that the AMA's concern for scientific method in patient care could have been adequately satisfied in a "manner less restrictive of competition and that a nationwide conspiracy to eliminate a licensed profession was not justified by the concern for scientific method."

Some legal experts feel that a large majority of what the AMA did was not really covered in this ruling, which left the door open for the AMA to continue its illegal boycott and conspiracy on another level. The other illegal activities may have gone unnoticed, but its doubtful. It is more likely that this was the best that the chiropractic profession could achieve in this forum. The fact remains that the AMA conspired with other health-care groups, associations, and government agencies in a much broader sense than just not allowing doctors to associate with chiropractors. Anyone reading the documents or minutes of the meetings of the CCHI and Committee on

Quackery can clearly see that the AMA's conspiracy was more widespread than what was addressed in the final court order and injunction against the AMA in September 1987.

Some AMA observers feel that this opinion accomplished little, other than driving the AMA underground in its activities against the chiropractic profession and other alternative targets they fought so hard against all those years. It is very unlikely that the AMA would simply throw in the towel and walk away after this ruling by the courts. After having spent millions of dollars and hundreds of years of man hours fighting its real or imagined enemies in the alternative health-care movement, those involved are nothing if not determined.

The Court stated that the AMA's boycott and conspiracy ended with its revised version of the Principles of Medical Ethics, voted on and passed at the mid-June 1980 AMA Annual Meeting, which basically stated that medical physicians "shall be free to choose whom to serve, with whom to associate, and the environment in which to provide medical services."

This can hardly erase all of the years of AMA propaganda spewed at its members, not to mention the resultant prejudice against chiropractic acquired in medical schools. The court specifically stated that the injury to chiropractors' reputations which resulted from the boycott has not been repaired. Judge Getzendanner stated that, although the conspiracy ended in 1980, there are lingering effects of the illegal boycott and conspiracy.

Documents obtained in 1987 clearly show that just *after* the AMA's convention in June 1980 another plan was drawn up which was much more covert and ambitious than anything the Committee on Quackery or the CCHI ever thought up. In the last week of June 1980, a group of AMA doctors received a report entitled "The Chiropractic Dilemma." It was put together by the staff of an AMA state association. This, according to law, *is* in fact the AMA, because it is just one of many associations and societies that make up the AMA; what a state or county medical society does officially is the same thing as the AMA doing it, because the state and county medical societies *are* the AMA.

A memorandum was sent on June 25, 1980, from Donald C. McCallum, M.D., to the members of the Ad Hoc Committee on Liaison with the Health Related Professions, which was made up of six doctors who were members of the AMA. The report was requested by the Ad Hoc Committee on Chiropractic. The report stated, in part:

- Some chiropractors still cling to the original theory of Daniel David Palmer that misalignments of the vertebrae, or "subluxations" are the principle cause of disease.
- However, chiropractic stresses that mechanical disturbances of the nervous system are what impair the body's defenses.
- Many physicians continue to view practitioners of chiropractic with deep suspicion.
- Clearly the scope, quality and length of chiropractic education cannot provide the depth of diagnostic training a physician receives. Even more fundamental, however, is the validity of what the chiropractor learns. If its basis is unsound, more training might only compound the error.

The report clearly pointed to the inevitable conclusion that chiropractors were here to stay, despite the AMA's opposition to them over the years. In its final recommendations, the medical staff stated, "It would appear that the traditional opposition and tactics of the medical profession and others to limit the scope of chiropractic practice have failed." It further revealed that the new tactics included developing a campaign "that would educate the public. . ." They stated that this campaign "should be an ongoing and continuous one. . .It must be strongly emphasized to the practicing physician that he or she must assist the campaign with additional dollars and effort to educate patients in putting a halt to practices that can be harmful to health." The report in essence directed its campaign to educate the public of the harmful practices of chiropractic and how this would harm their health.

The heart of this report on chiropractic was disclosed in the final recommendations:

Since chiropractors are here to stay, an adjunctive alternative, revolutionary in concept, is to establish a membership category or section within the structure of the medical association for those chiropractors who are ethical. . .The profession could utilize the strengths of this section in dealing with the overall chiropractic dilemma. Thus, any campaign against chiropractic by the medical profession could not be interpreted as an effort by the profession to "corner the market" in health care delivery as often has been the case in chiropractic strategy. . .Perhaps then, the most viable option is to encourage the gradual. evolution of chiropractic to a "limited" medical profession. The most familiar examples are dentistry, podiatry, optometry, psychology, speech therapy, andrology,

etc. Unlike chiropractic, however, they do not challenge orthodox medical theories of disease and therapy. Hence, they
are able to co-exist with organized medicine.

In other words, because traditionally the chiropractic profession
has been opposed to medical theory and practice, and because
chiropractors have challenged orthodox medicine, and because orthodox medicine does not control chiropractic as it does other
branches of medicine, there was a need to create a group of
chiropractors who would act on behalf of their medical lords in a
campaign directed against chiropractic. In such a campaign, the
medical profession would hide behind the chiropractors they
selected to front the campaign for them, so that they could not be
accused of trying the corner the market in health care. This, according to their own words.

Ultimately what the AMA group wanted to do was to reduce
chiropractic and thus control it. They said:

> Chiropractors can function satisfactorily as "portals of
> entry" into the health care system without being the providers
> of total primary care that medical doctors are (and that some
> chiropractors claim to be). . .As a result, chiropractors have
> the potential for evolving into "limited" or "limited medical"
> practitioners even though many of them would deny
> it. . .Thus, the "limited" practice model could be the basis of
> accommodation between chiropractic and organized
> medicine.

This may all sound very reasonable. However, this is, in fact, a
further attempt to control, and thereby contain, the profession of
chiropractic. By reducing chiropractic to a role of limited practitioners in health-care, serving the public at the portal of entry into
the health-care system, this plan would make it the role of the
chiropractor to refer patients to doctors. It would not work the other
way around. It would be a one-way street. Such an arrangement
would also reduce the effectiveness of chiropractic as a preventive
measure in health care, which is one of its functions today. It would
also drastically reduce the number of chiropractors in the health-care
system, as well as the number of patients seeing chiropractors.

With medicine dictating the terms and definitions of what a
chiropractor could and could not do as a "limited practitioner," the
public would miss out on a wide variety of benefits offered by most
chiropractors. For example, in the case of a serious car accident, a

patient with neck and/or spine injuries could conceivably need to see a chiropractor more than 30 times. Possibly twice that over a two-year period to totally repair the injury. Under the definition of a "limited practitioner," most chiropractors would be limited to 12-20 adjustments per patient. (Such restrictions are currently imposed on chiropractic services under many insurance plans as a result of medical influence in the insurance industry.)

At about the same time as the birth of this illegal anti-competitive "revolutionary concept" of utilizing chiropractors to front a medical campaign directed against chiropractic, the National Association for Chiropractic Medicine (NACM) was formed. Was this just a coincidence? Nothing in the Articles of Incorporation of the NACM shows any direct link between this chiropractic group and the medical society's plan to use chiropractors to front an attack by the medical profession. There is, however, a long series of activities which parallel the anti-chiropractic campaign. There *are* direct connections between this group of chiropractors and the National Council Against Health Fraud, which has been vocal in attacking the alternatives, including chiropractic.

When the Pharmaceutical Advertising Council and FDA came out with their survey of alternatives (October 1984) they named chiropractic as one of the Big Three in the campaign. On July 30, 1984, a small group of minority chiropractors in Texas filed their corporation known as the National Association for Chiropractic Medicine. Article IV of that groups Articles of Incorporation stated that the general purposes and powers of the corporation included the following:

> Members of this Association have joined together to set a self-imposed professional standard for members of the Association. It is our purpose: 1. to restrict our practice of Chiropractic strictly to neuro-muscular-skeletal conditions in a manner consistent with the world body of scientific knowledge regarding health sciences, and, 2. through ongoing educational pursuits, to broaden our use of therapeutic agents useful within the scope of neuromuscular treatment, and 3. clarify legal recognition and responsibility of the practice of chiropractic medicine, unrestricted by any philosophical dogma or subluxation complex theory.

One of the key points that opponents and critics of chiropractic have used for years against chiropractors has been the contention that it is unscientific, since orthodox science does not recognize it as a valid approach to disease. Since organized medicine, and therefore organized science, opposes chiropractic theory, it is very unlikely that there would be a "world body of scientific knowledge regarding health science" that could be said to validate, or recognize, the "scientific" merits of chiropractic theory.

In its February 14, 1985, Position Paper on Chiropractic, the National Council Against Health Fraud touted the NACM as "a more progressive-minded group" whose views "are in harmony with science and consumer protection." The Position Paper then revealed the following about the NACM: "Using guidelines set forth by the NCAHF Task Force on Chiropractic, NACM has openly renounced the 'subluxation' theory and unscientific practices." The NCAHF goes on to further reveal that the NACM does not present itself as "an alternative health-care system to medical science." The paper stated that the NCAHF was asked by a chiropractor (unnamed) to form a Task Force on Chiropractic to describe what, in the view of the NCAHF, would "constitute acceptable chiropractic practices." The Task Force was mostly comprised of chiropractors who share NCAHF's beliefs in science and consumer protection. The following further outlines the NCAHF's position on acceptable chiropractic practices:

1. Advance only methods of diagnosis and treatment which have a scientific basis.
2. Openly disclaim the non-scientific "subluxation" theory.
3. Restrict the scope of practice to neuro-musculo-skeletal problems loosely defined as Type M conditions [ie: muscle spasms, strains, sprains, fatigue, imbalance of strength and flexibility, stretched or irritated nerve tissue and so forth], recognizing that some Type M problems will fall outside the scope of even a scientific chiropractor.
4. Work closely with medical practitioners consulting with them on cases involving possible pathology and readily referring when reasonable and prudent.
5. Use conservative methods of manipulative therapy.
6. Avoid exposing patients to unnecessary radiation.
7. Work to increase public awareness about abuses by non-scientific chiropractors.
8. Help other chiropractors become more scientific in their approaches to health care delivery.
9. Work to prohibit unqualified practitioners of all kinds from performing manipulation.
10. Aid in the prosecution of alleged malpractice.

The NCAHF Position Paper goes on to explain what a scientific chiropractor will *not* be or do. One of the points they made under this heading was the following:

A scientific chiropractor will not. . . utilize unproven, disproven or questionable methods, devices and products such as adjusting machines or instruments, applied kinesiology, chelation therapy, colonic irrigation, computerized nutrition deficiency tests, cranial osteopathy, cytotoxic food allergy testing, DMSO, gerovital, glandular therapy, hair analysis, herbology, herbal crystallization analysis, homeopathy, internal managements, iridology, laser beam acupuncture, laetrile, magnetic therapy, Moire contourographic analysis, Neutrothermograph, orthomolecular therapy, pendulum divination, pyramid power, "Reams" test, reflexology, sclaraglyphics, spinal column stressology, Thermography, Thermoscribe, Toftness device, and so forth.

The NCAHF Position Paper on Chiropractic did not spell out exactly what NCAHF's relationship with the NACM is and what role it had in preparing this Position Paper. Who exactly was the chiropractor who came to the NCAHF and asked them to look into chiropractic to determine what were acceptable chiropractic practices? A deposition taken in Akron, Ohio, from the Secretary of the NACM involving an insurance case in Michigan obtained the following information, which is most revealing. The deposition picks up a line of questioning of Charles DuVall regarding the NCAHF's Position Paper on Chiropractic. The questioner, Ms. Tyner, was the attorney for a chiropractor whose insurance claim came into question. Charles DuVall was a consultant for an insurance company denying the chiropractor's claim, in part as a result of DuVall's opinions.

Ms. Tyner: "I have something attached, the Position Paper that you referenced early in your deposition. There is this, that physician paper that you're referring to?"
DuVall: "Yes."
Ms. Tyner: "And I assume you got the positions contained in this paper?"
DuVall: "Yes."
Ms. Tyner: "Did you prepare it or assist in its preparation?"
DuVall: "I assisted in its preparation."

This leaves little doubt as to why the NACM's position on chiropractic is so similar to the NCAHF's Position Paper on Chiropractic. The Secretary of the NACM helped prepare the NCAHF's position on chiropractic. The NCAHF states that the NACM has adopted the NCAHF's position on chiropractic.

The President of the NCAHF, William Jarvis, has stated that, in his opinion, "Chiropractic per se is nonsense." ("Patients Who Seek Unorthodox Medical Treatment," *Minnesota Medicine,* June 1990.) The NCAHF has been attacking chiropractic for years. In its May 1986 list of Available Resource Materials, it listed pamphlets, booklets, and articles on many different subjects dealing with alternative treatments, modalities, products, services, professions, and so on. Under "Chiropractic" it listed the following materials:

- "Chiropractic: How Much Healing," *Brown-Quad City Times* 1-36, 12/31/81. . .
- "Chiropractic Inching Ahead," Dr. Stephen Barrett, Private Practice, 5/82. . .
- "Chiropractors Knocking at Your Door," Dr. Stephen Barrett, Private Practice, 5/80. . .
- "Malpractice Inevitable Result of Chiropractic," Phil & Training Mode, LAMP 20-3, 2/79. . .
- "NCAHF Position Paper on Chiropractic," 2/85. . .
- "Rational Chiropractic Practice," Charles DuVall, OCCUP.
- Medicine & Legal Source Book, 21-32, 9/85.

The NCAHF's position against certain chiropractic practices is well known. What wasn't well known, and was kept from the public's eye, was exactly what role Charles DuVall played in putting this Position Paper together with William Jarvis or the NCAHF's Task Force on Chiropractic. Here we see one of the nation's most outspoken critics of chiropractic, whose statements are considered "expert opinion," linked up to this the new breed of chiropractor. They are working together to influence the insurance industry, bringing them more in line with what they consider is proper and "acceptable chiropractic practice."

The NCAHF Position Paper explains just how the Council feels about chiropractic overall: "NCAHF believes that a health care delivery system as confused and poorly regulated as is chiropractic constitutes a major consumer health problem." But even the NCAHF admits that all 50 states have licensing boards that regulate chiropractors. Perhaps it is felt that they should be regulated by

AMA doctors? In keeping with the old AMA party line, the NCAHF denounced chiropractic theory as "unscientific" and stated that "most chiropractors have not been taught to practice on the basis of the same body of knowledge about health and disease recognized by health scientists around the world."

That is no secret. Chiropractors are not trained in surgery, disease control and diagnosis, pharmacology, and other orthodox approaches to health care. The majority of their training does address 60% of what the body is made up of, which is the musculo-skeletal system. No chiropractor would ever say that he or she has the same education as a medical doctor. However, they take many of the same basic classes as medical doctors do with regard to the human body.

The NCAHF makes certain recommendations in its Position Paper which include recommendations to the insurance industry, legislators, consumers, basic scientists, educators, attorneys, law enforcement agencies, and medical doctors and "other scientific health care providers." To insurance carriers and third-party payers, it recommended:

1. Limit reimbursements to medically necessary services and to those practitioners who provide appropriate medical documentation that establishes the diagnosis and justifies the treatment.
2. Establish an independent commission financed by an insurance industry levy to investigate and curtail fraud and abuse in health care.

The insurance industry did just that in September 1985, just seven months later. This is the National Health Care Anti-Fraud Association (NHCAA). (See Chapter 7.)

The legality of the NCAHF's position on chiropractic may all be in question. The judge in *Wilk v. AMA* stated very clearly that what the AMA was saying to its members amounted to an illegal boycott and conspiracy to "eliminate chiropractic."The most important aspect of that case was the fact that the court recognized that the AMA had continually tried to hide behind its defense that it was concerned "for scientific methods in patient care" regarding chiropractic. The AMA's position, over and over, has been that chiropractic was "unscientific," but the Court struck this defense down and went so far as to conclude on the basis of "extensive testimony from both witnesses for the plaintiffs and the AMA that some forms of chiropractic treatment are effective."

If the Court determined that the AMA's conduct amounted to a boycott and conspiracy designed to "contain and ultimately, eliminate chiropractic," we can conclude that similar conduct by anyone else would also be a conspiracy to restrain and/or eliminate chiropractic. Whether that conduct includes denouncing chiropractic as "unscientific," or trying to eliminate certain practices, treatments, modalities, or chiropractic devices from being paid for by insurance companies, it is still a form of boycott and conspiracy. It certainly seems to qualify as a conspiracy in light of the connections between the NACM and the NCAHF and their position on encouraging insurance companies to refuse payment for certain chiropractic services, or to restrict the number of visits that they should pay for.

NACM'S Position on Chiropractic

On March 3, 1984, Charles E. DuVall, D.C., issued a Fact Sheet on Spinal Manipulation Therapy (SMT), which stated:

SMT is effective on a temporary basis, providing pain relief for a few minutes to several years. SMT does *not* permanently correct a joint dysfunction.

SMT is known to be addictive.

SMT is known to increase symptoms when used excessively and extensively.

SMT is *not* an innocuous procedure. There are many referenced cases of death, paralysis, rupture of intervertebral discs, etc., when performed incompetently, or when inaccurate diagnosis is concluded.

Some of this flies in the face of what many chiropractors employ in their practices. In addition to the these statements about basic chiropractic theory and practice, DuVall published a list of proposed NACM Advisory Board members for his new organization and their creditials:

Stephen Barrett, M.D.
Dr. Barrett is a psychiatrist and nationally recognized author, editor and consumer advocate. He is very knowledgeable about chiropractic, law, public relations, and political strategy. He is highly respected by the medical profession and *has excellent connections with the press and the insurance industry.* [Emphasis added.] Although reputed to be chiropractic's worst critic (James Parker has called him "the

chiropractic headhunter"), he is very supportive of NACM and has many ideas for our growth and development.

Michael Botts, Esq.

Mr. Botts is a former assistant state attorney general (Iowa) who worked in consumer protection division and was a member of the division's health fraud task force. [*Note*: What they didn't say about Mr. Botts is that he is also the legal counsel for the National Council Against Health Fraud.]

Stephen M. Levin, M.D.

Dr. Levin is an orthopedist who uses manipulation and has been active teaching chiropractors.

William T. Jarvis, Ph.D.

Dr. Jarvis is professor of health education at Loma Linda University and president of the 2,100-member National Council Against Health Fraud, with which NACM is an affiliate group. Dr. Jarvis wrote his doctoral thesis on chiropractic. He is very knowledgeable on this subject and is highly supportive of NACM.

Grace P. Monaco, J.D.

Mrs. Monaco is an attorney who specializes in health law and has many insurance industry connections.

Merlin Nelson, Ph.D.

Dr. Nelson, a pharmacist, teaches at Wayne State University School of Pharmacology and is president of the Michigan Council Against Health Fraud.

John H. Renner, M.D.

Dr. Renner is an official of the American Academy of Family Practice and is director of medical development at St. Mary's Hospital in Kansas City, Missouri. He is one of the country's top medical educators and is highly experienced in conducting educational programs and meetings. He writes columns for his local newspaper and a nationally circulated newsletter. He is also president of the Kansas City Committee on Health and Nutritional Fraud and Abuse and directs the Resource Center for the National Council Against Health Fraud. He can organize courses in diagnosis to help chiropractors avoid trouble.

If that line-up of Advisory Board members isn't slanted against chiropractic, then nothing is. Of the seven people named, five are known members of the NCAHF and four have worked with the PAC/FDA campaign from 1983 to the present.

The By-Laws of the NACM state the following:

Members agree to formulate and adopt a basic code of ethics as follows:

A. Base their practices on the knowledge accumulated by the world body of science. Toward this end, we acknowledge that we do not accept: a) D.D. Palmer's concepts of "sub-luxation," or other supposed spinal problems as "the cause" or a major cause of disease; and b) that chiropractors prevent or cure disease by the restoration of "nerve energy."

B. Restrict their scope of practice to neuromusculoskeletal conditions; to emphasize joint manipulation therapy, but to include all forms of orthodox therapy permitted by state and federal law.

C. Restrict their practice to treatment modalities which have been scientifically demonstrated to alleviate neuromusculoskeletal disorders.

D. Work closely with other licensed health professionals for the best interest of the patient both diagnostically and therapeutically; we acknowledge that chiropractic is not an alternative health system to medicine, but is allied therewith.

E. Work diligently with all licensed health professionals to establish safeguards and contraindications for manipulative procedure by unskilled persons.

F. Accept as a primary responsibility the upgrading of this Association through collaboration with scientists in education, research and development.

G. Establish and abide by a strict code of ethics that forbids unnecessary or excessive treatment.

H. Establish and abide by a strict code of ethics in advertising.

I. Rebuke practitioners who extol or utilize unscientific or unethical methods.

J. Inform the public of the standards and goals of this Association.

K. To rebuke overt commercialization and unscrupulous practice management schemes.

L. To establish peer review guidelines relating to third party payors.

Some of these points were repeated in the NCAHF's Position Paper on Chiropractic, so it is no wonder that the NCAHF touted this new "reform-minded" chiropractic group in that paper. The NACM also listed the benefits of membership with its association. There are said to be four ways that NACM "members can increase their income as a result of NACM's activities":

Personal Injury Evaluation
Attorneys and insurance companies can refer cases for independent chiropractic evaluations in personal injury cases.

Malpractice Evaluations and Expert Testimony
Attorneys can refer cases for evaluation of possible chiropractic malpractice.

Insurance Review
Insurance companies can refer cases for review of the appropriateness of treatment.

New Patients
NACM members can expect to attract new patients as the benefits of scientific chiropractic are explained to the public and to health professionals.

The NACM didn't incorporate until July 1984, and Charles Du-Vall, Jr., was not listed as one of the original officers of the NACM. He was listed as its Secretary sometime thereafter, and his father (now deceased) was listed as the Executive Director of NACM.

It's worth noting that the October Plan (See Chapter 5) was originally presented in October 1986 as a Proposal for Funding for the Public Issues in Health Care Choices Project of the Ohio Council Against Health Fraud. As it turns out, the Ohio Council Against Health Fraud was not even incorporated until April 17, 1987. That means they were already doing business using that name in October 1986 when they came up with the October Plan.

Inspection of the Ohio Council Against Health Fraud incorporation papers revealed the following Purpose or Purposes of this Corporation:

. . .Further, to engage in any lawful act or activities for which corporations may be formed (under Ohio Codes), including but not necessarily limited to the purpose of health consumer protection, combatting health fraud and misinformation, and conducting such other activities as are supplemental or incidental thereto, and are not in conflict with the purposes set forth in Section A. [Section A outlined its purpose as an IRS Tax Exempt organization under 501 (c).]. . .Activities related to health fraud include monitoring the information on health care publications and activities for acts that include the potential for insurance fraud or abuse. Information regarding such activities will be shared with state, federal, private and public agencies and consumer organizations involved in the detection, prevention or remidation [sic] of fraudulent insurance acts.

The Ohio Council Against Health Fraud apparently masterminded the October Plan to put together a study (the Emprise study) of the alternatives, apparently with the foreknowledge that such a study would not approve alternatives, nor find them safe or effective. The Council Against Health Fraud, the National office and all of their affiliates, chapters, and officials have worked endlessly to fight what they label "quackery" or "health fraud." They have worked to influence the public and private sector and the insurance industry against the alternatives, including chiropractic. They have worked to prosecute people in the alternatives and put them in jail. It is fairly certain that anyone involved with these groups is not a friend of chiropractic, or anything else in the alternative health care system.

Who then comprise the Ohio Council Against Health Fraud? The following names are listed in the Articles of Incorporation as the original incorporators of this anti-chiropractic, anti-alternative group:

William London, 1346 Stratford Drive, Kent, Ohio 44240
Charles E. DuVall, Sr., 2311 East Avenue, Akron, Ohio 44314
Charles E. DuVall, Jr., 2311 East Avenue, Akron, Ohio 44314

On one hand we have the National Association for Chiropractic Medicine, with Charles DuVall, Jr., as its secretary and his father the executive director, and on the other hand we see that he and his father are two of the three founders of the Ohio Council Against Health Fraud. We also see that the NACM is an affiliate group of the National Council Against Health Fraud. DuVall helped write the NCAHF's Position Paper on Chiropractic. The NACM has the color of a front group for the anti-competitive-type of activity that the NCAHF has been involved in over the years. It also appears that the NACM is exactly the type of group of chiropractors that the medical establishment had in mind to front a campaign against chiropractic.

NACM claims that among the benefits of membership is a means to increase a members' income by getting involved in insurance issues as paid consultants. It also highlights the fact that Advisory Board members of the NACM have either influence or connections in the insurance industry. These connections and influence in the insurance industry, by way of NCAHF officials, no doubt should open the door for any member of the NACM to act as a consultant in the insurance industry. These "ins" are claimed to exist in both private and governmental insurance programs. Could this adversely influence the insurance industry against chiropractic services now used?

Apparently the statements made by the NACM about the benefits of being a member were designed not only to attract new members, but to also make themselves financially attractive to the insurance industry. A goal such as "Establish and abide by a strict code of ethics that forbids unnecessary or excessive treatments" would most certainly attract the attention of the insurance industry, which is desperate financial trouble and is always looking for ways to cut corners.

It would certainly appear from this data that NACM promoted the connections into the insurance industry so as to get a foothold in that area. This seems to have been in order to make money and at the same time forward the mission of the anti-quackery campaign being directed against chiropractic and others. Should any of the members of the NACM manage to get involved in reimbursement and payment policy issues within the insurance industry, there could be no doubt that the remaining body of chiropractic would suffer economically.

It is not entirely clear whether or not the National Association for Chiropractic Medicine is one and the same as the "front" planned by the AMA group. What *is* clear is that this group has contributed to the economic downfall of chiropractic within the insurance industry. This is exactly what the medical campaign against chiropractic apparently postulated when planning to reduce chiropractors to being "limited providers" of health care, and this is the intention of the AMA's Committee on Quackery, the Coordinating Conference on Health Information, and the current campaign financed and cosponsored by the pharmaceutical industry, which has also influenced the National Health Care Anti-Fraud Association (NHCAA) and its health insurance company members, all 350 of them.

Medicare and the NACM'S Adverse Influence

In May 1986, the Office of the Inspector General of the Department of Health and Human Services, Richard P. Kusserow, issued a report entitled "Inspection of Chiropractic Services Under Medicare." It was prepared by the office of Analysis and Inspections in Chicago. The report stated that an Inspection was conducted from January through May 1985 on chiropractic services as provided for under Medicare. The inspection had among its four objectives: "To develop an understanding of chiropractic as a profession as seen by its practitioners, schools and associations, as well as representatives of mainstream medicine."

This "understanding of chiropractic" included discussion with 28 medical societies—and only 15 chiropractic associations. The inspection report stated that at one chiropractic college an official said that "subluxations are a minor part of chiropractic practice." The report goes on to state that "the term itself (*subluxation*) is out-of-date." In its final recommendations, the report stated that a legislative proposal to Congress should be considered; that proposal would include:

> Continue to limit Medicare coverage of chiropractic services to manual manipulation of the spine to correct a subluxation demonstrated by x-ray to exist. . .Cap the number of services for which a patient could receive payment at 12 per year. All covered services over 12 visits would be automatically denied. ($23.9 million savings in FY [Fiscal Year] 1987).

With regard to the "scientific validity" of chiropractic the report stated:

> Increased access to research funding by chiropractic colleges would provide one point of mutual interaction between chiropractors and other health professionals, and would serve to enhance the position of those segments of the profession that seek to improve the quality of chiropractic education and who would work to limit the use of questionable diagnostic and therapeutic techniques used by some chiropractors.

The report also gave some background on Medicare's history with chiropractic services. It stated that chiropractic was officially

included for coverage under the Social Security Act Part B, passed
in 1972. The report stated that:

> There was considerable controversy surrounding the pas-
> sage of this legislation which was adopted despite the recom-
> mendations and concerns about chiropractic as a form of
> treatment contained in the 1968 HEW Report, "Independent
> Practitioners Under Medicare." Almost every mainstream
> medical group also formally opposed passage.

It is ironic that this 1986 OIG Inspection report on chiropractic
would make reference to this 1968 HEW Report, which we now
know was totally influenced (via the Stanford study), financed, and
directed by the AMA. It is ironic because this 1986 report was also
adversely influenced in its final recommendations by another source
outside of government.

Prior to this report the Medicare Program was paying for up to 20
visits per year for chiropractic services. It currently pays only 12
visits a year per patient. The following passage from the report under
the heading "The Problem Side of Chiropractic" sheds light on this
change:

> During the study, discussions were held with reform-
> minded chiropractors who are in the process of forming a
> separate professional group of practitioners, the National As-
> sociation of Chiropractic Medicine, that would set strict stand-
> ards of ethical conduct and practice, and would actively work
> in cooperation with consumer groups and others to expose and
> rid the profession of questionable activities. . .The Department
> (HHS) should examine the ways in which it can further en-
> courage the submission of scientific research proposals by
> chiropractic colleges, which meet the standards applied to
> other projects supported by the National Institutes of Health.

This report touched on several things which the NACM and the
NCAHF have been saying about chiropractic and which, if followed,
would restrict the scope of practice of the profession of chiropractic.
The recommendations for limiting the number of visits to 12 per year
per patient is very restrictive of chiropractic, and definitely has
potential to have an anti-competitive effect and an adverse economic
impact on the majority of chiropractors in this country. The question
remains—was this by design?

Other Areas of Influence in Insurance

On April 5, 1988, Charles E. DuVall, Jr., conducted a training seminar for executives of Intracorp, a national company that supplies a billing review service for insurance-client companies. The seminar was called "How to Evaluate a Chiropractic Claim." Among the points of his seminar were two items entitled "Bad Backs/Big Bucks" and "Practice Promotion Programs Techniques." Both of these items were highlighted in the HHS Inspection Report on Chiropractic Services. Big Bucks was clearly an issue in the Inspection Report; the report made a big point about saving $23.9 million in one year by cutting chiropractic services to 12 per year, per patient. The Report also held up, as an example of how chiropractors are a problem, certain "patterns of activity and practice which at best appear as overly-aggressive marketing." The report included as examples of problem situations "practice-building courses." This example came directly after the paragraph above it mentioned the discussions that were held with the NACM.

The Intracorp seminar took a similar direction, with Charles DuVall, Jr., recommending to the executives that the following points should be looked for in chiropractic claims as are signs that a claim should be either denied or challenged:

- Treatment lasting longer than eight weeks
- Extended time lapse between trauma and initial treatment
- More than two modalities per visit
- Repeated or duplicate x-rays
- X-rays of unrelated areas
- Simultaneous treatment by a physician with a chiropractor
- Maintenance care
- Frequent comprehensive exams
- Redundant therapies
- Treatment appears unrelated to injury
- Moire Contourographic Analysis (Topography)
- Hair analysis, toxic metal analysis
- Thermoscribe, Thermodeltometer, Neurothermography
- Trigger point therapy
- Meridian therapy
- Accupressure
- Kinesiology, Muscle testing
- Activator
- Intensive day care, detentive day care
- Nutritional supplements

- Plethysmography
- Acupuncture
- Thermography

In addition, DuVall stated, "Any treatment of children (infant to 12 years) must be documented and medically necessary. Ask immediately for Doctor's records." In another instance of "promoting scientific chiropractic" he states, "If there is any question concerning *any* test, treatment, or procedure—immediately ask for scientific documentation and Doctor's records." In still another recommendation, which would further restrict a chiropractor's practice, he stated, "If the patient has been under treatment for extended period of time, i.e., 4-6 months, immediately ask for Doctor's records."

It is common knowledge that many chiropractic patients must see their chiropractors over an extended period of time for more serious injuries. According to DuVall this should be challenged, as it is a way for the insurance company to save Big Bucks. It is also in line with the NACM's position on what is "accepted chiropractic care" as well as in alignment with the NCAHF's Position Paper on Chiropractic.

During Charles DuVall's deposition in the insurance claim case, he was asked about the course he gave at Intracorp and his feeling about chiropractic SMT. The following is from that deposition:

Q: "Is it your feeling that spinal manipulative therapy, which you've referred to here at S.M.T., is a placebo?"
A: "It may be used as a placebo, yes."

Here we have a chiropractor, advising the insurance industry, who feels that SMT may be used as a placebo. He even stated that this was the case in 30%-40% of the cases that he reviews. Such an opinion must have caused many chiropractors to have been refused valid claims.

DuVall also included in his training seminar a section called "Facts on Spinal Manipulative Therapy (SMT)." He also presented these "facts" to the Ohio Association of Civil Trial Attorneys in Columbus, Ohio, on April 14, 1984. Making his views and positions known to the insurance industry and civil trial lawyers would surely improve the possibility of his being able to increase his income at the expense of thousands of other mainstream chiropractors. All of this, of course, is in line with the NACM's benefits for members. It is important to note here that chiropractors who set themselves up with an insurance company or third party payor as "chiropractic consult-ants" can make a lot of money. How this works is simple. The chiropractor consultant reviews claims coming in from chiroprac-tors. These consultants get paid so much for each claim. In some cases consultants even get a bonus for saving the insurance company money by denying claims.

There was a case in the Midwest of one chiropractor earning over $300,000 a year doing insurance reviews for an insurance company. It turned out that this chiropractor spent only 5-10 minutes on each case. He would make his recommended cuts and proceed quickly to the next case. He got $35-$50 per case. It would take a lot of case reviews at that rate to earn more than $300,000 in one year. A chiropractor who is consulting several companies at the same time, or sets up a "Peer Review" company for insurance claims, could make millions each year.

Combine that with receiving expert-witness fees from attorneys in insurance cases, or civil cases, or malpractice suits. That chiropractor could make a very nice living—at the expense of other chiropractors. This happens every day, and it is this means of earning extra income that the NACM promotes to new members. Using the connections mentioned in tandem with the NCAHF officials in the insurance industry certainly couldn't hurt either.

Making money from denying claims from other chiropractors is like acting as a henchman for the insurance industry. This only contributes to the further erosion of the chiropractic profession. For example, if one recommends arbitrarily that chiropractors get paid for only 12 visits per year, per patient, then the chiropractic profes-sion is losing future income. The worst thing about this is that the insurance company is not taking into account that this cap ultimately will cost them more. If patients are cut off at 12 visits, and they still have pain, then they will be forced to go elsewhere for less effective and more costly continued medical service. This would mean going to a medical doctor who might perform surgery or prescribe drugs on a month-to-month basis to handle the patient's pain. Because drugs do not address the cause of the pain, but only temporarily suppress the pain, the pain will persist and the problem may never get handled. This approach sells a lot of drugs, but doesn't really handle the problem for the patient or the insurance company. The insurance industry is being rather short-sighted in this regard. It is a fact that chiropractic services can *save* insurance companies money, not cost them more.

The insurance industry is not doing itself any favors by getting some "yes-men" as chiropractic consultants to deny claims and reassure the insurance industry that they are saving millions of dollars in claims. The insurance industry may itself become totally dependent on the opinions of these so-called experts. Why would the insurance industry do this, if they're really interested in saving dollars?

One must understand that within any given insurance company is a Medical Director—almost always a medical doctor—who is in charge of setting reimbursement policy for that insurance company. One has a medical doctor dictating to the insurance company what it should or should not pay for with regard to chiropractic services and other matters related to the alternatives. On top of that, these companies employ chiropractors to review chiropractic claims, but the chiropractors they hire are almost always in agreement with the medical doctors when it comes to cutting chiropractic services. A chiropractor who takes a position reviewing claims for an insurance company and does not cut claims, or allows certain "questionable" claims to be paid, does not last very long in that company.

Because the system is set up the way it is, many chiropractors have not bothered to deliver chiropractic services to people coming to them with Medicare or Medicaid. This of course just compounds the problem. No practitioner should allow "red tape" to dissuade him or her. There are ways, which will be discussed in Part Three, Solutions to the Problems, for denied chiropractors to challenge this system. It may be vital to the survival of the profession to do so.

Chiropractic Cuts in Payment Based on AMA Policy

Among the many items that Charles DuVall, D.C. listed that insurance companies should not pay for is something called thermography. Thermography is simply a means to an end. It involves a device which locates and shows the operator of the machine where an injury may be by indicating heat spots or hot spots. It is commonly agreed that where there is an injury along the spine there will be heat in and around that injured area. Identifying hot spots helps pinpoint the exact place that the chiropractor needs to adjust in order to alleviate the pain and correct the problem. There is even a national accreditation thermography school set up for training and certifying chiropractors to use the equipment in their practice. There are chiropractic colleges that have courses in thermography as well.

Mr. DuVall recommends that insurance companies not pay for this. His groups, the National Association for Chiropractic Medicine and the National Council Against Health Fraud, are also against thermography. As a matter of fact, DuVall feels about the whole of chiropractic much the way his colleagues in the NCAHF feel about it. His testimony in the Michigan insurance claim case included the following:

> Q: Is it fair to say that you feel chiropractic lacks a scientific base?"
>
> A: "That is true."
>
> Q: "The entire profession, then; is that correct?"
>
> A: "Chiropractic lacks a scientific base."
>
> Q: "And that would include everything encompassed within the profession? The practice of chiropractic, itself, has no scientific base?"
>
> A: "That's true."
>
> Q: "Is it your feelings, Doctor, that chiropractic is full of quackery?"
>
> A: "Yes, it is."

As in any medical specialty, chiropractors have a board in each state which oversees the licensed professionals. Should a chiropractor be found to be practicing outside his scope of practice, as outlined by chiropractic laws in each state, that board can call that chiropractor up on charges. The board can then either fine, revoke, suspend, or in other ways discipline that chiropractor. This type of peer review is designed to weed out incompetent practitioners. It works well as a system. However, DuVall is not in agreement with this system as it relates to chiropractors:

> Q: "And you would agree, would you not, that a board of— a state board of chiropractic, a state licensing board is not the proper means in which to define the scope of practice?"
>
> A: "That is correct."

DuVall is wrong on this point. The scope of practice of chiropractic is determined by laws, which are usually designed by the majority of chiropractic representation in each state. Should a law state that thermography, or nutritional counseling is acceptable, then that is the law. Should the laws state otherwise, the chiropractors in that state have to abide by the law. It is just that simple.

The litigation which included this testimony centered around a chiropractic claim involving the use of thermography, on which DuVall was employed as insurance consultant. He denied payment for the treatment, and when he was asked about this directly he responded as follows:

A: "Yes, the treatment parameters are excessive and have not been justified with appropriate medical documentation."

Q: "You do not feel that thermography should have been used in a treatment mode?"

A: "Thermography is not used in a treatment mode. It is a diagnostic tool and it is not scientifically validated for the treatment of neuromusculoskeletal problems."

Q: "Is it your opinion that it was used in the treatment?"

A: "It was apparently used as a diagnostic mode."

Q: "I thought you said there was no diagnosis?"

A: "Well, all I know is they may have run a neurothermograph, or whatever it is, which is supposed to detect subluxation; it is not a scientifically valid scientific instrument."

Q: "Doctor, I want to be clear: Are you saying that you don't know what thermography was used for in this file?"

A: "That's correct."

Here we have an "expert" working for an insurance company, making determinations on what should be paid for and what shouldn't be paid. He didn't even know what thermography was being used for in the case he was supposed to be evaluating for payment. He says that it was used for diagnostic purposes, yet he explains that it is "not scientifically validated for treatment." Then he goes on to say that it was used as a diagnostic mode. When asked specifically why he felt that thermography should not even be used as a diagnostic tool, and on what particular scientific study he was basing his opinions, he stated:

A: "The one by John McCulla."

Q: "Any particular work done by McCulla?"

A: "The work that he did in about 1908, I believe but there have been others that—and I don't remember their names offhand, Counselor, that have not confirmed the use of thermography for neuromusculoskeletal conditions."

DuVall was basing his opinion, in part, on a study that is almost 90 years old. Additionally, DuVall revealed the fact that he didn't feel that instruction on thermography taught to chiropractors by the American Chiropractic College of Thermography was adequate. He stated:

Q: "Are you familiar with the American Chiropractic College of Thermography?"

A: "Yes, Ma'am, I am."

Q: "And, you don't consider that to be adequate instruction on the use of thermography?"

A: "No, Ma'am."

Q: "And, again, that is because you haven't been presented with what you say are any scientific or clinical studies; is that correct?"

A: "That's correct."

Q: "So no matter what they instructed, in your opinion, that would not be?"

A: "That's correct."

The deposition gets down to DuVall's opinions about thermography:

Q: "Are you relying on the A.M.A. report?"

A: "I am aware of the A.M.A.'s position, yes, ma'am."

Q: "Was that part of your basis for your opinion?"

A: "Yes, Ma'am."

Q: "Do you consider that A.M.A. to have adopted or rejected the report, Scientific Affairs?"

A: "Yes, Ma'am, I would accept that."

Q: "What would you accept?"

A: "That, their report from the Committee on Scientific Affairs."

Q: "The report on the Committee of Scientific Affairs endorsed thermography; did it not?"

A: "And then they rejected it."

Q: "The House of Delegates did not endorse and did not reject the report from the Scientific Affairs Committee; is that correct?"

A: "That is correct."

Q: "And you interpret that to mean that they rejected it?"

A: "Yes, Ma'am."

Q. "Is it not a more accurate characterization that they didn't state a position one way or the other?"

THE ASSAULT ON MEDICAL FREEDOM

A: "If one chooses to take that [position]."

He was also asked more about his knowledge of thermography and the training that a chiropractor goes through:

Q: "Are you familiar with the Thermographic Society?"
A: "Yes, Ma'am, I am."
Q: "Are you familiar with the course taught by Clinical Ther-mography Associates, focusing on thermography?"
A: "I am aware of the Association."
Q: "Are you familiar with the course that I have just given you?"
A: "No, I am not."
Q: "Are you aware of the fact or not aware of the fact that there is a course taught on thermography by Clinical Thermog-raphy Associates."
A: "There may be."

Overall, DuVall's answers appeared to be evasive and misleading as well as self-serving with regard to the AMA's position on ther-mography. In addition, he also demonstrated a clear lack of knowledge about thermography and training courses on thermog-raphy. The bottom line with regard to his opinion about thermog-raphy was that he would not approve it for payment in an insurance claim. This was not based on anything other than his opinion and some studies that he selected to use as his basis for scientific opinion. It was certainly not based on his personal investigation:

Q: "What do you mean by that, your personal observations?"
A: "Personal observations and also the training that it provided as to a chiropractic in accredited colleges of chiropractic."
Q: "By that, you have personally used thermography and found it not to be scientifically valid; is that what you're saying?"
A: "No, it is not taught as a diagnostic procedure in the chiropractic colleges, today."

Here we have an insurance consultant making decisions on chiropractic insurance claims who:

1. Bases his opinions about thermography in part on a 1908 study.

2. Is not familiar with courses that are taught on the subject, and has never taken such a course.

3. Is aware that the AMA Committee for Scientific Affairs wrote a report that did in fact validate thermography but dismisses that report because it was not endorsed by the political body of the AMA.

4. Does not consider that thermography is taught at a chiropractic college as a valid reason to use it in practice.

5. Has never personally used thermography.

6. Has admitted in sworn testimony that he didn't even know how thermography was being used in the case that he was reviewing as a consultant.

Later in the deposition, DuVall explained a little about why he considers chiropractic quackery when he stated:

> The problem in chiropractic is its promotion. Chiropractic is an adjective and it means by the hands. And chiropractic has been used as a fence. Behind this fence is a promotion in which chiropractors are stating that they may treat problems that have no relation, whatsoever. . .Chiropractors continue to absorb the subluxation theory of D.D. Palmer, that is gospel and that the promotion from within chiropractic is unbelievable.

This position is, of course, totally aligned with the National Council Against Health Fraud's Position Paper on Chiropractic, as well as the position of the National Association for Chiropractic Medicine. It is the very basis of the attack against chiropractic that the A.M.A. attempted unsuccessfully to use in its defense in *Wilk v. A.M.A.*

This chiropractic insurance consultant's opinion about chiropractic is not an isolated case. There are many such "experts" with with these opinions who consult the insurance industry on a daily basis on issues of payment and reimbursement to chiropractors. There are many consultants who are also members of the National Association for Chiropractic Medicine and who are forwarding the anti-chiropractic party-line in the insurance industry. And they're well rewarded financially for their efforts. It is little wonder that chiropractors are hanging onto their practices by the skin of their teeth in many cases.

The adverse influence that members of the National Council Against Health Fraud and the National Association for Chiropractic

Medicine have had on the insurance industry is quite evident. The insurance industry has been losing billions of dollars each year in covering health-care costs created by inflated medical charges for surgery/operations, unnecessary medical testing, over-priced medical equipment and devices, over-prescribed drugs, and outrageous medical doctor fees. With medical doctors acting as policymakers within the insurance industry, it is not surprising that they have been cutting chiropractic services.

The insurance industry is desperately seeking a way out of its financial crisis. Under the guise of cost-containment programs, utilization review, peer review, and outside independent insurance consultants, the insurance industry is looking for ways to save money. It is apparent that the economic competitors of chiropractic have taken advantage of the insurance industry's crisis to help, direct, instruct, consult, recommend, advise, and otherwise influence the insurance industry to reject chiropractic claims and to restructure their payment and reimbursement policies to exclude these targeted treatments, modalities, services, products, and devices used in chiropractic.

The National Health Care Anti-Fraud Association must have greeted these "health fraud and quackery experts" with open arms. The stated goals and purposes of the NHCAA are very similar to those of the National Council Against Health Fraud and the National Association for Chiropractic Medicine: to improve the prevention, detection, and civil and criminal prosecution of health care fraud and to assist law enforcement agencies to prosecute health care fraud.

The influence of these anti-"quackery" anti-"health fraud" entities on the insurance industry has resulted in low payments, slow payments, or no payments for many chiropractic services. Such influence on the insurance industry is further evidence that the October Plan has, in fact, been carried out. DuVall's original plan in part, was to provide data on coverage as well as to provide information on "potential insurance fraud." It would appear that this October Plan is moving forward.

A good example of how NHCAA members have impacted chiropractic is the case of Dr. Paul Jondle, D.C., of Massachusetts. His insurance claims were being denied and he came under heavy attack by the Chiropractic Board of Examiners. Investigation determined that the board chairman overseeing his case was not only an "independent" insurance consultant with Aetna (which was denying Dr. Jondle's claims), but was also a member of the NHCAA. Other NHCAA insurance company members were also denying Dr. Jondle payment for his services. Such activity can really only be categorized as truly anti-competitive in nature.

Anti-Chiropractic Campaign in Review

1963-1975. The AMA carries out a campaign against chiropractic through its Committee on Quackery and the Coordinating Conference on Health Information (CCHI). During this period the AMA effectively and adversely influences private insurance companies and Medicare against chiropractic coverage. It "fixes" a so-called independent study commissioned by the Department of Health, Education and Welfare, done by Stanford Research Institute, to determine whether or not chiropractic services should be paid for by Medicare. It also works to influence Blue Cross/Blue Shield and other insurers against chiropractic.

June 1980. An AMA medical association assembles a report on chiropractic entitled "The Chiropractic Dilemma" which recommends using chiropractors to front a medical campaign against chiropractic.

1983-1984. The early plans for the Pharmaceutical Advertising Council/U.S. Food and Drug Administration's (PAC/FDA) Anti-Quackery Campaign are drawn up. Based on a survey done in October, 1984, chiropractic is officially named as one of the Big Three targets of the campaign. Experts on board in this campaign include doctors Victor Herbert, John Renner, Stephen Barrett, Mrs. Grace Monaco, and William Jarvis, Ph.D.—all with the NCAHF.

March 1984. Charles DuVall issues his "Fact Sheet on Spinal Manipulative Therapy (SMT)," which is used in his training seminars for insurance companies.

May 1984. The US FDA meets with the California State Food and Drug, Fraud Branch, the U.S. Postal Service, Federal Trade Commission, Board of Medical Quality Assurance of California, and a representative from the National Council Against Health Fraud (NCAHF). The NCAHF representative directs those present to the NCAHF's priorities, which includes chiropractic and other targets from the PAC/FDA campaign. This all parallels the old CCHI activity.

July 1984. The National Association for Chiropractic Medicine incorporates in Texas. Its platform parallels that of the National Council Against Health Fraud. It is an affiliate member of the NCAHF. It helps co-author the NCAHF's Position Paper on Chiropractic, and its Advisory Board is made up of NCAHF officials. It promotes these NCAHF's members as having influence in the insurance industry. Among the benefits of NACM membership is being able to become insurance consultants as well as experts for legal testimony in civil cases against chiropractors.

October 1984. The PAC/FDA Survey identifies the main targets of the campaign. The Big Three are vitamins, chiropractic, and psychological counseling.

December 1984. The Southern California Council Against Health Fraud changes its name to the National Council Against Health Fraud.

February 1985. The NCAHF issues its Position Paper on Chiropractic which was put together with the help of NACM official Charles DuVall.

September 1985. The PAC/FDA Anti-Quackery Campaign, which parallels the AMA's CCHI Congresses on Quackery, is launched officially at the Washington, D.C., Press Club.

September 1985. One week after the PAC/FDA Conference, the National Health Care Anti-Fraud Association (NHCAA) launches its first conference. The NHCAA is made up of insurance companies and federal and state government regulatory, enforcement and prosecution agencies, including the Department of Justice, FBI, U.S. Attorney's Office, FDA, Medicare, HHS, and others. This is the beginning of the Health Fraud Task Force.

December 1985. The NHCAA is officially incorporated in Washington, D.C. Its founding members include representatives from the Justice Department, HHS, and major health care insurance companies, such as Aetna, Blue Cross/Blue Shield, and others.

May 1986. Office of the Inspector General of the Department of Health and Human Services issues a report entitled "Inspection of Chiropractic Services Under Medicare." The report references the 1968 AMA-influenced HEW report on excluding chiropractic coverage. It also mentions that the HHS met with members of the National Association for Chiropractic Medicine. The final recommendations are to cut chiropractic coverage under Medicare to 12 services per year per patient.

October 1986. The October Plan is put together by the Ohio Council Against Health Fraud. It calls for chilling activities which include (1) monitoring alternative health claims, practitioners, modalities, and patients; (2) working with state and federal regulatory and enforcement agencies to prosecute alternatives; (3) conducting studies of alternative treatments, modalities, services, products, manufacturers, and therapies; and (4) sending these reports to the insurance companies and federal and state agencies to use against the alternatives, which they refer to as "health fraud/quackery" and/or insurance fraud.

April 1987. The Ohio Council Against Health Fraud incorporates in Ohio. Two of its founders are Charles DuVall, Sr., and Charles DuVall, Jr.

November 1987. The National Health Care Anti-Fraud Association (NHCAA) announces "First Computerized Network Designed to Combat Health Fraud Is Unveiled." The network is a central information system that monitors every single insurance claim from both medicare and private insurance companies that are hooked into the system. Florida is chosen as the test state, and the network is planned to go national in the spring of 1988. One of its first targets is a chiropractor.

February 1988. FDA issues a report on health fraud and a memo which outlines its progress in "fighting quackery." This includes a statement that the FDA "has placed a priority on the sharing of information among organizations working to combat health fraud." It also reveals that among those included in this sharing of data is Barnett Technical Services, which was part of the Emprise Grant Study of alternatives.

March 1988. PAC/FDA puts on a Health Fraud Conference in Kansas City, Missouri. As in most of the almost two dozen such conferences on "quackery and health fraud" that have been held in 22 different cities around the country, the speakers, panelists, and workshops are directed at targets from the PAC/FDA campaign.

Spring 1988. The NHCAA's computerized network, designed to track all health claims, goes national.

May 1988. FDA sets up a new unit, the Health Fraud Unit, in Kansas City, Missouri, headed by Gary Dean, Director of the Office of Compliance. Dean's responsibilities include the collection of information on health fraud and quackery to start up a data base for the FDA. According to Dean, he collects a great deal of data from John Renner, M.D. In addition, he receives at least 20 different targets for the FDA to pursue for regulatory actions, enforcement, and prosecution.

Summary

1. Chiropractic was targeted by the PAC/FDA Campaign.
2. Being a target translated into activity directed against chiropractic in the insurance industry.

3. The AMA medical society's plan to have chiropractors front a medical campaign against chiropractic has apparently been implemented.
4. The October Plan proposed by a small group of anti-chiropractic people, designed to adversely influence the insurance industry, has now come into being.
5. Anti-chiropractic consultants have been placed inside the insurance industry, and their actions as insurance consultants to the insurance industry have apparently moved the anti-chiropractic campaign directly into the economic arena, apparently by design.

The most significant piece of data to come to light is that apparently anti-chiropractic chiropractors were behind the NCAHF's Position Paper on Chiropractic. They founded the Ohio Council Against Health Fraud. The Ohio Council Against Health Fraud authored the October Plan. The National Association for Chiropractic Medicine (NACM), using its NCAHF Advisory Board members, apparently has placed agents into the insurance system to forward their philosophy. This has directly and negatively impacted the economic status of many chiropractors.

All of this, as well as other hidden factors, has had a tremendous economic impact on many chiropractors around the country. It must be emphasized that every state in the country is experiencing situations in which chiropractic payments are being cut. From all appearances, there is an organized, nation-wide campaign going on here.

Chapter 12

Chelation Therapy

"After further discussion, Dr. Sailer moved that Dr. Briggs' license be revoked. That motion was seconded by Dr. Towarnicky."
[Minutes of July 1987 secret meeting of the North Dakota Medical Association Board of Examiners, held without Dr. Briggs or his attorney present.]

"You engaged in public, unrehearsed deliberation. That's precisely what the law contemplates. It is the most effective protection that licensed physicians have from the collusion of a ruling clique of physicians that have garnered some political power for questionable purposes. It could happen."
[Letter from North Dakota Medical Association Board of Examiners' attorney to Board members who suspended Dr. Briggs on July 21, 1988, one year after the July 1987 meeting, apparently justifying the illegal meeting.]

The Case of Dr. Brian Briggs

Who is Dr. Briggs? To best describe this man I can only say that he is the epitome of what a good country doctor should be. In his 60s, healthy and happy. No matter what the adversity, his spirit is high. Having a practice that serves rural North Dakota, as well as patients from all over the state, and the country, he is what America used to know as a good doctor; he has a heart of gold. He has often taken on patients without getting paid for his work, and never complained.

He sometimes took payments in the form of I.O.U.s, food, animals, and time payments over an extended period. His dedication to his patients is sincere, and his successes are known nationwide. He is also a pioneer, in that he, along with his patients, pushed legislation in North Dakota to make laetrile and chelation therapy legal in that state. It's little wonder then that the medical establishment would go after him.

Dr. Brian Briggs' case is not only typical of what happens to doctors of medicine who employ this alternative approach in their practice, it is also an illustrative case of behind-the-scenes anti-competitive activity at work and the good-old-boy network being put into play.

Dr. Briggs' troubles began soon after he started to employ alternative treatments and products in his practice. After graduating from the University of Minnesota School of Medicine in 1954, he set up a conventional practice in family medicine in Minot, North Dakota. Up through 1976 Dr. Briggs was just another member of the medical staff at a local hospital in Minot. He headed up the drug dependency unit at this hospital and had no trouble until he started using vitamins and supplements. He was doing nutritional therapy and preventive medicine at the chemical dependency unit, and began using certain nutritional programs and supplements that are used in alternative medicine for cancer patients.

In October 1977, the hospital started to look into his patients records and his practice. They did not like what they found; substituting vitamins, supplements, and nutritional therapy for good old-fashioned pharmaceuticals just didn't cut it at the hospital. Dr. Briggs was forced to resign from the hospital staff, and in November 1977 he left the chemical dependency unit.

His problems persisted, and the hospital ordered him to discontinue his "new" type of therapy or face suspension of hospital privileges. At this time the North Dakota Medical Association started looking into Dr. Briggs. The president of the county medical society wrote to the executive director of the state medical association. His letter of September 29, 1978, dealt with Dr. Briggs' use of "laetrile and other questionable medications." There was a call for censoring Dr. Briggs because of his beliefs and practices in alternative medicine. Dr. Briggs resigned from the medical association and moved out of state to start over again in Illinois. The move proved to be a burden to his patients in North Dakota who traveled back and forth to him, so he returned to Minot a few months later. He re-applied for hospital privileges, but was officially denied on January 8, 1980.

Once again he left his home and went off to start again, this time in Minnesota, commuting from his home in Minot several times a week. His troubles from North Dakota followed him into the state of Minnesota. The medical association in North Dakota sent information about Dr. Briggs to the county and state medical associations in Minnesota, and they started a file on him in March 1980.

Three complaints about his use of alternative products and therapies were made within three months of his moving into that state. One complaint was from the National M.S. Society; the other two were from the county medical society and from an insurance company. Following these, the medical Board made a formal complaint to the Attorney General's office, which started to look into Dr. Briggs only after the medical association alerted it to the fact that it was looking at chelation therapy and Dr. Briggs.

From 1980 to 1984, the medical association conducted its "study" into chelation therapy. It turned over its findings, which were not favorable, to the Attorney General. He in turn began a case against Dr. Briggs. The Minnesota Medical Board also got into the picture and started collecting information on Dr. Briggs from the North Dakota Medical Board.

On April 19, 1983, the Minnesota Medical Board found Dr. Briggs in violation of its laws and rules because he employed treatments, prescriptions, and tests which were "not scientifically valid" or were "unapproved, ineffective and unsafe." He was also charged with "departing from or the failure to conform to the minimal standards of acceptable and prevailing medical practice." The board ruled to revoke his license.

An analysis of the medical society's files on Dr. Briggs revealed that the investigation and de-licensing procedures that took place in Minnesota were spurred on by a medical doctor who was in direct competition with Dr. Briggs' practice. This doctor stated in a letter to the Board at the very beginning of Briggs' troubles that he had lost two patients to Briggs' practice and he wanted chelation therapy and Briggs looked into. The file on his case, however, stated, "The record does not establish that Dr. Briggs made misleading, deceptive, untrue or fraudulent representation in his practice of medicine." It further revealed that the evidence presented in his case also showed that he never "treated cancer patients who may have benefited from conventional cancer treatment."

Following this decision to revoke his license, Dr. Briggs was forced to move back to North Dakota. Normally when an M.D. losses his/her license, that state medical board informs other states where that M.D. may also be licensed. Usually the other states revoke that practitioner's license based on the license being revoked in another state. North Dakota, however, has a law—a good law, which should be in every state—which forbids this type of action based on some other states findings and requires that if a medical doctor hasn't violated any North Dakota laws, then that license should not be revoked based on the merits of another state's actions.

Dr. Briggs was instrumental in getting two laws passed in North Dakota allowing a doctor to use both laetrile and chelation therapy, stating that they were accepted practice and valid treatment. This, of course, did not sit well with the medical establishment in North Dakota, and so, when Dr. Briggs returned, the wheels began once again to turn against him.

From the summer of 1983 through December 1985, the Medical Board, the Medical Association, and competing medical doctors worked behind the scenes to get something going against Dr. Briggs. They tried to find something to use against him, but there was nothing there. Nothing Dr. Briggs was doing was found to be inappropriate or out of agreement with the medical establishment with his practice. The Board even tried to get action going through the FDA, but to no avail. Even they could find nothing wrong with the products Dr. Briggs was using in his practice and they wrote the Board clearly stating that the items Dr. Briggs was using in his practice amounted to nothing more than food additives/supplements and not drugs.

According to all of the records contained in his files at the Board of Medical Examiners, there were no communications, letters, or complaints against Dr. Briggs. In effect, it appeared the Board backed off from taking any actions against him. From the time Dr. Briggs moved back to North Dakota in 1983 until October 1986, no actions were taken against him for anything he was doing with alternative medicine.

However, on October 8, 1986, a Board member (who had been involved in the 1983 action against Dr. Briggs) wrote the executive director of the Board about Dr. Briggs and instigated action against him. It appears that this doctor detailed to the executive director of the Board how he had attended a course on Health and Nutrition Fraud and Abuse at the American Academy of Family Physicians scientific assembly in Washington, D.C. He stated that the course was put on by Dr. John Renner. He said that he mentioned his name because "he is probably the most informed physician in this country on health fraud and quackery." He goes on to suggest:

> [Dr. Renner] would be a good resource for the Board of Medical Examiners if you ever needed anybody with his expertise. . .[Dr. Renner] handed out a book called the *Directory of Holistic Medicine and Alternative Health Care Services in*

the United States. . .I would get a coupy [sic] of this book because it really is a compendium of all the people in this country that are doing alot of quackery type items in the health care. Each state is listed and in North Dakota one name was listed, Brian E. Briggs. You know that he has an agreement with the Board of Medical Examiners in the state of North Dakota to enter into such type practices. As I said before, this book's edition says 1985 and this may be an area where he violated his agreement with the Board of Medical Examiners. If you can't get a hold of the book, I would call Dr. Renner and talk to him and may be he could even Xerox off the page concerning Dr. Briggs.

The Board's files revealed a note from Renner's office to the Board's chief investigator. The note stated that attached was a copy of the directory page which mentioned Dr. Briggs. The November 12, 1986, note also stated that the recipient should "feel free to contact Dr. Renner if you have any questions."

Following this note, the Board collected Medicare claims, some 15 of them, that involved Dr. Briggs while he was using EDTA chelation therapy and held, in July 1987, a secret meeting at which neither Dr. Briggs nor his attorney were present. According to North Dakota law, if a practitioner's license is under question and the Board plans to take any action against that practitioner's license, that doctor must be present during any such deliberations; but Dr. Briggs was not present, although the minutes of that meeting clearly show that the Board was briefed by their attorney on the "Dr. Briggs case." Dr. Briggs' use of EDTA was discussed and one of the Board members then moved to revoke his license, and this was seconded by another Board member present. It was then suggested that the Board, in an apparent attempt to create a case against Dr. Briggs, get a statement from the FDA on the use of chelation therapy. The minutes revealed that regardless of what the FDA stated, the Board would move forward anyway and conduct a hearing against Dr. Briggs' license. The minutes further revealed that they moved to bring on an action against Dr. Briggs once they got the information they wanted from the FDA.

Dr. Briggs had done nothing wrong by law in North Dakota. It would seem that the appearance of his name in a directory constituted serious wrong-doing on his part in the eyes of those wanting to take action against him.

In order to build a case against Dr. Briggs, the good-old-boy network began to work. On August 6, 1987, the Board sent a letter to the FDA in Minnesota stating they were "currently investigating a physician [Dr. Briggs] who is using chelation therapy for the treatment of hypertension and general arteriosclerosis." The letter stated that it was "understood that the FDA hasn't approved chelation for this purpose" and further asked the FDA to "please advise. . .whether or not [this] understanding is correct."

The FDA's reply was swift. On August 14, 1987, the FDA Compliance Officer sent a letter with attachments on chelation therapy. The attachment was stamped "Action Copy" and came from the office of Bruce Brown, who was the public relations officer for the FDA in the PAC/FDA campaign. The Action Copy was a press release which was a "warning to all Americans" urging them to "not use so-called chelation therapy capsules or tablets." This warning had nothing whatsoever to do with what Dr. Briggs was doing. But the routing on the Action Copy from Brown's office included in its routing other FDA people who were very active in the PAC/FDA anti-quackery campaign. They also attached an FDA paper on EDTA chelation therapy which basically stated that the FDA approved EDTA chelation therapy for removing lead only and not for anything else. Other attachments sent quoted AMA sources and other vested interest medical establishment groups.

This information on chelation therapy came from the same offices that were directly involved in the anti-quackery campaign in the FDA. It would appear that what happened to Dr. Briggs was therefore as a direct result of this campaign.

Almost one year after the Board held this illegal behind-closed-doors meeting, it called an official meeting and filed an official complaint against Dr. Briggs to revoke his license for one year—after having already decided to do so in July 1987. It's important to emphasized that this series of actions was a blatant violation of state law, not to mention the civil rights of Dr. Briggs, and possibly of RICO conspiracy laws.

Following the Board's official findings on Dr. Briggs on July 21, 1988, its attorney sent a letter to each of the Board members who participated in the hearings against Dr. Briggs. In his letter, he stated that the purpose of the letter "is to assure you that you did well." He then made a statement, which (knowing what took place one year prior) can be nothing more than a PR move on his part to hide from public view what really went on behind the scenes in the Briggs case:

> You engaged in public, unrehearsed deliberation. That is
> precisely what the law contemplates. It is the most effective

protection that licensed physicians have from the collusion of a ruling clique of physicians that have garnered some political power for questionable purposes. It could happen.

In light of the documentation uncovered in research into the Briggs case, what the good lawyer stated above is *anything but* what happened. The fact is that the Board *did* meet one year earlier. It *did* deliberate on Dr. Briggs' case, and it *did* discuss and propose to revoke his license. This is totally contrary to the intent of North Dakota laws governing how to conduct public hearings on a physician's license. A legal expert whom I consulted with this information stated that "...what occurred in Dr. Briggs' case was nothing short of a conspiracy to violate his Constitutional rights to practice medicine." But the attorney who wrote the Board members who participated in the Briggs case summed up the situation with this statement: "You were great. You really deliberated. That is not something of which you should be ashamed; feel good about it."

After he lost his license, Dr. Briggs took his case to the higher courts. He took it all the way to the State Supreme Court of North Dakota. His appeals were of no avail, and in the end the official time that he lost his license started when the courts denied his case. He was without a livelihood from March 1, 1990, to February 28, 1991.

On March 19, 1990, the Board sent the entire Briggs file to the Office of Inspector General of the Department of Health and Human Services in Denver, Colorado. The person receiving this information was part of the Task Force on Health Fraud and a member of the National Health Care Anti-Fraud Association.

It would appear that the Briggs case was considered a great success from the viewpoint of the anti-quackery campaign, because on May 3, 1990, the Office of the Inspector General contacted the Board about setting up a Health Fraud Conference in Fargo, North Dakota. The letter to the Board asked for its involvement at the Conference. The Conference did take place at the Blue Cross/Blue Shield of North Dakota headquarters, and Dr. Briggs' case was discussed. (Again, Blue Cross/Blue Shield is a member of the National Health Care Anti-Fraud Association and has actively worked behind the scenes against alternative doctors.)

During the course of research into Dr. Briggs' case, it was learned that an official of the North Dakota Medical Association had contacted Blue Cross/Blue Shield to have payments suspended to another physician in North Dakota because of his use of chelation therapy. The Blues denied claims from this doctor, and eventually the Board came after him as well. The Briggs' case is not an isolated one. The list is 1,000 names long. His case is typical of medicine's dislike and contempt for the competition.

The Case of Dr. Ed McDonagh

Dr. Ed McDonagh is one of the nation's leading chelation therapists, with a large and successful clinic in Kansas City, Missouri. His practice draws people from all over the world. A large man, with a heart of compassion and understanding for his patients, he, like Dr. Briggs, goes out of his way to accommodate his patients.

Dr. McDonagh's troubles began as a result of three factors: his success with patients, his pioneering attitude, and his location. Being in the Kansas City area put his practice directly under the monitoring and ridicule of one of the nation's leading anti-quackery spokesmen. Dr. McDonagh, known to his friends and patients as Mac, was also outspoken about his rights to practice. He stood up to adversity and went to bat for others in the field of alternatives, those less fortunate who could not fight back due to the financial hardships involved in attorney fees and the lost time in their clinics. With Mac it was the principle involved, freedom of choice in health-care, and his patients' rights to seek help from anyone they felt could help them. He did help them. His practice came under attack in the local media over the years and he fought back in the courts.

His chelation practice came under attack in earnest on November 7, 1985, two months after the PAC/FDA campaign was launched nationally. As a matter of record, there was a Tumor Conference at a local hospital, part of which was a presentation called "Health and Nutritional Quackery, Fraud and Abuse" by Dr. John Renner, the head of the Kansas City Council Against Health Fraud and Nutritional Abuse, headquartered in Kansas City, Missouri. Quoting Dr. Victor Herbert, a medical doctor from the Bronx V.A. Hospital in New York who was also associated with the PAC/FDA Anti-Quackery Campaign, Dr. Renner outlined "how to spot a quack." He listed nine indicators of a "quack," including:

> • Has credentials not recognized by the scientific community.
> • Espouses the Conspiracy Theory and its twin, the Controversy Claim.

The first criterion makes for some interesting debate; practitioners with "credentials not recognized by the scientific community" include chelation therapists who belong to the American
College of Advancement in Medicine (a national group of doctors
who employ chelation therapy, all of whom are licensed, and some
of whom are former members of the AMA); the American Holistic
Medical Association; the American Academy of Environmental
Medicine, and many others.

What each of these not-recognized-by-the-scientific-community
groups have in common is that they are associations of doctors who
believe and practice alternative medicine. Of course they wouldn't
be "recognized" by the "scientific community" because the "scientific community" is made up of the mainstream AMA doctors, all of
whom have a vested interest in seeing that these holistic/alternative
doctors receive no recognition and are put out of business. This
criterion is nothing more than an anti-competitive name-calling ploy
to further restrict the trade of those involved in the alternatives by
putting the label of "quack" on them and their practices. Calling a
licensed doctor a "quack" is nothing more than furthering the campaign against the competitors of the medical/pharmaceutical industries.

Now let's discuss the point of labeling a doctor of alternative
medicine a "quack" because he says there is a conspiracy or organized campaign directed against what he believes in. Documented
evidence indicates that it would be fair to say that there is a very good
likelihood that there *is indeed* a conspiracy directed against the
alternatives. Whether it's the "big picture" conspiracy with the
PAC/FDA Campaign, or something as small as a clique of good old
boys getting together to get rid of their competition in a small town
in North Dakota or Kansas or Missouri, it amounts to conspiracy any
way one looks at it. Alternative practitioners who say there is a
conspiracy or campaign against them may be making an astute
observation. Instead of indicating that they are paranoid or "quacks,"
the observation, on the contrary, makes them appear to be an intelligent threats to those involved in hiding such a campaign or conspiracy.

"The medical quack," Dr. Renner said in his presentation, "often
seems legitimate, usually having a license from the state to practice
medicine, osteopathy, chiropractic or naturopathy." Such a statement
has all the earmarks of propaganda and serves no other purpose then
to assign such practitioners the derogatory "handle" of *quack.* A
more accurate definition of *quacks* as used by Dr. Renner and others

in the Campaign would be "practitioners of a brand of medicine that does not espouse the use of surgery, drugs or radiation therapy, and who do not come under the control of organized medicine or organized science." Put more simply, they are "those practitioners who are in direct competition to organized medicine, which has resulted in a professional jealously which is the motivating force behind orthodox medicine's campaign against such practitioners, solely for economic revenge."

During the conference, information was presented on subjects which appear to have come directly from the PAC/FDA campaign list of targets. These included gerovital, cellular therapy, royal jelly, health foods, organic foods, vitamins, herbs, and food supplements. Under the listing of "FDA Categories of Health and Nutritional Fraud and Abuse," nine separate categories and examples were listed, all of which were directly from FDA documents used in the PAC/FDA Anti-Quackery Campaign.

Of the items listed in a section about harm that is done by "quacks," one of the first listed was "Is usually quite expensive." That is getting down to the true motivation: money that could be spent on orthodox medicine is paying for alternative therapies. Ironically, contrary to what the opponents to the alternatives say about how expensive alternative treatments are, there is simply no comparison between the costs of, for example, chelation therapy and open-heart surgery, bypass surgery, or balloon angioplasty. The alternatives are much more *inexpensive,* and are generally less risky than orthodox treatments for such things as hardening of the arteries.

In his presentation, Dr. Renner listed those sources of help for the problem of "quackery." These included:

A. FDA—If drugs, nutritional supplements or a medical device is involved.

B. FTC—For complaints regarding false or misleading advertising.

C. Better Business Bureau—If drugs, nutritional supplements or a medical device is involved.

D. Postal Inspector—If the product was promoted through the mail.

E. State Licensing Department—If the fraudulent remedy was promoted by a licensed doctor or other licensed practitioner.

F. State or County Prosecuting Attorney—Most have special branches to investigate consumer fraud complaints.

G. Local Health Department—For information about the reputation of the product.

H. Malpractice Litigation—Malpractice suits are being filed in increasing numbers.

Of these places to go for "help," the FDA, the FTC, the Postal Service, the Better Business Bureau, and prosecuting attorneys are all involved in the Anti-Quackery Campaign. These are logical choices to present to an audience, and it fits into the overall campaign against the alternatives.

Dr. Renner also listed many different practitioners, products, clinics, and modalities which he described as "recent developments in the Kansas City area." These "developments" amounted to a listing of entities, apparently being brought to the attention of those in attendance at this Conference so that they could be aware that these were the "quacks" in the Kansas City area. The listing included the following:

A. Herbalife

B. General Nutrition Health Food Stores (oil of Primrose)

C. Chiropractors
  • Sam Walters, D.C.
  • David Beaulieu, D.C.

D. Rudolph Alsleben, D.O.

E. Brenda Owens

F. Kay Smith (Neo-Life) [Smith was a distributor of alternative products in the Kansas City area.]

G. Bridgeport University

H. Harold Manners (metabolic theory) [Manners also had a clinic in Mexico where he helped thousands of patients who had been failed by orthodoxy. He was named in the PAC/FDA Campaign also.]

I. Parts of the Women's Health Expo [The list did not specify which part of the Expo was offensive; one can only speculate that something there met with Dr. Renner's disapproval.]

J. Alfalfa [Another product on the FDA's list for the campaign.]

K. Bee Pollen [Still another product targeted by the FDA in the campaign.]

Most, if not all, of these came under some form of attack after this point in time. Coincidence or not, it amounts to an apparent attempt to restrain the trade of those entities which came under attack. If it was not planned that way, the end result was that such an effect was created.

In addition to these, Dr. Renner listed 11 individuals "currently doing chelation therapy in the state of Missouri" and four "currently doing chelation therapy in the state of Kansas." Was this perhaps to give the impression that these doctors were all "quacks"? Although they were not listed as "quacks" specifically, the entire presentation was about this subject. One can only assume that because these names were listed that they somehow were being associated with "quackery" because they were chelation therapists.

In the presentation there was a list of questions that related to "quackery" which appeared to be some sort of a test for the participating audience. Included in the 22 questions was a section on chelation therapy. It read as follows:

Chelation therapy is:
(a) a recent miracle treatment
(b) good for atherosclerosis, diabetes and arthritis
(c) going to exceed laetrile in cost and misuse
(d) uses EDTA (FDA approved for lead poisoning)
(e) costs $3,000 to $10,000 per course of treatment

At the bottom of the questionnaire were the "correct" answers listed for each of the questions. For this question on chelation therapy, the "correct" answers were (c), (d), and (e). What is missing here is all of the data that one would need to make a clear and intelligent choice between chelation therapy and, say, bypass surgery. For example, bypass surgery could cost as little as $75,000 or as much as $250,000 in the case of a double or triple bypass operation. In some cases, charges have exceeded $250,000. Also missing are the comparative statistics related to patient mortality after bypass surgery and chelation therapy. Also missing is the risk factor having a bypass, compared to the risk factor of having chelation therapy. None of this relevant data is being presented.

To label anyone who uses chelation therapy as a "quack" is neither fair nor accurate. It apparently serves no purpose other than to spread the propaganda and falsehoods that are being distributed to the public through the PAC/FDA Anti-Quackery Campaign. I am not sure whether or not Dr. Renner, Dr. Victor Herbert, Dr. Stephen Barrett, Dr. William Jarvis, and the others involved in this Anti-Quackery Campaign are sincere in their presentation of what is or is not "quackery." Perhaps they are. However, this campaign appears to be directed exclusively at the practices of those people in the alternatives. The results have been that their trade and livelihoods have been affected in a negative way. Whether or not that is the intent of this campaign doesn't really matter. What does matter is that such effects amount to unfair competitive practices, and may very well be in violation of federal laws.

Extensive research on the subject of chelation therapy and the practitioners of it in the states of Kansas and Missouri sheds some light on why the medical boards in these two states came after practitioners of chelation therapy. Since Kansas and Missouri are next to each other, each state has patients that visit practitioners in the other state. Dr. Ed McDonagh's clinic is near the Kansas/Missouri border, and he has patients coming to him from both states. It is therefore relevant that the Kansas Board of Healing Arts would take any actions related to chelation therapy, which they did. The history behind the Kansas Board's ultimate position on chelation therapy is most revealing. It goes something like this:

1982 and prior. The Board had absolutely no complaints or data on chelation therapy at all.

September 6, 1983. Donald G. Strole, General Counsel for the Kansas Board of Healing Arts, forwarded a newspaper ad for oral chelation (which has nothing to do with EDTA chelation therapy) to Wayne Hundley, Chief of Consumer Protection Division of the Kansas Attorney General's office. He stated that he thought the ad was "downright false and fraudulent." Strole asked Hundley to let him know "whether your office wishes to take action." Nothing more appeared to come out of this at that time.

November 1983. The American Board of Chelation Therapy wrote the Kansas Board regarding its function as a Board for chelation therapists, apparently in reply to a request from the Board writing to them for information about chelation.

January 26, 1984. Two letters with this date, both to Dr. John Renner, were placed into the Kansas Board files on chelation therapy. One was from a cardiovascular surgeon from Chevy Chase, Maryland, regarding a phone conversation he had with Dr. Renner about chelation therapy. The letter contained this doctor's opinion about chelation therapy, which was best summed up in his closing statement on the subject: ". . .one of the reasons that I am not currently aware of any controlled studies which demonstrate benefit from chelation therapy is most likely the lack of application of the scientific method, including appropriate standards for documentation of its efficacy." (Considering he was a heart specialist, it is no great surprise that he would speak out against chelation therapy.) The other letter was a reply to Dr. Renner from the pharmaceutical company that manufactured Sodium Versenate (EDTA). This letter also denounced the use of EDTA for arteriosclerosis, and the author attached a statement from the American Heart Association on the subject of EDTA for this use.

February 6, 1984. Kansas State Senator Richard Gannon wrote the Kansas Board stating that one of his constituents asked him about chelation treatments. The Senator asked the Board if this procedure was authorized in Kansas, and asked if the procedure was "widespread" (as if it were some sort of epidemic disease) in Kansas. He even asked about any "fatalities connected with the procedure," and if there were any "substantiated cures associated with the procedure."

February 8, 1984. The Board's reply stated, "At the present time the Board is attempting to gather materials on chelation therapy. . .and, consequently, have not made a judgment." The letter also praised the use of chelation therapy, stating, "Some chelation therapy has a very valid medical usage, one area is the realm of lead poisoning, the other is in mercury poisoning, and a third is iron overdosage poisoning." The Secretary of the Board added that "I have the impression that this therapy is rather expensive, but I do not have actual data on this."

February 18, 1984. The American Board of Chelation Therapy sent the Board material on chelation. The Kansas Board took the material and sent it for analysis and evaluation to the University of Kansas.

February 20, 1984. The University of Kansas evaluated the materials and sent a letter to the Board. The evaluation was both positive and negative, but only that portion of the letter that was negative was ever used in any future correspondence by the Board to anyone asking about chelation therapy. The Board even sent copies of this evaluation to practitioners who used chelation therapy.

February 25, 1984. The Board files reveal that the Board members met on this day to discuss how to reply to the state legislator regarding his query on chelation therapy. It was recommended that the Board contact the FDA for more data on EDTA chelation therapy.

Late February 1984. The Board received the data from the FDA and the FDA's position was made known to the legislator. [Note: It should be pointed out that the materials sent from the FDA came from Julia Hewgley, FDA Kansas City office, who was associated

with Dr. John Renner's Committee in Kansas City.] In its letter to
Senator Gannon, the Board stated, ". . .there is considerable question
as to the value of the treatment of atherosclerosis by chelation, and
until adequate controlled investigations are done the Board cannot
endorse this form of treatment."

August 18, 1984. Board files reveal an entry in the chronology of
events on chelation therapy to include an entry which stated, "Any
complaints concerning chelation therapy should be referred to the
disciplinary counsel."

> (*Note*: There was no still position statement one way or the
> other officially recorded or published by the Board to this
> point. Then Dr. Renner once again got involved, and his
> involvement apparently led to the Board's decision and
> statement about chelation.)

September 10, 1984. The Board received another letter that was
sent to Dr. John Renner, this one from the American Heart Association, which contained an enclosure of its position statement on
EDTA chelation therapy. (Contained in the Board's files behind this
letter was the title page and pages 226, 228, and 229 a book written
by pro-alternative author Dr. Morton Walker. Dr. Walker's book
was entitled *The Miracle Healing Power of Chelation Therapy.*
These pages listed chelation therapists in Indiana, Iowa, Kansas,
Kentucky, Michigan, Minnesota, Missouri, Nevada, and New Jersey. *The names listed under Kansas and Missouri were the exact
names later listed in Dr. Renner's presentation at the Tumor Conference in November 1985.*)

September 28, 1984. A note on Board stationery indicated a
phone conversation with a Dr. Forrest Pommerenke, M.D., regarding
chelation therapy. The note stated to invite Dr. John Renner to "the
December meeting." (As in the situation with Dr. Briggs, however,
the Kansas Board met earlier than the scheduled December meeting
to make a determination on chelation therapy without anyone from
the "pro" side of chelation present to add any input.)

October 6, 1984. Without any proponents of chelation present,
the Board met to decide the fate of chelation and formulate an
official policy statement on this issue. Those present included Dr.
Pommerenke and Dr. John Renner. According to the former Board
attorney, Don Strole, these two doctors were largely responsible for
authoring the Board's position statement. The Board files reflect the
following took place:

- John Renner, M.D., from Kansas City, Missouri, appeared before the Board as requested by Dr. Pommerenke, to comment upon chelation therapy and the widespread and growing use of this therapy. Dr. Renner cited statistics and case examples of the harmful side effects of chelation therapy and the rising use and cost in the United States. He stated that the following Kansas doctors were using this therapy in Kansas: Drs. Acker, Cohnberg, Hunsberger, Thiemann and Riordan.
- The Board held discussion on this issue and appreciated the input of Dr. Renner.
- Dr. Pommerenke presented a draft of policy statement regarding Chelation Therapy to the Board.
- (Knackstedt-Uhlig) Remove words "dangerous and" from the first paragraph of draft. Carried.
- (Uhlig-Knackstedt) Adopt statement last two paragraphs, as submitted by Dr. Pommerenke with amendments. Carried. The statement will read:
  "The KSBHA believes that the use of EDTA and chelation therapy for every condition not approved by the F.D.A. is at best experimental. It is our unanimous opinion that the use of EDTA in the State of Kansas for any purpose other than therapy approved by the F.D.A. be considered investigational and that any physician who uses EDTA for any other than F.D.A. approved purposes should obtain prior approval from the F.D.A.
  "Failure to obtain a permit from the F.D.A. may be grounds for referral to the Disciplinary Counsel for appropriate action."

Almost immediately the Kansas board sent out a letter to the Missouri Board, dated October 16, 1984. The letter contained the entire statement as printed above from its behind-closed doors meeting on October 6, 1984. In addition, it stated, "We have had information that several Kansas residents received chelation therapy in Kansas City, Missouri, by physicians licensed in Missouri." No doubt, they were referring to the list of names that were given to them from the Walker book, which apparently had been disseminated by Dr. Renner the following year in Kansas City, Missouri, and were listed in his paper on quackery a year later at the Tumor Conference.

Following this meeting held in October, the Board in Kansas sent out a letter to all Kansas physicians, as well as physicians from

Missouri, asking them to attend a Board meeting in Topeka, Kansas, on the subject of chelation therapy. The letter stated that the Board would discuss chelation therapy and stated invited recipients to be present and present their views.

This letter to the proponents of chelation therapy did not state that the Board had *already* made a determination on the subject. Nor did it mention that it was based on a draft put together with the help of Dr. John Renner, or that it was negative. The letter also failed to inform those being invited that the Board had already sent out a copy of its position statement to the Missouri Board. On December 3, 1984, the Montana Board wrote asking for a copy of the statement as well. The word had gotten out to other States that Kansas had taken a position.

On December 7, 1984, the Board held its "open" meeting with the chelation therapists voicing their opinions and views about chelation therapy to the Board. Apparently this meeting in December was a PR gimmick designed to give the appearance that the Board was being objective and open in coming to its conclusions about chelation therapy. With the chelation therapists present, the board members discussed it, according to its file records, ". . . so that the 'pro' side of chelation therapy could be heard by the Board."

However, the damage was already done. Although as a result of this discussion the Board voted to strike the last paragraph of their earlier statement (Failure to obtain a permit. . .etc.) it had already sent out its previous position statement to at least two other states, Missouri and Montana. It is worth noting that the FDA *doesn't issue* permits authorizing *any* treatments, let alone chelation therapy.

Following the meeting with the chelation therapists, the Board sent out letter thanking them for their attendance and input. One such letter was sent to Garry F. Gordon, M.D., President of the American Academy of Medical Preventics (AAMPS), the national group for chelation therapists. The letter stated, "Most members of the Board I talked to felt that it was a very informative and extremely interesting subject." It thanked him for his presentation, which was almost two hours.

What the Board did not tell Dr. Gordon was that they had sent out the unrevised version in October, stating that disciplinary actions would be taken against any physician using chelation without prior FDA approval. The Kansas Board apparently did not correct this with the states it had sent the first version to in October.

All of these events played a role in Dr. McDonagh's case in Missouri. Missouri is where Mac had his practice set up, and Missouri had a copy of the original Kansas position on chelation therapy. His clinic is also the one closest to Kansas. Most likely it was the one referred to in the Kansas Board's letter to Missouri alerting them to patients from Kansas going to a clinic in Missouri.

In addition, other factors influencing the public, the media, and professional associations against McDonagh were in play. Some were in the open, and some were behind-the-scenes activities directed at McDonagh. Mac is a Doctor of Osteopathy, not a medical doctor, so all actions directed against him would have to come from the state osteopathic board or from the American Osteopathic Association in Chicago.

Mac started running a one-minute ad promoting chelation on local radio in the Kansas City area in January 1984. On January 26, 1984, one day after the radio spot was aired, someone wrote a letter of complaint about Dr. McDonagh's radio ad to the American Osteopathic Association. The writer, a woman with a newly established practice in the Kansas City, Missouri, area, stated that she and her colleagues at the University of Health Sciences "abhor this form of advertisement" and called for both the national and state osteopathic associations to take action against this type of activity.

On February 6, 1984, Dr. Marvin Meek, president of the American Osteopathic Association, wrote back. Although a copy of his letter was not contained in the files, it was mentioned in the next letter about Dr. McDonagh. On February 25, 1984, Dr. McDonagh appeared on a program called "Town Meeting" on Channel 9 in Kansas City, Missouri, to discuss chelation therapy. Dr. John Renner was on the same show as a noted critic of chelation therapy and rebutted Dr. McDonagh on the subject. Following the show, the same osteopath who complained in January sent another letter to the American Osteopathic Association to give an "update" on Dr. McDonagh's "embarrassing activities." The complainant pointed out Dr. McDonagh's defense of chelation therapy on the air, and his attempts to counter "the astute cross examination of John Renner, M.D." Once again the letter complained about how Dr. McDonagh was on a local radio station on a daily basis promoting chelation therapy in his paid advertisement.

The tirade in this letter goes on to strongly request that the American Osteopathic Association take a stand by submitting a radio announcement disassociating the AOA from chelation therapy. The writer goes so far as to state that "permanent damage is being done to our reputation which our forefathers had worked so hard to dispel." (Here she is talking about the founders of osteopathic medicine and its early organization which also came under the criticism of the AMA in its early days before they gave in to orthodox medicine.)

The Missouri State Osteopathic Association then wrote this D.O. and basically stated that its hands were tied with regard to chelation therapy, as the Supreme Court ruled that ethical codes restricting advertising are illegal. It appears that the State Association and the National Association of Osteopaths did not take a stand at this time against chelation therapy.

There were no complaints against Dr. McDonagh's practice and nothing in the files indicated that they took any actions against his license or right to practice, even though he was continuing his practice of chelation therapy.

A very successful tactic that has been used around the country against targeted practitioners has been to attack them in the media. A devastating article in the press can often do more damage to a practitioner's business than an actual court battle. The FDA knows this and those involved in this anti-competitive campaign are also well aware of what they can do to someone's practice with well-placed articles. This was to be the next phase of the attack against Dr. McDonagh.

The attack against Dr. McDonagh took on the color of a propaganda campaign. Dr. McDonagh and chelation therapy received national press when, on September 4, 1984, *The New York Times* ran an article on both. The article highlighted McDonagh's clinic and quoted Dr. John Renner as stating that it was his opinion as a spokesman for the Kansas City Committee Against Nutritional Fraud and Abuse that "chelation therapy has no medical value and is dangerous because it delays people seeking conventional treatments." He added, "People are being grossly ripped off by this chelation therapy business."

On November 16, 1984, the FDA sent out a survey letter regarding chelation therapy to all commissioners and directors of state health departments. The letter came from the Division of Federal-State Relations, Office of Regulatory Affairs, in Rockville, Maryland. (This is the office from which the health fraud unit was later run and where the FDA eventually housed the Health Fraud Tracking Computer System, after it was moved from its Kansas City, Missouri FDA office where it got its start.) The survey asked six questions related to chelation therapy, including these two:

Does the State have any reports of injury or death associated with the practice of chelation therapy?

Are State officials aware of proposals for reimbursements by "third party payers" for chelation therapy or any special tax allowance?

This letter showed up in the Board files, as well as at the State Health Department and the local office of the FDA in Kansas City, Missouri.

In the meantime, the media blitz against chelation therapy, and specifically Dr. McDonagh, continued. On December 9, 1984, two days after the Kansas Board met with the chelation therapists, an article appeared in the Des Moines *Register*. The article quoted Dr. John Renner, as head of the Kansas City Committee Against Nutritional and Health Fraud Abuse, directing his statements against Dr. McDonagh, his clinic and chelation therapy.

On December 18, 1984, the head of the Missouri Association of Osteopathic Physicians replied to the Missouri Division of Health's letter and the FDA's survey questions on chelation therapy. The letter stated that: (1) the association's office was aware that several physicians in Missouri were using chelation therapy; (2) they had received no reports of injury, deaths, or complaints of dissatisfaction from individual patients; (3) they were not aware of any malpractice suits in Missouri regarding chelation therapy; (4) patients had said that third party carriers have not provided coverage for expenses incurred with chelation therapy but have received indication that Medicare Part B carriers in other states have provided coverage; and (5) their office receives inquiries from potential patients, as well as current patients, and complaints from licensed physicians about chelation therapy. They also enclosed some literature about chelation therapy and sent this to the Health Department.

Another article appeared in a magazine on May 30, 1985, quoting Dr. John Renner on chelation therapy. In this article he was asked, "What do you tell a candidate for bypass surgery who wants to undertake chelation therapy instead?" Dr. Renner stated, "First, don't get angry when trying to dissuade the patient." The article included the usual anti-chelation therapy statements.

In an article in a Kansas City local newspaper, Dr. Renner said that as part of his operation against health fraud and quackery he runs "sting operations." He said his people "pose as gullible patients to gather information about quacks." This article ran on September 19, 1985, just a few days after the kick-off of PAC/FDA Anti-Quackery Campaign, at which Dr. Renner was a key speaker, was officially kicked off in Washington, D.C..

Apparently as part of a campaign against chelation therapy, and following the Kansas Board's position on chelation therapy, the Missouri State Board of Registration issued a five-page position statement on the use of EDTA chelation therapy on September 21, 1985. The statement basically denounced the use of chelation therapy for anything outside the use for which the FDA approved it. The statement also announced that it was contemplating state regulations to limit the use of chelation therapy in Missouri.

About three weeks later, a Kansas City newspaper ran an article on "health quackery" which extensively quoted Dr. Renner on the subject. Again, Dr. Renner disclosed in this article that he was involved in running undercover work in gathering up information on "quacks" in Missouri and Kansas. He stated that he uses the information he gathers to pass on to the Kansas and Missouri Healing Arts Boards.

A week later another article appeared in the same newspaper in the form of a weekly column by Dr. Renner called "Health Bulletin." In this article Dr. Renner once again denounced chelation therapy, using quotes from orthodox medical groups on the subject. Although he didn't single out Dr. McDonagh's practice or clinic in this article, according to Dr. McDonagh, it still had a direct economic impact on his practice at that time.

Two days later, on October 22, 1985, the Kansas City newspaper ran its own article on chelation therapy which included the usual propaganda against it. In the name of "balancing the article," it also included favorable quotes on chelation therapy from Dr. Charles Rudolph, an associate of Dr. McDonagh at his clinic. This article on chelation therapy preceded the November 7, 1985, Tumor Conference in Kansas City, Missouri, at which Dr. Renner was a key speaker.

During this whole period of time, there was not one single complaint filed against any chelation therapists by any patients of Dr. McDonagh's. However, he did lose patients as a result of this propaganda campaign against him and chelation therapy. He also had patients being denied payments or reimbursements for chelation therapy from insurance carriers during this period.

Paralleling the media campaign against chelation therapy and Dr. McDonagh, which appears to have its roots in the PAC/FDA campaign, the insurance industry also entered into the picture.

In early 1986, one of Dr. McDonagh's patients from South Dakota sent in a request for payment to the Farmland Insurance company in Des Moines, Iowa. His claim was denied, and the letter he received from the insurance company stated that his policy stated that major medical expenses would be covered only for the usual and customary expenses for coronary artery disease. They stated, "Since the treatment is not recognized by the American Medical Association or the federal FDA as medical treatment for your condition, we cannot consider it as usual or customary treatment."

The obvious contradiction in this denial letter is the statement that the policy "will cover the usual and customary expenses." What the Life and Health Claims Administrator said in the letter dealt with "usual or customary treatment" which the policy did not state, according to their own letter to the patient.

In May 1986, the PAC/FDA Campaign took its show on the road and held another Conference on Quackery, this time in Kansas City, Missouri, sponsored by the FDA, the FTC, the U.S. Postal Service, the Better Business Bureau, and the Missouri Attorney General's office. Dr. Renner played a large role in this conference. He headed a panel which included officials from most of the these agencies. He also spoke on the subject "Suggestions for Forming a Local Group to Combat Health and Nutritional Fraud and Abuse." Also presented was a paper which was entitled "Estimated Wasted Dollars for Fraudulent Health Practices." In this paper, Renner stated, "Chelation therapy seems to be the fraudulent treatment today for heart disease, although nutritional supplementation and megavitamins are also used. Estimated dollars wasted yearly on fraudulent heart disease treatment is $3 billion."

Almost immediately after this conference, another article appeared in the Kansas City newspaper. Once again, Dr. Renner was quoted on chelation therapy. The article stated that the Missouri Board of Healing Arts was planning to take steps to prevent the practice of chelation therapy. Dr. Renner stated that chelation hasn't been accepted and that studies have not been conducted by "recognized research organizations." In essence, he said that any published research on the subject of chelation therapy (many such papers are positive) is not acceptable because "orthodox science/medicine" did not conduct these studies. In reality there is little hope that any "recognized research organizations" would ever publish a positive report on chelation therapy. Doctors of medicine and osteopathy who are involved in chelation have done their own studies and have gotten them published. Stating that no "recognized" body of organized medicine or science has ever done a positive study on chelation is apparently just another propaganda ploy to further invalidate this very workable therapy.

Because the American Medical Association controls all of the major medical journals, it is very unlikely that a positive report, article, or study would ever appear in any of their publications. Additionally, the likelihood of any such report being published in something like the *New England Journal of Medicine* is also highly unlikely, since these journals and medical publications are almost exclusively supported by drug advertising.

The bottom line is economics. In this regard, Dr. McDonagh's practice suffered a great deal. It isn't known exactly how much he lost over the years, but what is known is that the campaign succeeded to the degree that his practice was affected. Chelation therapists all over the country have come under similar attacks. Something must change. It's up to these practitioners and you to determine whether chelation therapy has a future in America.

Chapter 13

Naturopathy

"Naturopathy is a nature-cure hodge-podge with a decided antipathy to drugs. The teachers in their schools are untrained in, and antagonistic to, medical science."
[American Medical Association Report on Naturopathy.]

"This was obtained surreptitiously from the records in the [Atlanta] State Capitol here, and I would be unable to refer you to the source or to furnish you with a similar photostat..."
[Letter from Executive Director of the Medical Association of Georgia to head of Jackson Medical Society in Kansas City, Missouri, with attached confidential records on a naturopath.]

A Case Study: Georgia

To appreciate and understand what happened recently to naturopathic medicine, in Georgia and other states, one has to first take a look at what *naturopathy* actually means. Then one must look at the roots of organized medicine's campaign, spanning over forty years, against this harmless alternative modality. All this information is based on documentation obtained from inside the medical establishment in the course of undercover investigations in Georgia and Florida on naturopathy.

Naturopathic medicine is a primary health-care system emphasizing the curative power of nature, treating both acute and chronic illnesses in all age groups. Naturopathic physicians sometimes hold licenses as chiropractors, medical doctors, and osteopathic physicians. They work to restore and support the body's own healing ability using a variety of modalities including nutrition, herbal medicine, homeopathic medicine, and oriental medicine. They do not use drugs, radiation, or surgery and are very outspoken critics of orthodox medicine's efforts to suppress medical freedom. Naturopathic doctors are currently licensed in Alabama, Arizona,

Connecticut, Hawaii, Montana, Oregon, and Washington. Licensing is a process requiring a rigorous educational and internship program.

How the American Medical Association depicts naturopathic medicine is entirely different. In the book *The AMA and U.S. Health Policy Since 1940*, they were referred to as cultists or sectarians. The book described naturopathic practitioners as those who "did not employ drugs but relied on such natural elements as water, heat, and massage for the cure of disease." The AMA was instrumental in successfully rolling back licensing laws for naturopaths in many states as part of its campaign against holistic medicine.

Most of the actions that the AMA was involved with occurred at the turn of the century, as part of its campaign against "quackery" described in earlier chapters. From 1940 to 1963, it was very busy going after its competition, including naturopathy. According to file records from inside the medical camps, these actions were usually in the form of letters written from AMA officials to government officials and private groups, asking them to take actions against naturopaths based on AMA reports and letters and complaints the AMA said it received on the targeted subject.

Between 1944 and 1956, in Georgia and Chicago, the medical attacks against naturopathy were grouped with attacks against chiropractic, mainly because many naturopaths held dual licenses. In January 1944, the AMA's Bureau of Legal Medicine and Legislation wrote a report and analysis on schools of naturopathy, with the help of its Bureau of Propaganda.

The report said that the AMA perceived that what was being said about "chiropractic schools applies with equal or greater force to naturopathic institutions." The AMA's concern with these schools was that professionals who were teaching courses were "untrained in and antagonistic to medical science." Well, even to a casual observer, any system that approaches illness with a "natural" method would be both contrary to and in direct opposition to orthodox medicine. The AMA's position against naturopathic medicine is understandable. It represents a form of competition to drugs and surgery.

Once this 1944 report was completed, the AMA entered into a campaign against naturopathy in Tennessee. Using this report, it was able to make use of the local state medical society to influence state legislators. In 1947 it succeeded in outlawing naturopathy in Tennessee.

Just prior to the legislature passing laws against naturopaths, the medical interests were able to get their allies to hold a grand jury to investigate naturopaths in Tennessee. The findings of that grand jury included an indictment against naturopathy, stating that they were granting licenses to naturopaths after attendance at just one lecture on the subject. This resulted in many naturopaths moving out of Tennessee and setting up practice in Georgia. True or not, the indictment was then used as the basis for a nationwide campaign of propaganda against all naturopathy on a state-to-state basis calling for legislation to be passed against naturopathy.

The AMA conducted more studies between 1944-1950 on naturopathic practice laws in each state which licensed them. In 1950, Georgia enacted a law which created the Georgia State Board of Naturopathic Examiners. Despite the protest and campaign of the Medical Association of Georgia (MAG), the bill passed in the Senate by a margin of 28 to 18 and the House passed it 104-23. Even though the medical interests could not get the Governor to veto the bill, he did state, "If the conduct of the members who practice naturopathy in this state is not in accord with the Act passed by the General Assembly, I shall do my utmost to repeal the Act in its entirety." Whether he said this to appease his allies in medicine or not isn't clear. What is clear is that this eventually happened.

The year 1950 was a good one and a bad one for naturopathy in Georgia. That year, the AMA in Chicago conducted a major campaign behind the scenes to go after a naturopathic practitioner in the Chicago area. This naturopath was attacked in newspaper articles influenced by the AMA, resulting in prosecutors charging him with 17 counts of practicing medicine without a license. In March 1950, the naturopath pleaded guilty to 10 of the 17 charges.

In the summer of 1951 he appeared on the doorstep of the Naturopathic Board of Examiners seeking a license to practice in Georgia. In the process he deliberately withheld from Board members the fact of his conviction in Chicago. He may have submitted false information on a state form for licensure to the Naturopathic Examination Board in order to deliberately hide his past.

It wasn't 18 months after he set his practice up that he brought the Attorney General down on his practice, thus putting all of naturopathy in the media and bringing it to the attention of the governor and the legislature. It started with a complaint sent to the Better Business Bureau by the son of one of his patients in February 1953. The BBB then sent two undercover agents into this doctor's office to gather information and evidence of wrong-doing. In turn they passed this information over to the Attorney General, who began an investigation.

The first thing he did was to write the Attorney General in Illinois, in April 1953, whereupon he became aware of the Georgia naturopath's earlier convictions and troubles. On May 7, 1953, the Georgia Naturopathic Examiners met, the Board held a hearing and declared that the naturopath's license was issued illegally by reason of fraud, and they apparently withdrew his license.

However, he continued to practice in the state without approval of the Naturopathic Examiners. He performed an abortion on one of his own assistants, resulting in hemorrhage, and she died of complications. This was the straw that broke the camel's back. The result was the end of naturopathy in Georgia as a single licensing board.

This, expectedly, brought the entire medical establishment down on *all of naturopathy* in the state. The officials of the Medical Association of Georgia didn't waste any time in lining up their allies in the Better Business Bureau, the Georgia Heart Association, the Cancer Society, and the Attorney General's office to begin their campaign to repeal the 1950 Act. In that way they erased naturopathy from the state of Georgia. At the time, there were 82 naturopaths licensed in the state, with 52 actively practicing in Georgia. (Today there are fewer than 10.)

The executive director of MAG began his campaign by writing to medical doctors around the state directing them to gather up as much data as possible about any naturopath operating in their areas. Once MAG had this data in hand, the names of every naturopath in Georgia was sent to AMA headquarters with a request for data on any of these people or the schools they had attended. The AMA responded by sending MAG articles, reports, and information that could be used in the campaign against naturopathy in Georgia. They enlisted the BBB to issue a resolution announcing its intention to fight naturopathy, which was published in November 1955. In December 1955, with the legislative session scheduled to start in January, MAG started contacting its allies at the State Capitol, readying them for the coming campaign. Using "key medical doctors" with close contacts in the Capitol, MAG effectively influenced someone in the Bill Drafting Unit of the Georgia House to review the earlier 1950 Act. This medical ally reviewed the 1950 Act, wrote his opinion, and sent it to the MAG executive stating that the Bill was possibly unconstitutional.

The MAG official wrote an ally at a local law firm. He sought the opinion of an attorney who was also a state legislator. This attorney reviewed the Bill and also stated that it was "passed illegally" and could be "attacked on Constitutional grounds."

What the medical interests apparently did then was to contact their allies in the Capitol. A grand jury was called, to investigate not just the one naturopath who had caused the trouble, but all of naturopathy. During November and December 1955, the grand jury met and recommended that the Georgia General Assembly introduce and support legislation to repeal the 1950 Naturopathy Act.

The grand jury's report was published on January 2, 1956, just before the legislature went into session. It appears that the sole purpose of this maneuver was to manipulate the legislature against naturopathy. This appeared to be a conspiracy directed against naturopathy, with the medical interests working behind the scenes to set it all up.

The medical association then contacted the AMA and had Oliver Field, of the AMA Bureau of Investigation, send everything the AMA had that could be used in the coming session. Field sent them a 17-page outline of everything the AMA had on naturopathy. He expressed his concern that this information reach MAG in time to be used for "any presentation before legislative committees." The data got to MAG on January 20, 1956, just days before the hearings.

Hearings on the 1950 Naturopathy Act were set for January 26, 1956. MAG officials wrote every medical doctor in Georgia to get them to participate in MAG's efforts to pass their House Bill which would repeal the Naturopathy Act of 1950.

It didn't take long. On February 10, 1956, the Governor signed into law House Bill 121, and the naturopaths no longer had their own board of examiners. In effect, they then came under the watchful eyes of their medical competition and adversaries. They were put under the Board of Medical Examiners, which was totally controlled by MAG member M.D.s.

Behind the scenes, the executive director of MAG worked to obtain control of, and/or copies of, all the Board of Naturopath's files on every practitioner they had licensed. He then wrote Oliver Field of the AMA, telling him his plans to obtain these files, which, he said, he knew would "be of invaluable use in [Field's] office."

The MAG official took the list of all naturopaths in the state and sent them to the Solicitor General, along with a copy of House Bill 121 which was now law. He told the Solicitor General that after having called several naturopaths himself he had determined that "they seemed to be still doing business as usual." This move was to influence action by the Attorney General's office against naturopaths. On February 29, 1956, the A.G. issued an opinion on

House Bill 121, stating that any violation of this law falls within the criminal courts to handle.

Other states were also influenced by the Georgia action against naturopathy. The Ohio State Medical Association wrote MAG asking for any information it could pass on which could be used to promote repealing the Ohio naturopathic law.

It appears that all of this was being coordinated by the AMA in Chicago, which was collecting data from Georgia and sending it on to other state medical associations, encouraging them to contact MAG in Georgia so as to get similar actions going in their own states.

Oliver Field wrote MAG and reported to them that South Carolina had passed a law against the naturopaths. MAG officials then got onto Florida and sent the medical association there information on the successes they had in Georgia.

On February 23, 1956, the MAG executive director wrote Field at the AMA and said he wished to thank him for the assistance in the campaign to repeal the Naturopath Law. He said, "You certainly had a world of information, and I was able to use some of it at the public hearing."

During March 1956, the covert campaign against naturopathy continued. Some of what was going on behind the scenes surfaced in a letter dated March 13, 1956, from the Director of the Crime Laboratory, Department of Public Safety, State of Georgia, to the Executive Director of MAG. In his letter, the Crime Lab Director stated that he felt that perhaps they didn't make the Naturopath Law quite strong enough and that perhaps some county "will make a test case out of it and clear the situation."

The director stated that he had contacted the Solicitor General on Saturday afternoon, apparently at his home, to discuss the matter of a test case with him. He identified the significance of this conversation with the Solicitor General:

> He stated he was just as much in favor of making a test case on this law as we were, however, he feels that we will have to have definite evidence. It is his opinion that you and members of the medical profession should be on the look-out for evidence that would be worthy of a test case.

This amounts to a conspiracy against naturopathy. Here we see the director of the crime lab stating that the Solicitor General was "as much in favor of making a test case on this law as we were." This would certainly appear to mean that the MAG official and the Director had already discussed and decided that they needed to get a test case to test this new law.

According to the MAG files, they didn't get a test case until 1960. Once again, it was a naturopath doing the work for the medical interests, whether by choice or not. This time a naturopath was charged with prescribing narcotic drugs to patients. He had allegedly obtained the substances from over 120 drug companies under the pretense of being a licensed medical doctor.

Like any practitioner charged with wrongdoing, that physician does not represent all of his/her profession, and is innocent until proven guilty. Quickly, MAG jumped at this opportunity for a test case with its allies in government so as to use it as an instrument to indict all of naturopathy.

The naturopath was indicted for a misdemeanor, after which the Solicitor General obtained copies of the court transcript and sent it to the secretary of MAG. The secretary wrote the Solicitor General and suggested that he get in touch with MAG's attorney, who might have some suggestions and comments on the strategy of the case against this naturopath.

The two talked, and the MAG attorney did in fact provide the Solicitor General with information and suggested strategy that "should certainly fortify" the Solicitor General's brief in the case against the naturopath.

MAG then proceeded to line up its ducks against naturopathy and for the Solicitor General's case against the practitioner. It requested that a professor of pharmacology at the Medical School of Georgia study and analyze the substances used by the naturopath so as to make a statement that these were in fact drugs. The strategy was to use this analysis and professional opinion in the case when the naturopath moved for for acquittal notwithstanding the verdict. Furthermore, MAG lawyers worked out a strategy wherein if it appeared that the state might lose on the motion, then they could "certainly help the Solicitor General by providing qualified expert evidence on this point."

The reference to getting "expert evidence" apparently referred to getting the professor to testify as an expert witness that the substances used were narcotic drugs, thus reinforcing MAG's campaign against all of naturopathy.

In an April 19, 1960, letter from the MAG attorney to the Solicitor General regarding the professor's analysis, the lawyer stated, "We trust this letter will be of service to you in preparing your brief for presentation to the Judge when he considers [the naturopath's] motion. . ."

All of this behind-the-scenes activity on the part of MAG officials and their attorney was not simply a case of them filing an Amicus (friend of the court) Brief to support the state's case against naturopathy. It was in fact an attempt to influence the outcome of a trial and a court decision against their competition. . .naturopathy. The MAG attorney continued, "If we can be of further service, please do not hesitate to call on us. If the case should have to be tried again, I believe we can obtain [the professor of pharmacy's] services as an expert witness. . ."

In the end, however, the naturopath won the case. The Solicitor General wrote the MAG officials on July 1, 1960, and stated that the judge denied a motion for a new trial and that the state would appeal the decision. According to file records, this never went the way the state wanted it to. Once again MAG's efforts to totally rid Georgia of naturopathy failed. But the failure didn't stop them.

Once the 1960 naturopath's case was laid to rest, MAG worked behind the scenes to get other allies in government involved against naturopathy. In June 1961, MAG turned over all of its files on naturopathy to the federal Food and Drug Administration. Apparently the FDA was conducting an investigation into the same naturopath the state had indicted. This type of cooperation between the FDA and the medical interests of the AMA and its members has continued up to the present time. However, coincidentally or not, 1961 was the same year that the AMA formed an alliance with the FDA, the FTC, and the U.S. Postal Service to combat quackery. This was the first year they jointly sponsored their Congress on Quackery, the forerunner of today's Conferences on Health Fraud.

At any rate, the naturopath began to have troubles now with the FDA, with the help of MAG. There was nothing in the files to indicate the outcome of these problems. What is known is that the medical association cooperated fully with the FDA and may very well have influenced the FDA to go after the naturopath to begin with. The absence of any FDA follow-up data in MAG files would seem to indicate that the FDA had no success against the naturopath.

The records kept by MAG on "quackery," naturopathy included, contain nothing more on any of its activities from the point that its efforts to "get" naturopathy failed in 1960 up through early 1980. That does not mean it wasn't active against its competition over those twenty years. It simply means the information was not there to obtain, and there is an explanation for this absence of data.

It seems that the chiropractors' 1975 lawsuit against the AMA (*Wilk v. AMA*) put the medical establishment on the alert and on the defensive. Apparently the AMA sent out a memorandum to all of its state and county medical associations and societies that they should cease any collection of records, recording of minutes of meetings, and memoranda so that these could not be used against them in any antitrust lawsuits by the chiropractors or others.

The Fulton County Medical Society and the Medical Association of Georgia, for example, both purged their files of any data that could possibly implicate them in antitrust, anti-competitive charges. The years that were missing from the file records were 1961-1975. These also happened to be the most active years of organized medicine's anti-competitive campaign against their competition. These were the years that such activities constituted violations of federal laws for which they were sued. However, the minutes of the CCHI were obtained in full for every meeting ever held during the years 1963-1975. These minutes make it obvious that the AMA didn't stop its national campaign even at the state level.

Between 1961 and 1965 in Georgia, the only major event related to naturopathy that occurred was that on November 11, 1965, the Georgia Attorney General issued an official opinion that naturopaths could not do any obstetrical work, and that no naturopath could practice who was not licensed prior to 1956. It appears that the medical interests had a hand in this opinion. Such a opinion would result in the profession dying on the vine, with no new naturopaths being issued licenses from this point forward.

Keeping in mind that many of the naturopaths who were issued licenses were also chiropractors, and that the medical establishment treated naturopathy and chiropractic as the same, the tactics used against each stemmed from strategies developed by the AMA to eliminate both from the health-care system.

This strategy is best summarized in a memo written by Robert Youngerman to Doyl Taylor, head of the AMA's Department of Investigation, regarding chiropractic (but also applied to naturopathy). He stated:

> The Committee (on Quackery) agreed that State Medical Societies' activity to encourage legislation rescinding State Chiropractic Licensing Laws should be held in abeyance until more information is obtained in regard to implementation of Section 141 [Social Security coverage of chiropractic services] previously mentioned.

On the other hand, the Committee still adheres to the basic policy that chiropractic licensure should be made so difficult that eventually more chiropractors are dying than new chiropractic licenses are granted. This would create the situation of a "profession withering on the vine" and dying an eventual death.

This was the exact strategy that MAG used on naturopaths, many of whom were also chiropractors, making it more difficult for them "to either become licensed or to continue practicing in the State" as Youngerman stated.

From 1965 forward, all of naturopathy in Georgia was affected by this opinion, although not very much was going on up until 1981 or so. Since the naturopaths did not have their own board of examiners (as a result of the 1956 conspiracy to repeal the 1950 Act), they decided to create their own private board.

In 1981 they formed a corporation whose purpose was to issue licenses to naturopaths. They called themselves The Georgia State Board of Naturopathic Examiners and Registrars, Inc. Their stated purposes included creating a system to better regulate the practice of naturopathy in Georgia, including issuing licenses. This non-profit corporation went along doing just that until it was noticed by the medical association, the Attorney General, and the Board of Medical Examiners.

Just prior to the forming of the corporation, the Director of Student Services at the National College of Naturopathic Medicine in Portland, Oregon, sent out a letter to the Georgia State Health Department. Her October 1980 letter asked if the state had any prohibitions on naturopaths wishing to practice in Georgia. She also asked about any pending legislation that would affect the future of the profession in Georgia.

No sooner was this letter received than it was sent over to the Joint Secretary of the State Examining Board, who then passed it down the line to the Executive Director of the State Board of Medical Examiners. A little more than nine months later, the Director of the Medical Examining Board was made aware of the new naturopathic corporation. On July 22, 1981, three weeks after the naturopaths published the public notice announcing the formation of their corporation, the Board director wrote the Attorney General's office about the notice. He asked the Assistant Attorney General to take "appropriate action on behalf of the State to request an injunction against this business. . ." He called what the naturopaths had published "deceptive advertising" and sent a copy of his letter to a member of the medical association.

In November 1981, he followed up with a letter asking the AG for a written opinion based on the information he sent. There was no action, so in December 1981 he wrote again. This time he claimed he was "getting increasing numbers of calls from the public inquiring about the legal status of these people."

It is of interest and importance to understand the relationship between the head of the Board of Medical Examiners and the medical association. The lobbyist for MAG had worked very closely with the Director of the Board on many occasions on key pieces of legislation. One piece was a proposed bill to take the Medical Board out from under the control of the Composite Board so that they could have their own board and therefore be free to solicit their own financing from the state legislature.

On this occasion, the MAG lobbyist met with the head of the Medical Board in the hallway of the legislature. Together they huddled over the proposed draft of the bill, out of sight of those who might see them. This little spectacle took place just outside, and down the hall from, the Medical Association of Georgia's office in the heart of the Capitol building. (Note: Just as a point of interest, the MAG office in the Capitol was a central point from which free pharmaceutical drugs were dispensed to legislators who came into the office with various ills, pains or other ailments requiring remedies. A most unusual arrangement to say the least, a pharmacy which amounted to a bizarre and brazen PR move on the part of MAG to influence state legislators.)

This little meeting of the medical interests with the Director of the Medical Board wasn't something that either one wanted publicly known. It would have created a scandal, shedding bad light on several political moves that were being planned behind the scenes at the time involving the head of the Composite Board of Examiners (who was over every licensed profession in the State, from hair dressers to plumbers to medical doctors).

At any rate, the naturopaths inspired another campaign against themselves by forming their own private corporation/board to issue licenses. Nothing came out of all of this until March 1982. After more requests for action from the Director of the Medical Board to the Attorney General, the A.G. published an official opinion on the issue of naturopathy which the medical people had been pushing him to do. The opinion, which was later challenged, basically stated that naturopathy was in fact the practice of medicine. Since there was no board of examiners specifically set up for naturopaths, they came under the direction and control of the Medical Examiners Board. The exception to this was anyone who had received a license prior to 1956.

The Board Director sent a copy of the A.G.'s opinion to every member of the Board, stating, "This item (naturopathy) would be on the agenda for the April Board meeting. . ."

Once the A.G.'s opinion was published, it drew a strong protest from naturopaths, their patients, and students of naturopathy. Letters of protest bombarded the Capitol, and legislators from all over the state heard the cry of injustice. The letters were routed to the head of the Composite Board of Examiners for reply. He, in turn, sent the letters over to the Director of the Medical Examiners Board for reply and comments. The Director simply reiterated the A.G.'s opinion that practicing naturopathy was against the law unless one was licensed prior to 1956. He stated in his letter: "Hence, until the law is changed, we must continue to refer violations to the appropriate local prosecutors."

Note that the opinion of the State Composite Board, the Attorney General's office, and the private medical interests (MAG), that practicing naturopathy was illegal, all hung on the 1956 repeal of the 1950 Naturopathy Examiners Board Act. However, there is a distinct possibly that the 1956 Repeal Act was passed as a result of an illegal conspiracy and the manipulation of the grand jury which recommended the repeal of the 1950 Act. This being the case, any legislation that passed was legally a sham.

In antitrust law, under the Noerr Doctrine, "lobbying activities are not illegal, even if undertaken for anti-competitive purposes." This is based on the constitutional right to petition, and this right to petition is also extended to influencing administrative agencies and the courts. However, there are limitations in the law regarding such activities. For example, there may be situations in which an "attempt to influence government action"' is nothing more than "harassment of a competitor or a mere sham," and, in such cases, the courts might find an unlawful combination or conspiracy in restraint of trade. The point in the antitrust law that dictates whether such attempts are illegal is whether or not these attempts were made to interfere directly with the business relationships of a competitor. If so, these actions would be actionable under the antitrust laws.

It appears in this case that the medical interests did in fact attempt to influence government agencies against their competition. Additionally, these attempts to influence were for the purpose of interfering directly with the business of a competitor. It was designed not only to interfere with the business of naturopaths, but also to place the competition directly under their own control by placing them under the Medical Board. Once the Naturopathy Board was abolished, that is what did happen.

Further interfering in the business of naturopathy, the head of the Medical Board sent a copy of the A.G.'s opinion to the phone company in an attempt to prevent naturopaths from advertising in the yellow pages ever again.

The head of the Medical Board was involved in a cover-up of behind-the-scenes actions against naturopaths by the state and the legislature. In a letter dated April 20, 1982, to one of the most outspoken consumer advocates in the country, living in the Atlanta area, the Director stated the following: "First, I am not sure that there is error which is due to legislative action in 1956. . .it appears that the Naturopathic Board was deliberately terminated, as was done in a number of States." He also stated, "Our legislation had no such language [a grandfather clause], and this was the reason a clarification of the law was sought." What the Director failed to reveal and disclose to the recipient of his letter was:

(1) The "deliberate termination" of the Naturopathic Board was as a direct result of a major campaign designed and carried out by officials of the medical association and their allies in the Health Department and the Solicitor General's office. It was apparently their behind-closed-door maneuvers that resulted in a grand jury being called to begin with, and the follow-up campaign to repeal the 1950 Act which was carried out in 1956.

(2) The efforts that apparently went on behind the scenes between MAG, the Solicitor General, and the Public Safety (Health) Department to "make a test case out of it and clear the situation," back in 1956.

(3) It was the fact that the naturopaths had found a loophole in the law and had set up their own private corporation, creating their own Naturopathic Board of Examiners, that sparked off the current opinion.

The Director further stated in the letter, "We are only empowered to do those things which we are specifically authorized to do pursuant to the Georgia Code." The question is then presented. . .Was the Director over-stepping his authority when he pursued a covert attempt to influence the phone company into not accepting advertising from naturopaths in the yellow pages? Or was that something the Board was empowered and authorized to do by law?

His next statement makes some very obvious contradictions about naturopathy and the state's role. He said: ". . .neither this Board or any other state agency can take on the task of determining who is qualified and who is not qualified to practice Naturopathy when the law does not specifically authorize the practice nor does it specifically authorize a state agency to do such screening."

Note his words: . .neither the Board nor any other State Board has such authority over Naturopaths. This statement is contradicted by the actions the Director took against naturopathy when he wrote the Assistant Attorney General asking him to issue an injunction against the naturopaths.

The Director ended his letter to the consumer advocate for alternative medicine by stating that he couldn't "bend the rules" and added, "However, this Board is not making any special effort concerning the practice of Naturopathy."

This last statement is anything but the truth in light of the actions that the Director did take. These include: (a) calling for an injunction against Naturopaths regarding their advertising and private corporation, (b) calling for a Special Meeting of the Board to review naturopathy, (c) unduly influencing the phone company against accepting naturopaths ads in the yellow pages, and (d) reporting to the Attorney General that the Board was "receiving increasing calls from the public" about the legal status of naturopathy, resulting in the AG issuing his Opinion putting Naturopathy under the control of the Medical Board.

There definitely appears to be a coverup of what really happened behind the scenes against naturopathy involving the Director of the Board of Medical Examines and others. Evidence exists which shows the plan to adversely influence the trade and business of naturopathy.

Three months after the A.G.'s opinion was issued, on June 18, 1982, the non-profit corporation of naturopaths filed suit against the Attorney General, the Solicitor General of Cobb County, and the Medical Board in Federal District Court.

On June 22, 1982, the Attorney General wrote a memo to the Director of the Medical Board outlining the suit. In this confidential communication ("attorney-client privileged") letter, the A.G. stated that if the Director had any questions to call him, and that he could share this information with the Board members.

On the same day that the naturopaths filed their suit, a woman who worked for the state filed an affidavit regarding an undercover infiltration of a naturopath's clinic in the Atlanta area. The affidavit showed that this "undercover agent" had visited the naturopathic clinic back in October 1980, at the time that the state had received a letter from the Naturopathic College in Portland, Oregon.

The naturopaths' law suit was dismissed on August 4, 1982, for failing to meet the prerequisite of presenting a substantial federal question for the court to address. In other words, it wasn't a matter for the federal courts to decide.

The attorney for the naturopaths was successful in getting an injunction against any actions directed at the naturopaths pending a decision by the Federal Appeals Court. The August 1982 stay from the Court was in effect until a final decision was reached by the Courts.

In the meantime, the state managed to get a report on naturopathy written by an assistant professor of *history* from Southern Technical Institute. The report was labeled "Eyes only" and the author told the Director of the Medical Board that it could be sent to other members of the board. The Director then wrote a letter, dated December 6, 1982, to the Assistant Attorney General with a copy of the history professor's report on naturopathy.

It is of interest to note here that *after* the head of the Composite Board of Examiners worked with the Director of the Medical Board (who was junior to him) to pressure the A.G. into issuing an opinion against naturopathy, the Composite Board Joint Secretary went on to become the Executive Director of the Medical Association of Georgia.

In January 1983, the new, but temporary, Joint Secretary of the Composite Board of Examiners requested a summary of the files on naturopathy from the Director of the Medical Board. With the new legislative year starting up, it appears that more activity was being planned against naturopathy. The Director sent the files and stated in his cover letter, "The Board received numerous inquiries about the legal status of naturopaths."

He didn't say whether or not those "numerous inquiries" were made by members of MAG as part of a campaign against naturopathy. This is a tactic the medical people had used in the past. He added that, as a result of board investigations of complaints, it was evident that certain people were practicing naturopathy without a license. No patient complaints against any naturopaths, however, were to be found in their files.

A form of deceit through omission has played a role throughout this campaign by the medical interests against naturopathy. Whether by omitting information or masking true intention or covering up behind-the-scenes activity, manipulation, and adverse influence, all of the actions directed against naturopaths have had the color of conspiracy.

Another example of this was contained in a March 2, 1983, memorandum from the Executive Director of the Medical Board and the President of the Board to the MAG lobbyist regarding naturopathy. The lobbyist had requested a summary of all actions taken by the Board related to naturopathy, along with their position on naturopathy. In the memo, the Board stated, "It would appear that if a clarification (of the naturopathic issue) is needed, it would certainly be helpful to get one from the Georgia General Assembly. . .The General Assembly repealed the Naturopathic Examining Board in 1956, partially in response to a presentment of the Fulton County Grand Jury."

This was not entirely true; some behind-the-scenes manipulation was going on at that time by the medical interests, which apparently included calling a grand jury as part of the anti-naturopathy campaign launched by MAG.

The Director's memo also referred to other factors going on at that time: "At the same time, other legislative bodies were repealing similar naturopathic laws. This was done in Florida at the same time. . ."

He neglected to say that the Medical Association of Georgia, working with the American Medical Association in Chicago, which was coordinating actions on a state-to-state level, had been involved in influencing actions in Florida against naturopathy. Arizona, Missouri, Ohio, Utah, and Florida had all contacted officials of MAG and asked for its "blueprint" for repealing naturopathic laws in their states based on the success MAG had in Georgia. This was all coordinated by the AMA, which encouraged other state medical association executives to contact officials at MAG at that time.

This wasn't "something that just happened." It was a campaign—thought up, coordinated, and executed by medical interests against their competition. The campaign's purpose was to generate the appearance that the public was interested in clarifying the question of the legal status of naturopathy, when in fact it was the medical interests creating and stirring up the interest. The result was to pressure the Attorney General into issuing an opinion based on the interests of the medical establishment in Georgia.

Once again, the medical establishment moved to enact legislation against naturopaths in Georgia, this time in the form of Senate Bill 212. The Director of the Medical Board, along with executives from MAG, felt that this bill would further "clarify" the naturopathic issue. While the bill was still on the Governor's desk for his signature, the medical interests apparently got a friendly reporter to do an article slanted against naturopathy. The article appeared on April 8, 1983, and included statements from the Executive Director of the Medical Association which were inaccurate and deliberately omitted important facts about the anti-naturopathic campaign going back to 1950 and 1956. For example, he was quoted in the article as saying, "The fact that naturopaths were even licensed in the first place was the result of strong politicking and a close vote of the General Assembly."

This is simply not true. In passing the bill, the General Assembly vote was 104-23, and the Senate voted affirmatively 28-18. There was no "close vote" in either legislative house back in 1950.

Another point in the article that omitted important data was a statement attributed to the MAG official, who stated, ". . .the big push for naturopaths in Georgia came after South Carolina and Tennessee clamped down on their practices." Yes, Tennessee had a Grand Jury going in 1947, and it led to laws against naturopathy. Yes, South Carolina passed a law repealing its act, which Georgia used in their State. What was omitted was the fact that it was *the AMA* who was collecting data up from different states and then putting state executive directors from its medical societies into communication with each other for the purpose of coordinating the state-to-state anti-naturopathic push to either repeal already existing laws or to abolish the practice altogether.

What was also omitted was any information about what role the medical association had in both the grand jury of 1956 and the eventual repeal of the 1950 Act. Obviously missing from this article was any mention of an organized campaign by the medical interests against their competitors, the naturopaths.

The article was apparently timed to influence the state legislators when the Bill was being considered for passage into law. Once again, however, the naturopaths used their patients, students, and allies to write letters to the Capitol to defeat the bill, and in the end they won that small battle.

Following the Federal Court of Appeals decision in June 1983 against naturopathy, naturopaths took their case to the Supreme Court of the United States. On October 11, 1983, the U.S. Supreme

Court denied their petition to hear the case before the Court, thus upholding the lower court's ruling against the naturopaths.

Following this decision, Judge Charles Moye, Jr., lifted the injunction against the state that had prevented it from taking actions against naturopaths, opening the door for charges to be filed against naturopaths in the state.

It wasn't long after that the Attorney General's office wrote the Director of the Medical Board notifying him of the Supreme Court decision. It appears that the Board and the State Attorney General's office waited for their opportunity to strike; they didn't make any significant moves until November 1985, almost two years later. They sent a cease-and-desist order to a naturopath named Seneca Anderson. Anderson responded by filing a suit against MAG, the Board, and others involved against naturopathy. The medical interests moved to dismiss the case against them. In the meantime, the naturopath's attorney fell ill and couldn't make the deadline of answering the Motion for Dismissal within the 10 days allowed by law. So the case was dismissed on May 6, 1986.

The attorney responded with a motion to keep the case going based on his illness. In a final ruling on September 19, 1986, the Court ruled to stay the dismissal. But this wasn't the end. The state moved to recover court costs, and on October 15, 1987, after motions and appeals, the naturopath had to pay $2,256.17 in fees and costs pending the ruling of the appeals court.

To his credit, Anderson persisted in fighting for his right to practice naturopathy. He appealed and the appeals court sent his original case back down to the lower state court to be reheard. The lower court in DeKalb County ruled that Seneca Anderson could practice as a naturopath under the supervision of either a medical doctor, a doctor of osteopathy, or a chiropractor. This was a tremendous win for all of naturopathy in the state, because it opened the door for others to practice naturopathy untouched by the medical interests or the state.

The troubles against naturopaths have not ended. In the last six months of 1993, the State Medical Board and the Attorney General came after three other naturopaths. One simply moved to DeKalb County, where, according to the Court ruling, a naturopath could practice under supervision. The other two naturopaths are still undergoing attack at this writing. One is a naturopath who was devastated by charges brought against him, and the other is fighting back in the courts. Both are in communication with people who can help them, and hopefully they will prevail.

Chapter 14

Acupuncture and Holistic Dentistry

"The new report calls acupuncture 'unproven, based on primitive concepts that are totally out of step with present scientific knowledge.'"
[National Council Against Health Fraud's Position Paper on Acupuncture, 1991]

"Acupuncturists should tell patients the treatment is experimental and has not been proven."
[Dr. Dean Edell, January 25, 1991, KGO-TV, San Francisco.]

Acupuncture

Acupuncture is not new to the health-care system. It has been around for almost 5,000 years. Its proving grounds were in ancient China, in an environment that accepted it as a workable system. Today it is even used to replace pre-operation drugs given by anesthesiologists in the Orient and in the United States and other Western countries. Such a practice is not received with open arms by the pharmaceutical companies who make the drugs or by the medical doctors who administer them in the operating room.

Acupuncture as an alternative health-care system came under fire early on after it was introduced in this country. It wasn't long after it first became popular in the U.S. in the 1970s that federal courts were reviewing cases involving its use in medicine. In one very famous case, (*Andrews v. Ballard*, 498 F. Supp., 1038 Southern District Federal Court, Houston Division, 1980) the judge made an astute observation about this practice. He said:

Acupuncture has been practiced from 2,000 to 5,000 years. It is no more experimental than is the Chinese language as a mode of communication. What is experimental is not acupuncture, but Westerns' understanding of it and their ability to use it properly.

Even with this federal court opinion on the books as law, the opponents to the alternatives have not let up on their attack. As early as 1973, only a few years after acupuncture came into use in the United States, the American Medical Association, working behind the scenes, directed the governmental members of the old Coordinating Conference on Health Information (CCHI) against acupuncture. (See Chapter 2.) The AMA reported in a later meeting that the FDA was successful in getting an injunction against the importation of acupuncture needles from Hong Kong. There was even a move on the part of the FDA to have acupuncture needles labeled.

The AMA's history of fighting the alternatives includes its stand against acupuncture. Although its early roots are back in the CCHI/AMA era, they continue today in this present campaign against the alternatives.

As outlined in Chapter 5, acupuncture was among the alternatives to be studied by panels of "experts," who included most of the spokesmen involved in the anti-quackery campaign who are also members of the National Council Against Health Fraud (NCAHF).

Informing the public, media, government agencies, and insurance companies about acupuncture is one of the activities of the NCAHF. Its May 1986 list of resource materials on health fraud and quackery listed several items on acupuncture:

> "Acupuncture Hoax Admitted." Author Earnshaw. *The Australian.* 10/26/80. . .
>
> "Acupuncture Treatments for Pain Relief." Author Ulett. *JAMA (Journal of the American Medical Association).* 2/20/81. . .
>
> "Statement Regarding Acupuncture." Medical Council, Academy of Sciences. 1982.

In June 1989, an article appeared in the medical magazine *Postgraduate Medicine,* entitled "The Health Fraud Battle: Education is the Best Defense." The article drew on information from the FDA, the FTC, the U.S. Postal Service, the AMA, the American Cancer Society, and the National Council Against Health Fraud. It described some of the "problems of health fraud" and how to "recognize health fraud." Among "health fraud" products and treatments it cited:

> ACUPRESSURE and SELF-ACUPUNCTURE—
> Acupressure and Self-Acupuncture devices are claimed to promote healing through application of pressure, needles, or

electric stimulation to an area of the body, such as the leg, which in turn cures migraines or digestive problems. Acupressure devices sometimes have magnets as their components, as in the case of insoles for the feet with specially designated sections to control health or well-being of other parts of the body.

Omitted is information regarding the history of the use of acupuncture needles in China and its validation as useful therapy by the federal courts in Texas. The other forms or devices mentioned are simply adaptations using modern Western technology. These variations are being applied to what is already known to work using ancient principles of acupuncture. Whether it's applying pressure or electrical impulses to the acupuncture points on the body, it all amounts to some form of acupuncture. All of these approaches are used in alternative medicine and with varying degrees of success.

This ancient approach to healing takes away from the sale of drugs, so it is understandable that the pharmaceutical companies would be involved in some way in attacking it. It is also understandable that medical doctors who make a living by drugging patients just prior to an operation would be on the defensive. Anesthesiologists are among the highest-paid medical specialties in the country.

An article published in *Minnesota Medicine* in June 1990, entitled "Patients Who Seek Unorthodox Medical Treatment," attacked acupuncture, along with a myriad of other alternative practices, as "health fraud or quackery." (The others included chiropractic, homeopathy, massage therapy, visualization, spiritual healing, and herbal medicine.) The article quoted William Jarvis, Ph.D., as saying:

". . .The modern medical model says that the mind is the body. . . There are a number of systems around today that are nothing more than mind-body dichotomies, from chiropractic, which manipulates the spine but insists it's treating the life force, to Chinese acupuncture. . .The notion of a mind-body connection goes back to the Greeks, who believed in an ethereal spirit that inhabits the body. I call that spook medicine."

The National Council Against Health Fraud's Position Paper on Acupuncture listed a variety of procedures used in acupuncture, including:

- Low-voltage current applied to needles (electroacupuncture), a relatively recent development...
- Manual pressure (acupressure)...
- "Touch for Health," developed by a chiropractor using acupressure points and an unreliable muscle-testing method (applied kinesiology). The therapist claims to diagnose nutritional and glandular "deficiencies" that are then "corrected" by manipulation or nutritional supplements.

For the most part, acupuncture is based on oriental principles and practice that have been used successfully for almost 5,000 years. Every state allows its use, and many insurance companies pay for its use. Traditional acupuncturists were for the most part Asian practitioners, although more and more Westerners are now involved in its use.

In every ethnic culture, there is some form of traditional medicine that has been passed down from one generation to another. Thus ancient practices have been brought into the 20th and 21st century. Such practices as African herbal medicine, Native American sweat lodges (detoxification and cleansing), Chinese herbs, and acupuncture are now a part of Western alternative health-care systems. They are not under the control of orthodox medicine, nor are they a part of the pharmaceutical industry. This doesn't mean that they are any less effective. Some would argue that because they are a part of ethnic medicine, rich in tradition and culture, they are irreplaceable. They are a part of the free-enterprise system in health-care and should be allowed to continue to exist as competitors of the drug industry. However, a very startling statement about "medical customs" of ethnic groups, made in the NCAHF's Position Paper on Acupuncture, appears to be at the least prejudicial and offensive:

> Every ethnic group has its own set of medical customs not supported by science. Some proponents argue that Asian populations should have access to their traditional remedies, however ineffective and unscientific they may be...
>
> Cultural activities are generally tolerated provided they do not conflict with laws for the general population and are not dangerous. Chaos would result if the populace could not be protected from misrepresentation, and if insurance companies were forced to pay for all traditional foreign methods.

One must understand that a person who believes that spiritual healing, or the presence of the spirit/soul, is nothing more than "spook medicine" could not possibly grasp how most alternative, or holistic, medicine works. Considering that most of science dismisses the presence of the spirit or soul such a statement is understandable. Is the statement bigoted? It stands on its own for the reader to decide.

Also in this Position Paper is the following statement regarding acupuncture and science:

> The World Health Organization has listed forty conditions for which claims of effectiveness have been made. They include acute and chronic pain, rheumatoid and osteo-arthritis, muscle and nerve "difficulties," depression, smoking, eating disorders, drug "behavior problems," migraine, acne, ulcers, cancer, and constipation. . .

The Paper goes on to state that "scientific evidence supporting these claims is either [dubious] [this word was apparently edited out of the Position Paper] or nonexistent." What they didn't state was whether or not the World Health organization position on acupuncture was positive or negative.

They also stated that all states allow it to be used, that practitioners can be licensed in 18 states, and that insurance companies pay for its use. Additionally, the American Academy of Medical Acupuncture of Berkeley, California, "sponsors courses for physicians given under the auspices of medical schools, including UCLA, Jefferson Medical College, and Temple University. The University of Hawaii also sponsors a course." Even though the Paper acknowledged all of these facts, it went on to say in its recommendations:

> The National Council Against Health Fraud believes that after more than twenty years in the court of scientific opinion, acupuncture has not been demonstrated effective for any condition.

The Paper also lists recommendations for physicians, consumers, and legislators. To physicians, it recommends, in part, the following:

> . . .most reports claiming positive and statistically significant results for acupuncture are flawed by biased patient selection, poor controls, lack of blinding, or insufficient numbers. There is no physiologic rationale for why acupuncture should work other than for its placebo or counterirritant and distracting effects. For these reasons, acupuncture should not

be offered without full informed consent, reminding patients that acupuncture is experimental, and has not been proven more effective than a placebo, and has some risk of complications. . .

As the judge in the federal case in Texas stated, the only thing that is experimental about acupuncture is Westerners' understanding of it. Some of what is referred to as "spook medicine" may also play a role in the body healing with the use of acupuncture. It is wildly assumptive to say that the spirit has nothing to do with healing; just because science cannot find one in the body does not prove that one doesn't exist or that it doesn't play a role in healing the human body. Even medical science recently acknowledged that an individual's "mental attitude" and "spirit" does help in the recovery from illness. This appears to be what is meant by the statement that "there is no physiologic rationale for why acupuncture should work. . ."

The Paper addressed the following recommendation to consumers:

> Acupuncture cures nothing. It may relieve symptoms with frequency of a placebo. It may be harmful. Consumers wishing to try acupuncture should discuss their situation with a knowledgeable physician ["who is not a proponent" was edited out in the original version of the Paper]. . .

There appears to be a bit of prejudice against acupuncture in this statement. The statement that acupuncture "may be harmful" appears to be speculation without any supporting reports, studies, scientific evidence, or case law. Such a statement could have a deterrent effect on anyone thinking about using acupuncture, giving them the impression that acupuncture is dangerous. It is, however, less dangerous than many of the narcotic drugs that are prescribed by medical doctors to help alleviate pain . One is again looking at what amounts to nothing more than propaganda, apparently designed to take away the consumers' choice in the marketplace.

The following recommendation was made in the Paper to legislators:

> Acupuncture licensing should be abolished. Public display of unaccredited degrees by individuals offering any form of health care should be banned. And insurance companies, HMO's and government insurance programs should not be

forced to cover acupuncture unless scientific evidence demonstrates that it has value.

What we are witnessing here is propaganda designed to cut the competitors of the pharmaceutical and medical industries from the health-care system. Calling for licensing laws to be abolished, denouncing acupuncture as dangerous or causing harm, saying that insurance companies that cover it are being "forced" to do so, all appear to be little more than rhetoric. None of this serves the public. It serves only to restrict access to acupuncture or any other alternative practice.

Holistic Dentistry

Within the alternative health-care system are many dentists who practice *holistic dentistry*. This form of dentistry employs a philosophy which includes the removal of mercury amalgam fillings. These practitioners maintain that mercury amalgam may play a role in allergies and other problems related to mercury in the human body. Orthodox dentistry would argue that the amount of mercury contained in these old fillings is so minute that it doesn't make a difference and has no impact on a person's health. Proponents of holistic dentistry argue that this is not the case. There is evidence that there is such a thing as bio-accumulation with respect to mercury. If someone is allergic to mercury, whether it be a small amount or a large amount, the fact is that they are allergic to it.

This same principle of bio-accumulation plays a role in environmental medicine. If a person were exposed to 1 part per million (PPM) of DDT every year over a 15-year period, the theory is that he would have accumulated 15 PPMs of DDT in his body by the 15th year. Since oil-based chemicals are housed in the fat tissue, this accumulation of chemicals over many years may lead to physical problems, including cancer. It is postulated that eventually these chemicals may enter the blood stream in search of additional storage areas because the existing fat tissues are already full of previously stored chemicals. In a male body, the largest concentration of fat is either in the testicles or in the brain. In a female body the largest concentration of fat occurs in either the area around the breasts or in the brain. Eventually these chemical toxins may enter into organs and other areas in the body. Those involved in environmental medicine believe that these chemicals cause many problems related to allergenic reactions. Holistic dentists basically feel that same way about the mercury fillings. Their solution is to take out the old toxic mercury fillings and replace them with harmless fillings.

This procedure has not been accepted by orthodoxy dentistry and therefore has been attacked as a form of fraud or quackery. Those dentists who are practicing holistic dentistry have come under fire by their dental boards around the country. One of the largest concentrations of such dental practitioners is in California, and in that state the Dental Board and the Dental Association have come down hard on these holistic dentists.

In the Anti-Quackery Campaign, this form of dentistry has been targeted as "health fraud or quackery." Insurance companies have been alerted not to pay for it because it is not based on "any scientific evidence" that makes the removal of these mercury fillings necessary. Any dentist who sends in a claim to an insurance company for reimbursement or payment for the removal of mercury fillings could be charged with fraud because the insurance company, in turn, notifies the dental boards.

How this came about is simple and was outlined in Chapter 5. In the Grant Proposal to review every form of holistic/alternative practice, treatment, modality, service and product, the following was said about this form of dentistry:

> Many of the unproven treatments for cancer are claimed to work on other diseases. For example, proponents of metabolic therapy claim that the removal of mercury fillings for the cure of allergies should also be undertaken by cancer patients to reduce the burden of metal toxicities in order to free the immune system to focus on eliminating cancer. Similar rationales are articulated for cytotoxic testing, hair analysis, vitamin supplementation and the like.

The reader will recall that the purpose of the study was to develop reports that could then be used by licensing boards, insurance companies, and state and federal regulatory agencies in their "fight against health fraud." Evidently two things were included as part of the action plan to go after holistic practitioners. First, the medical, dental, chiropractic, osteopathic, and other licensing boards have received the names of those practitioners in their respective states who are practicing the targeted treatments. Second, they have received reports on the treatments themselves. Any licensing board then has the justification to go after anyone practicing any of the various forms of alternative/holistic treatments reported on. In this regard the proposed study stated:

One aspect of the project will be to provide data on coverage. Another aspect will be to provide information on potential insurance fraud or abuse and misrepresentations billings to appropriate state, federal and private agencies to permit the government and insurers to take appropriate action against documented health fraud. . .For example, some of the modalities that a state or state regulatory agency might require that information on are hair analysis for vitamin and mineral prescribing, chelation therapy for any use but the treatment of lead poisoning, DMSO for any use but interstitial cystitis, dental amalgam testing and cytotoxic testing.

It was further proposed to use these reports for "white papers" that could then be used to support initiatives including ". . .legislation or regulatory proposals on a national or state level dealing with credentialing."

These plans for action against alternative practitioners most probably have been initiated in many, if not all, states; but since California is the "hub of alternative medicine and dentistry" in the country, actions against those practicing in that state would have received a high priority. Many dentists who employ the principles of holistic dentistry also use acupuncture, supplements, homeopathy, and the removal of mercury amalgam fillings. I know of several cases that came before the dental board in California, which resulted in both good and bad results for the practitioners.

One case involved a very humble man who practiced in central California near the Napa wine country. I met him at a meeting of holistic dentists and alternative physicians. His story is typical of what can and does happen to alternative practitioners. He was brought before the Dental Board more than five years ago on charges related to his removal of mercury amalgam. The Board voted to put him on one-year suspension, during which time he was to re-train. At the end of this year suspension he was to reappear before the Board and would be allowed to go back into practice under terms outlined by the Board, including "spot checks" on his practice to make sure he was no longer holistic methods. Since his livelihood depended on meeting these terms, he followed the Board's ruling for one year. He then appeared before the Board, and, contrary to the original ruling, the Board extended his suspension. This time he was ordered to do more training and reappear at the end of another year. Once again he complied with the ruling and did what he was supposed to do. At the end of that second year he appeared before the Board again, and again they extended his suspension. This went on for almost five years.

By this time he was at the end of the proverbial rope. It was to his credit that he had persisted as long as he had without any source of income. Needless to say, this situation put a tremendous stress on his personal life. Ultimately he had to sell his house. His wife divorced him. He had to sell all of his dental equipment, which had been sitting, unused, in a storage shed on his property. As a result of all of this, he ended up selling fruit at a roadside stand in Napa County in order to make enough money to exist and to send money to his ex-wife and children. I spoke with him after all of this happened. He was a broken man. It was a pathetic situation, but not an uncommon one. I know of practitioners who, after losing their licenses as a result of this campaign, have had to begin new careers as diverse as commercial fishing in Oregon or driving cabs in New Mexico. In one case, mentioned in an earlier chapter, the victim committed suicide. There are hundreds of such cases around the country where practitioners have been persecuted for their beliefs and practices. Their civil rights have been denied, and their lives have been ruined.

Some are more fortunate. Dr. Vaughn Harada, D.D.S., of Santa Monica, is an excellent example of a practitioner who fought back and won. He too was called before the Dental Board. Dr. Harada is a very likable man who believes in what he is doing. He is soft-spoken, has a flair for drawing in people, and as a speaker is very articulate. He cares about his patients and is also a courageous fighter. In honor of his Japanese/American heritage, I refer respectfully to him as a Holistic Ninja. He quietly goes about taking on his enemies, and in the process many of them are transformed into allies.

He went to his Dental Board hearing knowing that they were operating from a preconceived idea. He was aware of the existence of a pre-determined adjudication on his case which had been decided upon by the Board before he even entered the room. Fortunately he was well-equipped to present his case. Armed with Bill Moore, one of the most dedicated and outspoken attorneys for alternative medicine in the country, Dr. Harada approached the hearing ready to do battle.

After Mr. Moore presented Harada's case, the young assistant attorney general who was representing the Board was not only impressed by what Moore had to say, but actually took it into consideration. Part of what Mr. Moore presented to the Board was a detailed account of the overall campaign and conspiracy being directed against alternative medicine, in which holistic dentistry was targeted along with many others. When the assistant attorney general read Mr. Moore's account of this campaign and conspiracy, she commented that she had no idea that this was going on. The Board dropped the whole matter within two or three days.

Several more of Mr. Moore's clients were similarly fortunate in having him at their side before Board hearings. The results was basically the same as in Dr. Harada's case. Unfortunately, not all alternative practitioners have had such success. If these practitioners had known what was going on behind the scenes and had been able to present a report with a full chronology and supporting documents in their defense, they might have had better success.

The attack against holistic dentists is part of an organized assault that threatens the very principles upon which this country was founded. It is the responsibility of the American people to fight any such efforts to erode or diminish the freedoms that are meant to be enjoyed by us as citizens of the United States.

Chapter Fifteen

Homeopathy

"Dr. Dan Clark has lost his license in the State of Florida. . .This kind of quackery needs to be eradicated. I have notified the FDA, the Attorney General of Missouri, the FBI, and the St. Louis Post."
[FAX Transmission from Dr. John Renner to Missouri Attorney General, February 26, 1992.]

"It has been difficult in this country over the past 60 years for any innovative physician to try to introduce a new form of therapy without harassment from fellow physicians, FDA, AMA, and the American Cancer Society."
[From Dr. Clark's letter of resignation from the Volusia County Medical Society, November 2, 1981.]

The case of Daniel J. Clark, M.D., is a classic example of how a doctor who was taught orthodox methods and converts to a holistic/alternative practice can be destroyed. Dr. Clark is a mild-mannered, humble, and deeply religious man who sincerely believes in the alternative methods. His beliefs and practice of the alternatives cost him his license and thus his livelihood. His case is similar to that of Dr. Brian Briggs of North Dakota, as well as that of Dr. Ed McDonagh, with behind-the-scene activities playing a role in his demise.

Dan Clark's problems began soon after he graduated from medical school. He received his medical degree from the Medical College of Georgia, and in 1978 he completed a three-year residency program at University Hospital in Jacksonville, Florida. Licensed in both Georgia and Florida, he set up his practice in Ormond Beach, Florida. According to Florida records on his case, ". . .initially his practice included gynecology, family practice, and general nutrition."

However, Dr. Clark began to practice metabolic (nutritional) therapy soon after setting up practice in 1979 and used it to help treat cancer patients. The state's files said:

The purpose of such therapy is to enhance the immuno-
logical and biological capacities of a patient—nutritionally,
immunologically, and physiologically—in order to improve
the patients performance in combating cancer. This cancer
treatment includes the administration of Amygdalin (Laetrile),
vitamins, herbal teas and detoxifiers, and the application of
salves and packs to cause localized hyper-thermia. . .It is not
conventional, orthodox, or widely practiced form of cancer
treatment. No other physician in Volusia County uses it. Most
accredited medical schools in the United States do not teach it.
The American Medical Association (AMA) considers it to be
experimental. Eventually, [Dr. Clark's] metabolic treatment of
cancer patients began to account for 15% to 20% of his practice.

This was all in 1978-1979, and his practice began to catch on and
become very popular with patients from around the area and
throughout the state of Florida, and then from outside the state. His
practice was growing rapidly and this didn't sit very well with the
powers that be, including those doctors in his area who were losing
patients to Dr. Clark's practice.

One key to why they eventually came after him is contained in the
statement "No other physician in Volusia County uses it." In other
words, Dr. Clark drew the attention of his peers because he was the
only one using this treatment in the county, resulting in many
patients who had gone to other physicians going to Dr. Clark. A type
of professional jealousy led to some covert anti-competitive activity.
This behind-closed-doors plotting led to actions being directed
against Dr. Clark.

Dan Clark is a man of integrity who is not one to run away from
a fight. He is not afraid to stand up for what he believes in. In an
effort to convince the members of the medical society that what he
was doing was worthwhile and helpful to people, Dr. Clark met with
members of the society in March 1981. He brought with him Mr.
Robert Bradford, an expert on metabolic therapy from American
Biologics in Chula Vista, California. He did this at his own expense
with the expectation that his peers would welcome this new approach
to cancer treatment with open arms. Mr. Bradford explained the use
of laetrile in the treatment of cancer, as well as the role of a nutritional program in treating the disease. The society did not, however,
react with the enthusiasm that Dr. Clark expected.

His integrity was again demonstrated when, on October 2, 1981, he resigned from the local hospital staff with which he was affiliated in Ormond Beach, Florida. In his letter of resignation he stated:

> Throughout the history of medicine, one will notice medicine has been slow to accept new ideas and new methods of therapy until years after they were discovered. The same is true today, also, because doctors often oppose change and often harass pioneers in their field for endeavoring to discover new and better ways of helping people. With that I leave you with my resignation.

Following a series of confrontations with his peers, on November 2, 1981, Dr. Clark wrote another letter of resignation, this time to the medical society. Dr. Clark had been the subject of much ridicule from them about his newfound approach to cancer treatment. In this letter he stated his feelings about the unfriendly reception he and Mr. Bradford had received at the March meeting:

> You followed the usual routine and trend of medical men for the past 400 years by expressing doubt and disbelief over a relative new form of treatment which was different from the accepted norm. It has been difficult in this country over the past 60 years for any innovative physician to try to introduce a new form of therapy without harassment from fellow physicians, FDA, AMA, and the American Cancer Society.

With his closing statement, Dr. Dan Clark unknowingly opened himself up to a vicious attack from the medical establishment, an attack that would persist for more than ten years:

> With this, I will leave you with my resignation from the VCMS [Volusia County Medical Society], because I don't care for the harassment from the censor committee about future patients that I may treat.

What had occurred just prior to his resignation was something that no one could have prevented: one of Dr. Clark's patients died from cancer while under his care. As in orthodox medicine, alternative medicine may not help every patient all of the time. An alternative doctor may lose a patient. However, because it was Dr. Clark's patient, his orthodox enemies became determined to go after his license.

The patient the Board focused on was a woman with breast cancer, who chose to be treated with laetrile, diet, juices, enzymes, and other metabolic treatment. She was under Dr. Clark's care from October 1980 until her death on August 30, 1981. Until Dr. Clark made his presentation to the medical society and then resigned, there were no charges brought against him. It wasn't until he resigned from the hospital and the medical society that charges were filed. The counts included the treatment he gave the patient, the fact that these treatments were not accepted, and the allegation that "the treatment of [patient's name] by Respondent (Dr. Clark) was not medically beneficial, and to the exclusion of other forms of proper medical treatment, was harmful to the patient." The Board charged that the treatment he gave her was both "fraudulent and constituted misrepresentation."

The proceeding omitted a vital piece of information that played a role in the patient's death—her state of mind. What was going on in her life had a major impact on her overall well-being and health and on the outcome of her treatment. Whether treatment had been delivered by an orthodox doctor or by Dr. Clark, the situation was such that it probably would not have made a difference. The patient had lost her husband some years before. Although she had lived with that tragedy, it had almost destroyed her will to live. Her husband had died of lung cancer after having received radiation and chemotherapy treatments. When she learned that she too had cancer, she was horrified about the future and the thought of dying. She had personal doubts about any form of treatment working for her after having lost her husband and seeing that his treatment didn't help him. She appeared to have no hope of survival. She displayed moderate-to-severe depression during the entire time she was being treated by Dr. Clark. At Dr. Clark's recommendation, she received psychological counseling, which determined that she suffered from a deep depression which was seen as a probable block to her immune system response to treatment. At first she had responded to the treatment, but the depression took its toll and her disease progressively got worse.

As Dr. Clark put it, the patient had exercised her right to choose what form of treatment she desired, and any complaint against him for helping her exercise her rights was not justified. However, this didn't stop the medical establishment from coming after him.

In the end Dr. Clark's hearing recommended a one-year suspension. This was overruled by the state attorney on the case and changed to revoking his license altogether. The final ruling was on

April 21, 1983, almost eighteen months after he resigned from orthodox medicine.

Dr. Clark's attorney got the Board's decision put on hold, pending a hearing on August 13, 1983. The outcome was that his license was revoked anyway. Following this action, hundreds of patients and consumers supporting alternative medicine from around the country wrote the governor of Florida about Dr. Clark's situation. The letters were sent over to the Florida Board of Medical Examiners for reply. All of the replies simply stated that his license had been revoked and referred the letter writers to the final order.

Up to this point it seems that the motivating force and drive behind any actions against Dr. Clark was professional competition and medical prejudice against what he practiced and believed in. This is very common. Alternative practitioners run into prejudice against their practice all the time. Once Dr. Clark had lost his license, the medical orthodox machinery went into action. His name was posted in an information network which links all Boards in the U.S. with the Federation of State Boards of Medical Examiners in Texas, which informs every state medical board when a doctor has a disciplinary action taken against them. Should a doctor have a license in another state, that state usually follows the lead of the state that took the action against a doctor and takes action on the license in that state as well.

Dr. Clark was licensed in Georgia as well as Florida, so Georgia got involved. It seems that the people involved in the PAC/FDA Anti-Quackery Campaign are also linked into this system. When Dr. Clark had his license revoked, one of the principal anti-quack "experts" wrote the Florida Board asking for all of the file information on his case.

On April 2, 1984, eight months after the final order, the Florida Board sent 259 pages of Dr. Clark's files to Grace P. Monaco, one of the founders of Emprise and a member of the National Council Against Health Fraud. The State Board sent her a copy of the Investigative Report on him, a copy of the Administrative Complaint on him, and copies of all Final Orders on his case.

Apparently after Ms. Monaco received them she reviewed the information and on April 16, 1984, asked for additional information on Dr. Clark's case that the State Board had not sent. In a letter she requested:

1. The May 16, 1983, Motion of Respondent Clark for Reconsideration. [This was his motion to reconsider the Board revoking his license instead of just a one-year suspension.]

2. The Hearing Officer's Findings of Fact on the above hearing.
3. Dr. Clark's Motion for Exceptions to the Recommended order. [Which was denied. He had his license revoked regardless.]

She also asked for any information or data that they might have regarding Dr. Clark's action in the Fifth District Court of Appeals. Dr. Clark had filed an appeal regarding the Board's revocation order, but to no avail.

Apparently Mrs. Monaco had a hidden agenda regarding Dr. Clark. On June 20, 1984, she wrote the Board again about him, this time regarding an entirely different matter. Dr. Clark had gotten involved with a group known as the International Institute for Research on Metabolic Diseases and Cancer. He was listed in some of their promotional materials as the Vice Chairman of the group, along with a long list of other alternative practitioners from around the world. The group's purposes included:

1. Research in methods and theories concerning cancer disease, including special investigations on natural foods.
2. Study of all methods concerning research in preliminary stages of cancer.
3. Research work in laboratories authorized or appointed by the Institute to evaluate therapeutics coming from natural substances.
4. Publication of statistics and results of the research in the journal of the Institute and also in the "International Protocol Management of Cancer." This protocol would be sent to official health organizations including the Department of Traditional Medicine of the World Health organization (WHO).

The group's research facility and clinic was set up in Portugal. With alternative physicians from all over the world now having a place to go to both research and treat patients, it would seem this presented a potential problem for orthodoxy. Its U.S. headquarters was listed as the office address of Dr. Clark. Perhaps this is why Monaco got involved. Or, perhaps it was because one of her chief clients was the American Cancer Society. Whatever the reason, she saw fit to alert the Florida Board about it. She enclosed all of the printed materials on the Institute, including its objectives, the board members and their biographical histories, its articles, and a description of the group. In her letter to the Board she stated:

I pulled out my file on de-licensed physicians which showed a Daniel G. Clark (License No 26861) de-licensed in case No. 82-1220. [This is a typo on the middle initial, which should be a J.]. . .I believe that certainly members of the World Health Organization, the U.S. Congress and the major voluntary associations combatting cancer should be made aware that the Vice Chairman of this group is a physician who has lost his license in Florida.

Her letter was also sent to three other people: John Carbonneau, Joe Zavertnik, M.D., and Robert C. Seelman, M.D. It is of interest to note that Joseph Zavertnik, M.D., is an oncologist who served on the American Cancer Society's National Unproven Methods of Cancer Management Committee and is also on the Florida Cancer Council.

The very next item in Dr. Clark's Board files was a letter dated July 5, 1984, to Grace Monaco enclosing all of the Orders issued on Dr. Clark. Within six weeks of this letter being sent to Monaco, the Board received an anonymous tip by phone from someone stating that Dr. Clark was still practicing medicine. A memo dated August 20, 1984, indicated that based on this tip the state was to investigate Dr. Clark again, and another case was filed against him in 1985. In this case, however, there appears to be some involvement with oncologists from the Florida Cancer Council working behind the scenes against Dr. Clark.

In the new case, the Florida Medical Board relied almost exclusively on a confidential report regarding Dr. Clark dated October 2, 1985, from the Florida Cancer Council. That confidential report stated in part that one of Dr. Clark's patients ". . .was not treated in accordance with normal breast cancer treatment which is known to be effective." The report further revealed that the Florida Cancer Council felt that Clark had treated the patient with "ineffective remedies."

How the Florida Board got this confidential report is also of interest. Apparently a letter dated October 15, 1985, was sent to the Department of Professional Regulation from Dr. John Carbanneau. He had forwarded the confidential report that was sent to his office to the State Board.

Two doctors of oncology who were directly involved in this case against Dr. Clark were directly linked to Grace Monaco in her letter dated in June 1984. It was within one month after Monaco received the package of data from the Florida Board on Dan Clark that the Board received an anonymous tip about Dr. Clark. Following that came the investigation. Investigators used the confidential report on

Clark from the Florida Cancer Council against him in that case. Was all of this a coincidence, or was it something more? Although no documents present in the files say specifically to "get Dr. Clark," in the end they did. The following is a rough summary of what happened in the investigations of Dr. Clark:

- Case 0050076. This was a complaint filed September 9, 1984 (after the anonymous tip was given to the Board, just after Monaco contacted the Board about Dr. Clark). It was filed by a medical doctor complaining that Dr. Clark had practiced. It was investigated to March 3, 1985. Since he was already facing charges by the Attorney General, the Board "ordered that this complaint should be, and the same is hereby dismissed."

- Cases 0063790 and 0063702. These two complaints were filed by the Department of Professional Regulation after the preceding case was dismissed. In these cases, the Florida Cancer Council sent the confidential report on Clark to be used against him to help the state make its case. However, since the attorney general was already working on another case, this was dismissed also.

Although Dr. Clark had his problems, all of what was going on behind the scenes was not fully known at that time. It was determined that Grace Monaco had been to Florida before the Board earlier, with others, in what she described as ". . .our attempt several years ago to convince the Board that laetrile was harmful and that the statutory provision for repeal shall be exercised. I hope someday that success will meet us in that field."

Whether she was invited to speak on the subject as a direct result of Dr. Dan Clark's presentation to the medical society regarding his use of laetrile and how patients could benefit from its use is not known. What is known is that she was there to make a presentation against the use of laetrile. Present with her was Dr. Victor Herbert and Dr. Zavertnik, both later involved in the study of alternatives, and both outspoken critics of alternative treatments for cancer.

As we have seen, the NIH Grant progress report outlined how Grace Monaco would make presentations at conferences sponsored by the Florida Pediatric Oncology Committee, the Florida Cancer Council, and the Food and Drug Administration's Second Health Fraud Conference in March of 1988. She was apparently involved in

Florida prior to and during 1984, and then, in 1987-1988, Monaco made a presentation on "quackery" to the very group that got involved on the Clark case after Monaco had contacted the Board in 1984. Following all of this Dan Clark started to have a different kind of problems.

The FDA started up its own investigation of Daniel Clark in 1992. Several things occurred which may have played a big role in why he was under investigation and attack by the FDA. Dan Clark is educated in the use, operation, and application of what is referred to as EAV machines (electronic acupuncture Voll machine—so named after the inventor, Voll). There are many different brand names for these machines, including Vega, Profile, Dermatron, Interro, Computron, and many others. These devices are used by doctors of homeopathy and alternative medicine throughout the world. Dan Clark had been invited to speak before a group of chiropractors in Missouri on one of these devices.

Clark's visit was to take place in St. Louis, Missouri, in the early part of the spring of 1992. Dr. John Renner, after hearing about this visit, sent a FAX Alert from his Consumer Health Information Research Institute (CHIRI) in Kansas City, Missouri, about Dan Clark. His February 25, 1992, FAX went to Missouri Attorney General Terry Bell, as well as to the Missouri State Board. The following is the entire content of that FAX:

> From: John H. Renner, M.D.
> Dr. Dan Clark has lost his license in the State of Florida. My sources tell me that this involved the death of a patient. Please check with the Florida Licensing Board to get full details.
> The gadget being promoted is similar to Vega Profile, Interro, and other EAV machines. This is not an FDA approved diagnostic machine. The silly advice given with this kills patients. This is similar to the machine that was confiscated in St. Charles that was being used by an M.D. The Wisconsin Chiropractic Board has outlawed machines identical to this. This kind of quackery needs to be eradicated. I have notified the FDA, the Attorney General of Missouri, the FBI, and the St. Louis *Post*. I hope someone will prevent an accident rather than wait for a patient to die.

This FAX contained incomplete information about the death of Dr. Clark's patient. Since Renner boldly stated, "The silly advice given with this kills patients," his FAX alert might be better named an "alarm." The data in the FAX was unsubstantiated, lacked any evidence or documentation, and did not contain any cited cases where such "advice kills patients."

Included was a copy of an article on the Vega test for allergy diagnosis, which was not positive. Here we see that Dr. Renner alerted the FDA, the FBI, and the Missouri Attorney General, as well as the media, about Dan Clark coming to Missouri to talk about, and/or demonstrate an EAV machine. As a direct result of this propaganda action that Dr. Renner took, there was never any presentation by Dan Clark in Missouri.

What did happen was that the FDA became involved with his case. It started by collecting as much data as possible about Clark from the Florida Board. Its letter dated June 26, 1992, asked for all files on every case against Dan Clark. They were to be sent to the FDA offices in Orlando. The person making the request was a Melissa J. Hill, Investigator from the FDA.

The Board responded on August 7, 1992, and enclosed copies of his application for a medical license along with "his discipline file." The Board sent the FDA only one case file, the one that resulted in the revocation of his license. According to the letter, all of the other cases had been sent to the State Attorney's office and weren't housed at the Board offices any longer.

The FDA received the files during the first part of August 1992, and the "anti-quackery" machine went into gear. Having already been tipped off by Dr. Renner, the FDA began plans to investigate Dan Clark in Melbourne, Florida, where Clark now owned an alternative health product company, Bio-Active Nutritional. It wasn't long before Dan Clark's office started to get strange phone calls from people asking him about his "machine." He even had people writing him asking about the machine. In all cases Dan Clark told them the truth: he didn't have any such machine and didn't use one. He was in the business of selling supplements, not machines. There were reports of surveillance of his offices and of his staff being followed in an attempt to find out where he had the machines hidden. Toward the end of 1992, he received a visit from agents of the FDA's Orlando office, who came in looking for his machine. Of course, they didn't find one because he didn't have any. They left empty-handed. This wasn't the end of the FDA's activities on Dan Clark. He still got strange phone calls. People came to visit his office under the pretense that they were interested in his "machines." The FDA must have been disappointed with its hot tip about Dan Clark, because there was nothing there to find.

Apparently they didn't stop there. There were meetings and conference calls, letters, and memos generated around the Clark case. The Health Fraud Task Force got involved, according to one report. Meetings were quickly put together and state agencies were contacted, but it seemed that no one knew anything more about Dan Clark and his mysterious machines. Quite frankly, they didn't exist; The FDA got a bad tip. He was involved in selling homeopathic remedies and that was it. He wasn't seeing patients and he wasn't using an EAV machine. It was a situation that the FDA should have left alone.

Dan Clark is still in business, and for the time being it appears that they are off his back. He is still without a license, but has plans to get his license back. With what he knows about the situation now, he may have a good shot at success. After all those years of not having a license, and not having an income as a doctor, he may never recoup his losses, but the assault on medical freedom hasn't totally destroyed Dan Clark. He may be scarred up and have a few bruises, but they haven't taken everything away from him. He still has his honesty, his integrity, and his willingness to help people no matter what his enemies have done to him. He also has truth on his side, along with some very able legal experts. He has the advantage of having a lot of information about the conspiracy and campaign that he has been a victim of, and he is determined to use it. The outcome of his situation remains to be seen.

Chapter 16

The Case of Willem Khoe, M.D.

> *"A: '. . .these are measurements points along meridians, and to me I don't care which point—which measurement point along which meridian. The effect of acupuncture is the same no matter where in the human body you stick the needle.'*
> *"Q: 'Have you ever heard of diagnosis in the science of acupuncture by palpation of meridians?'*
> *"A: 'No.'*
> *"Q: 'Do you know what a trained person, physician trained, in acupuncture looks for when he observes the human body?'*
> *"A: 'No, I would not know the things he looks for.'"*
> [Testimony by the state's "expert witness" Dr. Joseph Boyle against Dr. Khoe at licensing hearing.]

The case against Willem H. Khoe, M.D., involved a lot more than just his acupuncture practice. It also involved the use of homeopathics, vitamin injection, the use of the Dermatron, treatment for TMJ, and the basic principles of acupuncture. These were all put on trial by the California Board of Medical Quality Assurance back in 1983. Dr. Khoe's case is an encouraging example of how a state licensing board can be challenged and defeated, resulting in a win for alternative medicine.

Dr. Willem Khoe is a leader in the field of acupuncture. His training and education show that he is highly qualified as a practitioner of both acupuncture and orthodox medicine. He graduated Loma Linda University School of Medicine and had a family practice in the Los Angeles area since 1955. He specialized in abdominal surgery until 1972, when he began studying acupuncture. He is a Fellow of the American Society of Abdominal Surgeons. He was also the Chief of Staff of Serra Memorial Hospital.

His experience is vast in both schools of medicine. He began his study of acupuncture at the University of Southern California (USC) and continued his studies in Japan, Hong Kong, and Germany. In his practice as an acupuncturist he had administered in excess of 50,000 acupuncture treatments and had published in excess of 30 articles on acupuncture medicine. He had been an invited lecturer on acupuncture at the World Health Organization, National Institutes of Health, and at many acupuncture symposia in China, Switzerland, Japan, West Germany, Austria, Australia, and throughout Southeast Asia.

He was the President of the Acupuncture Research Institute in Los Angeles, California, which is accredited by California and other states for qualifying students for acupuncture licensing examinations. His credentials also include being a faculty member of the Institute for Advanced Research of the World Health Organization. He has lectured on acupuncture at Loma Linda University School of Medicine, USC School of Medicine, and New York University School of Medicine, as well as many hospitals in the Los Angeles area.

Additionally, he was an Examiner for the Board of Medical Quality Assurance's Acupuncture Certification Program. On a *pro bono* (without pay) basis, he hosted physicians from around the world so that they could observe his office practice. Dr. Gerald Looney, an Associate Professor and Assistant Director of Emergency Medicine at USC School of Medicine, as well as a graduate from Johns Hopkins Medical School, said that Dr. Khoe has "treated more doctors and their families than any other physician [he knew]."

In addition to all of these qualifications, he is also known as "the doctor's doctor" amongst his peers. It is probably because of his impeccable credentials that the Medical Board of California went after his license. He must have been one of their biggest targets because he was so well trained and so popular. It would have been a feather in their cap if they could have succeeded in discrediting a man of his stature.

According to the records, the case against Dr. Khoe involved several major modalities and treatments used in the world of alternative medicine. The underlying theme of the proceedings against him was the question of what constitutes the standard practice of medicine by a physician using acupuncture in his practice—or, as the issues were framed and presented by the state against Dr. Khoe, what constitutes an "extreme departure" from that standard of practice.

At issue were several points that would interest any alternative practitioner who employs any of the following:

- Acupuncture
- Dermatron (or any other EAV machine)
- Homeopathic medicine

- Vitamin B-12 injections
- Acupuncture techniques to discover physical problems
- Acupuncture related to the issue of a patient wearing metal and how that may influence the energy flow.
- Vitamin therapy for patients
- Record keeping of patients which differs from allopathic record keeping.

Certain aspects of Dr. Khoe's case would apply to almost all alternative practitioners, regardless of whether they use acupuncture or not. One of these aspects is the process of being challenged by a State/Board witness (or insurance consultant or insurance claims adjuster). Of particular interest is a challenge by a witness who is either not trained, or doesn't practice, or is not educated in the particular aspect of alternative medicine in question.

During the course of the case against Dr. Khoe, one of the main issues that came up was the standard of practice of a physician using acupuncture in his medical practice. According to documents in this case there was an agreement among the physicians—both those who used acupuncture in their practice and those who didn't—involved in his case. They all agreed that a combination of traditional allopathic approaches can be combined with acupuncture diagnostic procedures in evaluating a patient for acupuncture treatment.

The prosecution's witnesses included Dr. Richard Kroening, M.D., who had been a licensed M.D. in California since 1963. (He graduated from the California College of Medicine.) He was in private practice before he studied acupuncture from 1969 until 1973. He was a faculty member at UCLA studying acupuncture. He had been the Director of the Pain Management Clinic at UCLA since October 1977 and had written and lectured on acupuncture for almost ten years. Since Dr. Kroening was an allopathic doctor, as well as being trained in acupuncture, the state felt that he would be a good witness for them against Dr. Khoe.

In his testimony he was asked about using acupuncture diagnostic procedures in evaluating a patient while combining this with standard allopathic approaches. The questioning went as follows:

Q: "Now does the—does the amount of diagnostic technique, traditional Western allopathic diagnostic techniques—all right?—Is the amount of that vis-a-vis the amount of information that is received from traditional acupuncture diagnostic techniques—can the doctor, depending on his experience, within the standard of practice use some of each without using all of both?"

A: "One could do that."

Q: "And as far as treatment is concerned, with respect to a physician licensed to practice in California, who has knowledge of acupuncture, can he, based on his training and experience in the presentation of a patient, combine traditional allopathic treatment with acupuncture treatment?"

A: "Yes, he can."

Q: "And can he, depending on the presentation of the patient and his training and experience, use one to the exclusion of the other, depending on the circumstances?"

A: "There are a lot of ways to Mecca, and if there—the choice—treatment of choice by your decision-making is acupuncture, it's acceptable. There may be an alternative way to do it in addition to acupuncture. To me that's a theoretical—that's a matter of your personal competence and style on how you carry out your therapy."

These statements by the prosecutor's witness is important for several reasons, the most obvious being that the decision as to whether to use allopathic or acupuncture is a matter of treatment of choice made by the practitioner, and that a decision to use acupuncture for a patient is an acceptable choice.

There was also agreement in the case that the appropriate manner of treatment in chronic cases in a primary-care setting when delay of traditional treatment (allopathic) would not endanger the patient is to give acupuncture a try and determine future treatments from the results.

In Dr. Khoe's case, several charges were brought against him by the state in the licensing hearings.

One of the charges brought against Dr. Khoe involved his use of vitamin B-12 treatments. The accusation charged that "there was no medical basis for the injection of vitamin B-12 and its use needlessly exposed them (two patients) to risk." The attorney for Dr. Khoe (G.T.S. Khalsa, of San Francisco) argued that this charge was a typical illustration of how an accepted procedure is alleged to be an extreme departure from the practice of medicine. He pointed out that the only physician who made an independent review of the records before the accusation was filed was Dr. James Boyle (not to be confused with Dr. Joseph Boyle, former president of the California Medical Association), who concluded that "there was no medical basis from the examination or history for injecting vitamin B-12 or any other fluid. . .and this is an extreme departure from standards of medical practice."

One has to take into consideration the fact that Dr. Boyle did not have a primary care practice, nor did he have any "continuing responsibility for patients" in his practice. He was a consulting gastroenterologist who did not use acupuncture in his practice and was of the opinion that a patient would get the same response no matter where an acupuncture needle is placed in the human body. This "expert witness" didn't understand anything about acupuncture, and was not in agreement with it, yet was testifying against it. Such has been the case in many instances where alternative practitioners have gone into hearings or court cases and the "experts" testifying against them had no knowledge about, didn't use, and/or didn't believe in the modality or treatment they were testifying about and against.

Another prosecution witness, Dr. Richard Kroening, had set forth "why a physician who was untrained in acupuncture is not qualified to make these kinds of judgments." The following is from his testimony:

Q: "Now, he [Dr. Khoe] with his patient also used two modalities. He used acupuncture and electroacupuncture with respect to the aquapuncture [injecting fluid into an acupuncture point]. Would that be an appropriate modality to use on this patient?"

A: "Local treatment of those tender points would be appropriate by injection techniques."

Q: "And would vitamin B-12 be an appropriate solution to use?"

A: "I think it would be appropriate."

Q: "Can a physician, though, practicing acupuncture in California, do that for his patient?"

A: "Yes."

Q: "Dr. Boyle reported and here is what he said—let me ask, do you understand that Dr. Boyle doesn't know anything about acupuncture?"

A: "That's why I'm here, I think."

Q: "All right. He wrote 'there is no medical basis from the examination or history for his injecting vitamin B-12 or any other fluid along the medial border of the scapula, and this is an extreme departure from the standards of medical practice'? From a traditional allopathic perspective, he's right, isn't he?"

A: "He certainly is."

Q: "Makes no sense whatsoever?"

A: "No, it doesn't."

Q: "But from an acupuncture medicine perspective, it makes all the sense in the world, doesn't it?"

A: "Yes."

Q: "And it's understandable, is it not, how Dr. Boyle, who doesn't know acupuncture, would come to this conclusion?"

A: "The information he has, that's an appropriate response on his part, yes."

Q: "But he's wrong, is he not, when he says it's an extreme departure from the standards of medical practice?"

A: "Not for a physician who does acupuncture, but for a physician who practices regular medicine it would be a very strong departure, yes."

Q: "For Dr. Khoe in this case, it is not?"

A: "I think that would be appropriate."

Here we can see that even the state's prosecuting witness made statements that support the alternative approaches in medicine. In this case these statements clearly drew the line on the issue of the standard of practice of acupuncture and the standard of practice of allopathic medicine. More importantly, it was demonstrated that the standards of allopathic medicine cannot be used as a valid measure against the practice of acupuncture, or for that matter, any form of alternative medicine used by a licensed practitioner.

Additionally, even the pharmaceutical industry and the American Medical Association have issued statements or published documents that support the use of injectable vitamin B-12. This also came out in this case.

Dr. Boyle had referred to the 1980 *PDR* (*Physicians Desk Reference*—a directory of all pharmaceuticals made), wherein the Squibb Company says that vitamin B-12 could be dangerous. Standing on its own, such a statement could be used against any practitioner using B-12. If not challenged, such testimony or evidence could be damaging to a practitioner. However, someone who does his homework and a good attorney who researches the area can usually come up with some other statement which would not only contradict the first statement, but also carry more weight. This was the case for Dr. Khoe. His attorney aptly pointed out the following:

He [Dr. Boyle] neglected to also state that in the same *PDR* edition the ELi Lilly Company concluded that although the possibility of sensitivity type reactions following administration of any parenteral [injection] preparation must always be kept in mind, there is no documented evidence that vitamin B-12 itself is toxic, even in large doses. Many thousands of injections of a 100-mcg dose have been administered to humans without toxic or allergic reactions.

Dr. Khoe's attorney also submitted the AMA's *Drug Evaluation* Book (1980 edition), which stated: "No serious toxicity has been reported following the use of either preparation [of vitamin B-12]. Allergic reactions to impurities in the preparation occur rarely. Injection causes little or no pain, and no adverse local effects have been reported."

All of the witnesses for Dr. Khoe also testified that his use of vitamin B-12 was totally appropriate.

A second charge against Dr. Khoe had to do with his use of Huneke neurotherapy, a new method of acupuncture treatment. Recalling that Dr. Boyle's testified earlier that in his opinion a physician would get the same results regardless of the placement of the acupuncture needle, he testified also regarding Huneke neurotherapy. Despite being provided an opportunity to review records which included an expert description of what these treatments were and how they worked, as well as text references on the subjects, Dr. Boyle testified that he was not familiar with Huneke neurotherapy and really "didn't want to take the time to investigate it." The following is from his testimony:

Q: "What is the Huneke method?"
A: "I only know what is said here. I do believe it's a method of acupuncture."
Q: "Okay. Did you make any investigation to find out what it was other than what was in the report [provided to Dr. Boyle from Dr. Khoe]?"
A: "I didn't really care whether it was or wasn't what he said."

It was also revealed in the case that this "expert witness" was unfamiliar with the criteria that a physician practicing acupuncture uses in determining an appropriate treatment plan:

Q: "Have you ever heard of diagnosis in the science of acupuncture by palpation of meridians?"

A: "Palpation of meridians?"

Q: "Yes."

A: "No."

Q: "Have you ever heard an acupuncture diagnosis by observation?"

A: "By observation of the patient or something particular? I've heard of diagnosis by observation in all branches of medical science."

Q: "Do you know specifically the kind of things in acupuncture that a trained person looks for in observing a patient?"

A: "No, I would not know the things they look for."

At one point in his testimony, Dr. Boyle described his understanding of how endorphines affect acupuncture therapy. His testimony revealed to those present his lack of understanding of acupuncture. Professor Tiller, former Chairman of the Department of Material Science at Stanford University, who studied on a Guggenheim Fellowship at Oxford University, was present during Dr. Boyle's testimony and explained in detail the role of endorphines in acupuncture. He concluded that Dr. Boyle "proved the adage that a little bit of knowledge is a dangerous thing."

Two expert witnesses for Dr. Khoe testified that, based on his testimony, Dr. Boyle was not competent to testify about issues regarding the use of acupuncture by a physician in California.

The Dermatron is a brand name for one of the many EAV machines on the market. These are used by practitioners in alternative medicine, especially by homeopathic physicians and homeopathic dentists. One of the charges in the accusation against Dr. Khoe referred to his use of the Dermatron in his practice. It stated that "the use of the Dermatron device in examination or treatment of the patient was not of any accepted medical value in the diagnosis of disease in general nor of the patient's specific complaints, and it was not proper for this to influence or to be used to support [Dr. Khoe's] diagnosis."

Dr. Khoe had used the Dermatron on one patient's first visit and on another patient during the second visit. He testified that he uses the Dermatron only after he has come to a conclusion by using traditional techniques of diagnosis and that he uses it only to confirm his diagnosis. He also testified that he never uses it for the treatment of patients. It was also pointed out that the prosecution did not present *any evidence* that the Dermatron is not a medically reliable instrument. Neither of the state's "expert witnesses" were qualified to give an opinion on the Dermatron due to lack of training, experience, or understanding of how it worked.

Professor Tiller was a qualified witness on the subject of the Dermatron. He was also a Distinguished Advisory Professor in Electrical Engineering at the University of Delaware, and had published in excess of 200 papers, 45 in the area of biomaterials and electrodermal studies, and he had studied acupuncture points and meridians for ten years. He had recently completed a paper entitled "An Analysis of Electrodermal Instruments for Skin Monitoring," which included a study of the Dermatron. In his expert testimony on the Dermatron, Professor Tiller explained how it operated and stated that in his opinion the instrument was scientifically reliable, safe, and effective. In an effort to dispel the standard attack against EAV (that they are dangerous because of the electrical current that passes through the patient's body), he explained that the amount of energy received by a patient is "less than the energy received by a person from the fluorescent lights in the hearing room."

In addition, three other doctors testified that the Dermatron was medically reliable, safe, and effective.

The only evidence that the prosecutor presented about the Dermatron was from Kenneth Baumgartner, a lawyer for the FDA, and James Veale, Director of the FDA's Bureau of Medical Devices. Even their testimony could not outweigh the testimony of the expert witnesses for Dr. Khoe. Mr. Baumgartner testified that the FDA has procedures to determine whether or not the Dermatron is an appropriate device to use but has not done so. He simply stated that the purpose of the FDA's investigators and compliance officers is to investigate devices and report findings to the Agency so that decisions regarding enforcement can be made. In other words, neither the investigators or the compliance officers in the FDA are equipped to, nor can they, make decisions about whether some medical device is appropriate for use or not.

Mr. Veale of the FDA testified that no application to the FDA for the use of the Dermatron was required. He also stated that the FDA has taken no action to ban the use of the Dermatron.

This all took place in 1982-1983, so the FDA's position at the time applied to Dr. Khoe's situation. The current situation is that the FDA has been receiving "expert" evidence, reports, and data from the "anti-quackery" people which hold that any form of EAV, Dermatron, Interro, Accupath, Computron, and so on are all "quack devices." Since it relies on this "expert" opinion, its current activity may be based on those opinions. This does not mean that the "experts" giving these opinions cannot be challenged. They most certainly can be. If one were in the position to do so, using the tactics and strategy used in Dr. Khoe's case, one would probably have success in negating and invalidating the "expert" opinion based on the fact that these "experts" have neither formal education in, nor training in, nor experience with the EAV machines.

In Dr. Khoe's testimony about the Dermatron he said that he had demonstrated the use of the Dermatron on many occasions at the National Institutes of Health and was never told there was any legal question about its use. The situation may vary from state to state, but the facts remain the same with regard to expert testimony about its use, effectiveness, and safety, as well as its application in medicine.

The point here is simply that if the opposition, prosecution or "experts" do not know what they are talking about, it is because they have no training in, education about, or understanding of EAV machines. It is also because they are using the standards in allopathic medicine to measure alternative modalities, which is like comparing apples and oranges. There is no way it can be done.

One of the charges alleged that "no standard medical techniques were directed toward the determination of the origin of the patient's back pain." In the course of this patient's treatment, Dr. Khoe determined that the patient had been in a bad motorcycle accident and that he may have suffered TMJ dysfunction as a result of the accident. He also determined that an interruption in the acupuncture meridian could be a contributing factor in his chronic complaints of headaches and upper back pain. He treated both conditions.

All of the expert witnesses, including three for the prosecution, testified that TMJ dysfunction can be a result of physical trauma and can cause a chronic problem of headaches. Two of the prosecution witnesses also testified that TMJ dysfunction could also be the source of upper back pain. Dr. Kroening testified that TMJ dysfunction was a likely source of the patient's headaches and that the manipulation that Dr. Khoe used was within the standard of practice. Dr. Khoe had adjusted (manipulated) the patient's jaw. He also gave him acupuncture treatment, both with injection of vitamin B-12 and needles, to alleviate the back pain. Both a prosecution witness and one for Dr. Khoe stated that this was standard and proper and was not evidence of gross negligence, incompetence, or an extreme departure from the practice of medicine.

One of the other charges alleged that "no adequate medical history or physical examination was taken or conducted." Again, the standards of allopathic medicine were being used as a measuring stick to determine that what Dr. Khoe did was not to their standards. However, a witness for Dr. Khoe testified that what he did was within the standard of practice and there was no evidence of gross negligence, incompetence, or repeated negligent acts.

As a matter of fact, the prosecution's witness, Dr. Kroening, testified that Dr. Khoe's palpation of certain acupuncture points on the patient's back was a valid diagnostic procedure to use in arriving at a treatment for pain. He also stated that Dr. Khoe had done a sufficient history and physical examination to begin treatment of the patient.

Q: "Okay. Now with the presentation of this history and everything we talked about, the next thing that Dr. Khoe did was to palpate acupuncture points from the top of the man's neck down to his waist. He had him strip down—take his shirt off, put him on the table and so on. Would that procedure, in acupuncture medicine, be a valid diagnostic approach in gaining information about how to treat the patient?"

A: "Examination of the associated or shui points on the back is part of the diagnostic system in acupuncture, yes. It would be appropriate."

Once again, the standards of acupuncture were shown to be the standards to be used in such cases, not allopathic standards of medical care. They are simply not the same and cannot be used to make determinations or uphold accusations against an alternative practitioner, in this case an acupuncturist.

One accusation against Dr. Khoe was that "there was no accepted medical basis for [Dr. Khoe's] advice to the patient to avoid wearing metal on his body as an aid to energy flow." During the testimony of two of the prosecution's witnesses, it was conceded that they knew little about acupuncture medicine, and that as far as they were concerned "there was no medical basis for advising a patient to stop wearing a metal watch band." However, Professor Tiller explained in some detail in his testimony why there is a scientific basis to support a physician who utilizes acupuncture in his practice to advise the patient to remove a metal watch band from his wrist.

Three witnesses for Dr. Khoe also testified that "the advice to remove the metal watch band is known and utilized in acupuncture medicine." The prosecution's witness, Dr. Kroening, was aware of the practice and stated that he knew of published reports on the subject and thought the advice "might be helpful."

Once again, the standards of orthodox medicine were invalidated in their application to acupuncture.

One of the other charges was that the "treatment which followed the initial diagnosis, including vitamin therapy, was ineffective and not reasonably designed to care for the patient's diagnosed ailments or to relieve the patient's discomfort." This is a point which has come up in the past with many alternative practitioners. In Dr. Khoe's case, the one prosecution witness who testified to this charge was Dr. Boyle. He stated that the diet given to the patient was not reasonably designed to help his condition. However, every other witness, for and against Dr. Khoe, testified that the treatment program of diet, vitamin supplements, and acupuncture that was prescribed was properly designed to treat the patient.

The outcome of the case involving Dr. Khoe was very important to acupuncture practitioners as well as other alternative practitioners. The bottom line was that Dr. Khoe won his case; the charges did not hold up. In the end his victory was a victory for any practitioner who employs any of the modalities, treatments, products, tests, and services that Dr. Khoe used in his practice. His case was a victory for all alternative practitioners, not just acupuncturists.

It serves as a beginning to a solution to the problems that confront all alternative practitioners, manufacturers, and patients as a result of the campaign against them.

The following chapters also address what can be done to address and handle these issues. The solutions are for anyone interested in health-care freedom of choice. The solutions are offered as tools which can and must be used in order to change the situation for the better. It's one thing to have data that could help. It's a "whole 'nother matter" to use it and use it effectively.

The following, then, is a start. The rest is up to you, your family, friends, associates, and allies.

Part Three

The Solutions

Chapter 17

Solutions to the Problems

"WASHINGTON (AP) State officials who violate someone's rights while performing governmental duties may be sued and forced to pay monetary damages, the Supreme Court has ruled.

"The 8-0 decision in a Pennsylvania case could expose officials to costly lawsuits when they are accused of violating a Civil War-era federal law aimed at preventing abuses of power."

[AP Wire story, November 5, 1991.]

"In a ruling that could give consumers a weapon to fight anti-competitive business practices, a split Supreme Court ruled yesterday that a Virginia woman may sue Blue Shield of Virginia for refusing to pay her psychologist's fees."

[Washington *Post*, June 22, 1982.]

Parts One and Two of this book outlined the many aspects of the problem that should be confronted and handled by the victims of this campaign against the alternatives. Victims include licensed professionals, unlicensed practitioners, manufacturers, distributors and sales outlets/stores, multi-level companies, consumers/patients, attorneys for alternative clients, insurance officials, and government officials.

These last two are included because in many cases they have been misled, duped, used, manipulated, misdirected, or adversely influenced, and in most cases were "just following orders" and trying to do their jobs. In many instances the people involved were simply tools of the campaign or conspiracy, and did not know the true nature of what was going on behind the scenes.

However, those who have been involved in planning this campaign/conspiracy *are* liable for their acts and should pay the price. They have known from the start what they are doing, and why, and for whom they are doing it. Those who have taken an active part in the campaign have knowingly pursued goals that were in effect illegal and in violation of the victims' civil rights. There have been violations of antitrust laws and RICO conspiracy laws and other wrong-doing. The remedies discussed in Part Three should be applied to them, along with the others who have conspired in this campaign.

The losses suffered by alternative practitioners are enormous, and those at fault should bear the burden of compensation. Consider, for example, the financial losses of chiropractors in this country during the time that this conspiracy has been in place, perhaps more than 30 years. An amount of $10 billion is not too far off when one considers that most chiropractors who have provided services under Medicare have not been paid for services that exceeded 15 per year. Over an eight year period (since 1986), that's a lot of unpaid services for a lot of chiropractors. Or consider a group of chelation therapists who cannot get paid for their services by insurance companies. This may have been going on over a twenty-year period. According to Dr. Renner there are about 1,500 chelation therapists practicing in the U.S. That being the case, 100 patients per therapist per year, that's 15,000 patients nationwide per year. Multiply that figure by twenty years and you have an idea of how much money these practitioners have lost from insurance companies' non-payment for services. You can see that there is a probability of about 300,000 patients not getting paid from insurance companies for chelation therapy. If we estimate top-end figure of $5,000 per patient, per year, times 300,000 patients over twenty years, we arrive at an estimate of $1.5 billion in services not paid by insurance companies as a direct result of the campaign against chelation therapists.

Additionally, consider all the patients lost as a direct result of the insurance companies' refusal to pay for chelation therapy. Many more are denied access to it (because of this campaign) than have received it. Many of these people have been forced to undergo bypass surgery or some other similar operation, which costs at least 30 times more than chelation ($150,000 compared to $3,000-$5,000). $45 billion has been paid out for heart surgery over the same time period by insurance companies.

How foolish the insurance industry is, really. It could save billions of dollar a year by allowing full chiropractic coverage, acupuncture, chelation therapy and others in the alternative health-care system into the marketplace. By seeing that their economic competitors are cut out of the economic insurance pie, these market manipulators are attempting to guarantee their own economic futures while depriving the American public of a fundamental right to choose.

The following, then, are various remedies and solutions, which could result in turning this situation around and putting an end to the assault on our medical freedoms.

Solutions for Practitioners

Fighting Insurance Denials

- Challenge every denial, especially where an insurance company has used an "expert" consultant on your case.

- Demand to know the basis of the denial.

- Demand to know which consultant was used.

- Challenge that consultant's credentials, training, education, and experience as it relates to the item for which the consultant denied payment.

- Where it is legal to do so, record every conversation between your staff, yourself and the insurance company. (Check with your attorney on your state's laws regarding taped phone conversations.)

- Put everything to the insurance company in writing. If you have a phone conversation with them, follow up immediately, memorializing (committing to writing what has been stated verbally) what was discussed.

- Always demand that *they* commit what *they* say to writing and send you a letter confirming such communication.

- Always demand a copy of the policy which they claim is the basis of their denial. Get it in writing. If you get no satisfaction, then. . .

- Use the state laws regarding your rights to petition your State Insurance Commissioner. Demand that the Commissioner look into why your claim has not been paid. State laws vary from state to state regarding the time period allowed by law during which a claim must be paid. In some states it is 30 days; in others it may be 45 to 60 days. Check with your State Insurance Commissioner's office.

• By law, the State Insurance Commissioner's office must look into every complaint when an insurance company has gone over the time allotted in which to pay a claim. (If, for example, insurance companies are not paying any chiropractors for their use of thermography, then every chiropractor in that state should write the Insurance Commissioner's office demanding an investigation into this practice of non-payment.)

If, after the State Insurance Commissioner's office looks into the nonpayment, you still don't receive satisfaction, then you could do one or more of the following to remedy the situation.

• Remind the State Insurance Commissioner that you are aware of the fact that State Insurance Commissioners may themselves have been influenced against the denied item as a direct result of anti-competitive outside influence. Remind the Insurance Commissioner that as a public servant he is obliged to carry out the law and pursue the case against the insurance company on your behalf regardless of what outside influence may or may not have entered into the decision.

• *If necessary,* inform the Insurance Commissioner that his office is not immune from civil suit if it is found that the office is involved in furthering any anti-competitive activity (reference recent Supreme Court case outlined below) or have been involved in violating your civil rights. Do not back off from making such statements. The situation cannot get any worse; you have already been denied payment, and in the process your civil rights may have also been denied. Stand up for your rights.

• File a Small Claims Court action for each insurance claim that has been denied. Each state sets different amounts that a Small Claims Court can address, usually below a certain figure. To find out the procedure, look up the phone number of the Small Claims Court closest to you in the phone book under County Government, and call them for instructions. In many areas the charge to file is very little; it can range from $12.50 to $50.00. If you wish, you can handle a small claim without the aid of an attorney.

If you have a large number of unpaid claims, and each one falls within the amount you can file for in Small Claims Court, you may want to hire an attorney, on a monthly retainer basis, to file for all the unpaid claims you have from all insurance companies involved in non-payment.

Be Prepared. In any Small Claims Court, each case is addressed separately. You should have all your paperwork together proving that the insurance companies have not paid you when by law they should have. This would include:

(a) All the paperwork on the unpaid claim;

(b) The State Insurance Commissioner's letter to the insurance company on your behalf and any replies;

(c) The state statutes showing that the insurance company has exceeded the allotted time period during which they were to pay;

(d) Supporting affidavits from patients showing receipt of service and evidence that their insurance policy covers your service.

(e) Any letters from the insurance company to you or your patient showing the denial of payment; and

(f) Any other documentation that you or your attorney feel would be relevant to the payment of the claim.

This practice is not an abuse of the legal system. It is in fact your right to use this avenue as a means to get paid when refused payment. I know of many practitioners who have used this with great success. In one such case, the person filing for unpaid claims hired an attorney on a monthly retainer basis, and his attorney succeeded in collecting as much as $15,000 per month on claims that were not being paid prior to using this system as a remedy. It does work.

According to practitioners who have used this remedy to obtain payment from insurance companies, the Small Claims Court looks unfavorably upon anyone who is obliged to pay a bill by law and does not. In most cases the Small Claims Court has ruled in favor of the claimant, providing that the documentation is good.

Also, in almost every case the insurance company is forced to hire, or pay for, an attorney *for every case* in which a representative must appear before the Small Claims Court to answer the claims filed.

For example, if every chiropractor in a state were to file for every unpaid insurance claim from every insurance company that had ever denied payment, and all concerned had a good case for payment— well, the consequences are obvious. The insurance companies involved would almost automatically start paying practitioners who had been taking them to Small Claims Court, particularly after the loss of a few cases. No insurance company wants to pay attorney fees on "petty" claims for which it is continually being taken to Small Claims Court. After a while legal costs could run into the hundreds of thousands of dollars, especially if a whole profession or group of practitioners started filing and winning Small Claims Court cases.

Of course, there is no guarantee of victory in Small Claims Court every time one files. However, it is a remedy that should be used more by those whose livelihoods have been assaulted and damaged by this campaign within the insurance industry.

Fighting Medicare/Medicaid Nonpayment or Limited Payments

Sometimes practitioners do not want to get involved with patients who come to them with Medicare/Medicaid insurance coverage because the payments are so much less than private insurance companies' payments. In many cases, Medicare/Medicaid restricts the number of visits or services that are eligible for payment. Yet most practitioners are uncomfortable turning away such patients— they are in the business of helping people lead better and healthier lives.

If a practitioner, a chiropractor for example, wants to be paid for Medicare services, remedies could be applied that could result in getting paid for more services than Medicare normally allows. The case of Dr. E.M. Nash is one example of what can be done.

Dr. Nash had filed a case before an administrative law judge to review his Medicare cases that were denied because they exceeded the limits of 12 services per patient over a one-year period. The following was taken from the proceedings of the Office of Hearings and Appeals of the Department of Health and Human Services, Social Security Administration:

During 1987, the claimant [Dr. Nash] provided chiropractic services to several Medicare beneficiaries.

The carrier [Blue Cross/Blue Shield of Michigan] allowed payment under Medicare Part B for the first 12 services rendered to each beneficiary. However, it denied coverage in excess of 12. The claimant appealed these denials and, in a few cases, additional visits were allowed, but in general, no more than 12 such services were allowed.

Section 1869(b)(2) of the [Social Security] Act provided for administrative law judge hearings in Part B cases where the aggregate amount in controversy was at least $500.00.

The specific issue is whether payment should be made for services rendered by the claimant to these beneficiaries for services in excess of 12.

. . .This depends, in part, on the nature of the carrier policy with regard to extension of chiropractic treatment parameters. . .

. . . In addition, the issue is whether payment should be made to the provider of services pursuant to the waiver of liability provision of section 1879 of Title XVIII of the Social Security Act.

It is the decision of the undersigned that the claimant, E.M. Nash, D.C., complied with all pertinent carrier policy requirements for documentation allowing for extension of chiropractic treatment parameters, that the services provided by the claimant constituted medically covered services, and that an allowance should be made for these services.

The administrative law judge in the Nash case also made some recommendations and brought out some issues that are important to any practitioner who has experienced similar denials from Medicare:

In December 1985, HCFA [Health-Care Financing Administration] mandated that all carriers implement a screen on chiropractic claims, to be set at 12 services per year. Carriers were required to make medical necessity determinations on all claims where these parameters were exceeded.

Although the 12-visit "screen" was mandated by HCFA, the development and implementation of standards for chiropractors were left to the carriers. A cap of 12 services per year per beneficiary was proposed by a study performed in 1986 ("Chiropractic Services Under Medicare") [See Chapter 11], but has not been implemented.

. . .Blue Cross/Blue Shield of Michigan published its 12 parameter screen in its publication, *The Record,* which was first sent to providers in February 1986.

...*The Record* for February 1986 went on to state that, effective for services rendered on or after January 1, 1986, a maximum of 12 chiropractic treatments per year was allowed, regardless of acute or chronic condition, unless support documentation indicating the medically necessary reason for exceeding the parameter was included with the claim.

...Blue Cross/Blue Shield of Michigan further delineated and expanded the supportive documentation requirements in *The Record* of June 1987. This article reiterated the information previously published in *The Record* of February 1986, adding that Medicare would not allow more than 12 treatments per calendar year *unless* there was documented evidence of a new injury or an acute exacerbation of a patient's condition. The supporting documentation necessary to validate the medical necessity of treatments that exceeded the parameter of 12 visits had to include:

(1) a demonstrated change in the patient's condition or symptomatology;
(2) a demonstrated change in the level of subluxation or an acute exacerbation of a current condition;
(3) documentation of the patient's complaints, explaining how the injury or change occurred.

...Carriers should develop parameters under which an extension in the course of treatment could be supported based on special documentation of need and under which coverage will be finally terminated for lack of reasonable expectation that continuation of treatment would be beneficial.

The Judge ruled in favor of Dr. Nash:

It is the decision of the administrative law judge that the services rendered by the claimant to the beneficiaries in this case were reasonable and necessary. The carrier shall make an allowance for those services, and determine the reasonable charge therefore, consistent with the findings and conclusions set forth herein, under Medicare Part B provisions of Title XVIII of the Act.

One key reason the case went his way was Dr. Nash's own testimony, which could be applied by any practitioner. Dr. Nash contended that the determination of whether the chiropractic care be provided was reasonable and necessary should be made on the basis of chiropractic standards, not the standards of the general medical profession. (*Note:* It was discovered in this case that the 12-visits-per-year guidelines set up by Blue Cross/Blue Shield of Michigan were set by a chiropractor, Dr. Freas, who was not only a paid employee of BC/BS of Michigan, but also a good friend of Dr. Charles DuVall.)

He also presented into evidence a section of BC/BS of Michigan's Medical Criteria Manual (MCM) published on January 2, 1985, which stated, "Necessary services are those services which are generally accepted by the profession as being appropriate diagnostic and therapeutic procedures provided to treat a specific symptomatic, neuromusculoskeletal condition."

Dr. Nash noted that this section referred to section 2251.5 of the MCM, which provides that the chiropractor should be afforded the opportunity to effect improvement or arrest or retard deterioration within a reasonable and generally predictable period of time. He stated that the length of time in which this can be achieved varies with each patient and some patients with a chronic or reoccurring subluxation pattern require continual correction. He argued that such treatment is not maintenance, but rather treatment for a reoccurring condition which is necessary to prevent the beneficiary's condition from further degenerating or deteriorating. He likened this level of chiropractic care to that of a diabetic who requires insulin on a life-long basis or an individual with hypertension who requires hypertension medication to keep blood pressure controlled. In his opinion, these are the same type of reoccurring conditions as are many subluxation patterns.

Dr. Nash's case provides an example for other practitioners to follow in challenging the 12-services per year limit in cases where the circumstances require more than 12 visits.

To follow Dr. Nash's example and challenge the Medicare/Medicaid programs a practitioner should shore up one's position in the following ways:

1. Have a copy of this book in hand and use those portions of the book that relate to your issue.
2. Have your attorney, if you are using one, read this book.
3. Get a copy of the Nash decision and review it for data which aligns and parallels your case before the review/hearing board hearing your case.
4. Present the same arguments that Nash presented in his own defense, if they apply.

5. Use information the Administrative Law Judge presented in the Nash case for your own.

6. Bring out the entire anti-alternatives behind-the-scenes manipulation of the Social Security Act. It relates to your profession as evidence that the figure of 12 visits a year was designed by the opponents of alternatives on an arbitrary basis. This would include everything presented in this book related to:

    (a) The AMA "fixing" the HEW study and the Stanford Research Institute report on chiropractic;

    (b) The data about the National Association for Chiropractic Medicine, the National Council Against Health Fraud, Emprise, the October Plan, and the plan to adversely influence the insurance industry, including Medicare and Medicaid; and

    (c) Data on how the Social Security Act was directly affected and influenced to limit visits to 12 per year by the very same people who have been attacking alternatives.

7. Place this entire book into the record as evidence that the government has been used and manipulated by your opponents.

These methods, with applicable modifications, apply not just to chiropractors, but also to any medical doctor using alternatives—chelation therapists, acupuncturists, homeopaths, naturopaths, dentists, and others in the alternative health-care system.

Using Other Legal Remedies

The following strategies can be applied to the insurance industry or any government agency (such as the FDA), that has, in some way, attacked one's practice, denied a claim, seized products, records, or data from one's office, and so on.

FEDERAL TRADE COMMISSION (FTC) LETTER OF COMPLAINT

Using the system to your advantage is a must for your survival. The FTC has been given the responsibility to enforce the antitrust laws of the United States. One way the FTC does this is to investigate and bring charges in the courts against anti-competitive activity. One tool that one can use is to petition the FTC to investigate anti-competitive activity. The petition is in the form of a Letter of Complaint.

A Letter of Complaint is a formal request made to the FTC to investigate charges of anti-competitive activity, whether it is about an insurance company, an insurance consultant, an enforcement activity being carried out by the FDA, or some other act, many of which are described in this book. One can easily put together a complaint that shows an anti-competitive conspiracy being directed against all of the alternatives or a selected portion of the alternatives. To file a Letter of Complaint:

1. Take the following preliminary steps:
   (a) Contact an FTC official in your regional area and establish a line of communication.
   (b) Let the official know who you are and that you are interested in filing a Letter of Complaint related to anti-competitive activity. Let the contact know that you are part of a group of professionals that have been wronged.
   (c) Find out what the FTC needs in order to respond to your petition.
   (d) Collect and assemble whatever is needed. Present it to the FTC in the form of your Letter of Complaint.
   (e) Maintain phone and letter contact with your contact throughout the entire process.
2. In your Letter of Complaint, show who is involved, what groups are involved, what acts of anti-competitive activity have been committed, what financial harm these acts have done, and the nature and scope of the conspiracy.
3. Make sure your Letter of Complaint is well-documented and includes (a) a concise chronology of events involving the conspiracy to restrain trade or other anti-competitive activity, (b) any and all documentation you have to back up the charges of anti-competitive activity, and (c) a summary put together by an attorney who is familiar with antitrust law. Do not employ an attorney who does not specialize in this area of law.
4. A Letter of Complaint should be presented by an entire group of professionals who have been harmed by the anti-competitive activity. For example, if it involves chelation therapists, it could be done representing the entire group through the American College of Advancement in Medicine (ACAM). If it involves chiropractors, it can be done either through the

state association of the International Chiropractic Association or the American Chiropractic Association. If it involves
manufacturers or sales companies, it can be done on behalf
of all similar companies.

5. Should more information be needed to back up your position
   in a Letter of Complaint, then you should seek out the
   assistance of a qualified investigator to collect additional
   documentation and evidence to help make your case solid.
   Depending on the circumstances, you may have to have this
   done before even beginning the Letter of Complaint.

If the FTC finds merit in your petition, a decision may be made to
investigate. It may take eight to twelve months for the investigation
to be completed. Should the FTC determine that there is in fact a
conspiracy to restrain trade, or some form of anti-competitive activity involved, it has the power to take those involved to court.
Should the FTC challenge the anti-competitive activity, you must
then "wait in the wings" to see what the outcome will be. If it is
positive, the FTC may rule that there is in fact an anti-competitive
conspiracy. Then, based on the FTC's findings, you can take other
actions, some of which follow.

DECLARATORY JUDGMENT

According to *Black's Law Dictionary,* a Declaratory Judgment is
a judgment of the court, the purpose of which is to establish the rights
of the parties or express the opinion of the court on a question of law
without ordering anything to be done. You file for a Declaratory
Judgment before a judge, who determines the facts at issue and
passes his opinion in the form of an order in his findings. If you want
to have the court pass judgment on, say, an anti-competitive conspiracy, or violations of the RICO Act, or Civil Rights violations,
you present your case to make this point. The opposition then
counters what you present, and eventually the judge rules on the
issues before the Court. It is different from a jury trial in that the
judge makes the determination of the outcome. If an anti-competitive
conspiracy case is presented and the judge rules that in fact such
exists, he may also impose a remedy of an injunction against those
involved. There are no monetary damages in a Declaratory Judgment. It simply stands on its own. A Declaratory Judgment may take
much less time in the courts, and cost less, than filing a Class Action
suit, or an antitrust conspiracy suit in a federal court.

When you file for a Declaratory Judgment, you should include all relevant information. Have the specifics of your situation investigated so as to tie that individual situation into the overall anti-competitive scene. Your specific situation is just one piece of a whole pie, and you may need additional data to show the connection and prove your case. Using the information contained in this book to make the general points you want to make is a big start, but you will need to provide evidence in your submission to the judge regarding the direct effects of the campaign upon your particular situation. Consult with your attorney.

Should you prevail with either a Declaratory Judgment suit or the FTC Letter of Complaint, you could then use the legal victory in an individual suit, a Class Action suit, or other action.

INDIVIDUAL AND CLASS ACTION LAWSUITS

A lawsuit is a remedy available to all practitioners. As in the preceding actions, you should have all the facts together before moving forward with a case. Whether the suit is against an insurance company, Medicare/Medicaid, Worker's Compensation, a government agency, or private parties or groups, you should have all the available documentation available for an attorney to work with before you start out.

Your preparations should include having an expert in the area research and investigate your specific situation, tying in the documentation and evidence uncovered with the larger picture.

What is happening on a state-to-state basis is simply one piece of a whole picture. The national campaign/conspiracy against all alternatives works its way down to the state and local level, but almost always ties back to the core plan to destroy the alternatives. That bridge between what is going on locally or state-wide must be linked back up to the national campaign in order to show the scope and nature of the conspiracy being directed against you. Taking your case to court as a separate action would simply be one more remedy.

You must have standing to bring an action. Present a solid case built on a foundation of documentation and evidence that will prove your case. This should be taken up with your attorney in terms of the merits of your case. If any of your previous actions have ended with a legal victory, it may be possible to plug in to that successful action, filing a suit based on that victory.

Some types of cases that individuals or groups could file include civil rights suits, RICO suits, and antitrust suits.

A Class Action suit is a suit that has been brought by representative members of a large group of persons on behalf of all the members of the group. The class must be something ascertainable, in that the members must share a common interest in the issues of law and facts raised by those bringing the suit (the plaintiffs). Other special requirements must be met before the trial court will specifically certify the action as one that could be maintained as a Class Action.

If the court determines that it is in fact a certified class, then all the members of the class must receive notice of the pending action, to give members an opportunity to exclude themselves from the class if they so desire. Anyone who stays in the class is bound by the judgment of the court in the action. Subclasses may be formed within the Class Action in order to reach an identifiable and manageable class size for the purposes of the litigation.

Over the past 50 years, many Class Action suits have been successful, and three of these dealt directly with the American Medical Association and its anticompetitive activities. The one that stands out, because of its relationship to the conspiracy against alternatives, is *Wilk v. AMA*, which dealt with issues involving violations of the trade laws of the U.S. (anti-trust laws).

Those who would possibly have standing in such a suit would include chiropractors, chelation therapists (D.O.s and M.D.s), acupuncturists, homeopaths, naturopaths, holistic dentists, holistic doctors, alternative product manufacturers, alternative product multi-level companies, health food stores, alternative clinics, and consumers/patients.

The amount of work that such a large case would require is tremendous. The fact remains that there is a such a large class of people who have a common interest in the fact that federal laws regarding antitrust have been violated and their civil rights have also been violated.

Victory may take years and can cost millions of dollars. In the case of *Wilk v. AMA,* the class represented all the chiropractors in the country who were damaged by the AMA's conspiracy against them. The case was filed in 1975 and it ended in 1987, 12 long years later. They obtained a favorable decision. However, it cost them millions of dollars. It is the opinion of many who have been involved in these issues that, in the end, the expected benefits have not been realized by the majority of chiropractors attempting to practice in this country. It appears that the conspiracy against the chiropractors, and others, has continued. Years past the point that the judge in the *Wilk* case said the conspiracy had ended, evidence exists to prove otherwise. So there is a down side to such suits. However, although it's a long hard road, a Class Action suit *is* another remedy. Additionally, should any of the previous remedies (such as a Declaratory Judgment or FTC Letter of Complaint) end with a victory, then a Class Action suit would be much more viable.

A Class Action can be filed on many different grounds, some of which include conspiracy to violate antitrust laws, conspiracy to deny civil rights, and RICO conspiracy. Each of these could also be filed as a separate suit, by an individual.

CIVIL RIGHTS ACTIONS

In a recent Supreme Court case, [*Hafer v. Melo*, S.Ct. 1991 WL 221067, (U.S.)] the Court ruled:

State officials may be held personally liable for damages under s. 1983 [Civil Rights Statutes] based upon actions taken in their official capacities. . .This Court has refused to extend absolute immunity beyond a very limited class of officials, including the President of the United States, legislators carrying out their legislative function, and judges carrying out their functions, "whose functions or Constitutional status requires complete protection from suit." State executive officials are not entitled to absolute immunity for their official actions.

. . .It has been settled that the Eleventh Amendment provides no shield for a state official confronted by a claim that he had deprived another of a federal right under the color of state law.

. . .Damage awards against individual defendants in federal courts are a permissible remedy in some circumstances notwithstanding the fact that they hold public office.

. . .We hold that state officials, sued in their individual capacities, are "persons" within the meaning of s.1983. The Eleventh Amendment does not bar such suits, nor are state officers absolutely immune from personal liability under s. 1983 solely by virtue of the "official" nature of their acts.

This ruling by the Supreme Court of the United States is very significant and relevant to any alternative practitioner, manufacturer, or clinic singled out for prosecution based on alternative beliefs and practices. It would appear that in such cases where medical boards, attorneys general, or state food and drug agencies (all of whom are state officials) have been involved in a conspiracy which in effect has resulted in a target being denied civil rights, that targeted victim may use this as a remedy. Consult your attorney.

RICO CONSPIRACY SUITS

The Racketeer Influenced and Corrupt Organizations (RICO) Act has been used—and misused—since it was passed years ago as an instrument for government to pursue organized crime. However, it is a very good tool that could be used by anyone who can show a pattern of racketeering activity on the part of those involved in such activity.

Such a pattern has been asserted to exist within the insurance industry. Aetna, Emprise, and others were sued under RICO, as discussed in Chapter 7. If a conspiracy can be shown to have continued over a period of time, and to be in effect at the present time, and if said conspiracy has violated several federal laws, that activity could be classified as a form of racketeering. It could therefore come under the RICO statutes. This is something on which only a good attorney who is familiar with the RICO laws as well as the anti-alternative campaign could pass judgment. However, it has been used. It is safe to assume that the type of activity documented in this book could be considered violations of RICO laws.

ANTITRUST SUITS

The purpose of the federal antitrust laws is important to understand, as they are there to protect the fundamental principles of the free-enterprise system. These laws are primarily concerned with controlling private economic power through competition, which is considered desirable for several reasons:

(a) *Efficiency in resource allocation.* Competition tends to keep costs and prices lower and to encourage the efficient allocation of economic resources.

(b) *Consumer Choice.* A free competitive market is also thought to be socially desirable because it provides greater opportunities to succeed and offers consumers a broader choice.

(c) *Avoidance of concentrated political power.* By preventing any single person or group from acquiring dominant economic power, the antitrust laws help to avoid undue concentration of political power as well.

(d) *Fairness.* Finally, the antitrust laws encourage fairness in economic behavior among competitors. Through competition, resources are allocated through market forces, rather than through favoritism or prejudice. Competition may also promote equitable distribution of income.

Concerted action among competitors that tends to create a monopoly is termed a *combination in restraint of trade.* Examples include limiting the output of any business or profession for the benefit of the parties to the combination (usually to the detriment of the public). The difference between a combination in restraint of trade and a conspiracy is simply this: Was there an intention to restrain trade or monopolize? If so, then the agreement may be punishable as a criminal conspiracy.

Early law held that if the subject of the agreement to restrain trade was a "necessity of life" (as alternative medicine and products are), then the agreement was punishable as a criminal conspiracy. This appears to be the case as outlined in this book.

A conspiracy is criminal if two or more persons combine for the objective contrary to the public interest, even where such acts would not necessarily be unlawful if done individually.

Group Boycotts and Concerted Refusals to Deal

As we have seen, there appears to be a boycott against alternatives going on in the insurance industry as a direct result of a conspiracy to restrain the trade of those practitioners involved in the alternatives. In looking at the law in this regard, the following is important to understand: "An individual is free to choose those they wish to deal with, except when such refusal amounts to monopolization or an attempt to monopolize." *(Gilbert Law Summaries)*

If the insurance industry is working from a list of practitioners, or a medical board is operating from such a list, or a government enforcement agency is taking actions from such a list, and that list was constructed with the help and direction of the chief economic competitors of those who have been affected by these entities, most certainly a conspiracy is going on.

Also, when a *group of competitors* (such as 350 insurance companies) agrees not to deal with a person or firm (an individual practitioner or a group of them or a clinic) outside the group, there is a *combination in restraint of trade*, in violation of the anti-trust laws.

Additionally, if a group of competitors (such as a chiropractic group formed to influence insurance firms and government insurance programs against their competitors in chiropractic) agrees to deal only on certain terms, or agrees to coerce suppliers (insurance carriers) or customers (patients) not to deal with the boycotted competitor (the targeted alternative practitioner, modality, service, product, or clinic), there is also a combination in restraint of trade.

Taking this one step further, if one applies the principles of the anti-trust laws to the pharmaceutical industry for its combination and criminal conspiracy against its economic competitors in the alternative health-care market place, then one could include that industry in any anti-trust law suit. Again, consult with an attorney who is familiar with these laws.

Disseminating Information Among Competitors

The central question surrounding the issue of whether or not the exchange of information is legal under the antitrust laws is answered by determining if the exchange of data constitutes an unreasonable restraint of trade and if it lessens competition. Where the exchange of information lessens competition, such activity has been found to be in violation of the antitrust laws. One might apply this concept of law to a group (Emprise) devising a plan (outlined in Chapter 6) designed to influence the insurance industry against paying for the services, products, and practitioners that were targeted. That October Plan was also designed to influence various state and federal agencies into taking actions against those targeted. This in effect would put those entities out of business, or reduce their impact on the marketplace as providers of health care, etc.

Furthermore, the law clearly states that where the exchange of information is aimed at *suppressing competition,* such exchange is illegal. In *Eastern States Retail Lumber Dealers Association v. United States* [234 U.S. 600 (1914)], the court held unlawful the circulation by an association of retail lumber dealers (substitute: an association of health insurance companies or some other anti-alternative group) of a list of names of wholesalers (substitute: alternative targets) who sold directly to consumers. The court reasoned that a conspiracy not to deal with such wholesalers could be inferred just from the exchange of such information.

Concerted Action by Competitors to Influence Government

Antitrust law also addresses a very important issue that has been detailed throughout this book: that is, any concerted action by competitors designed to influence government action. Now, the Constitution allows for the right to petition, which includes lobbying, attempts to influence administrative agencies (such as medical boards, the FDA, the FBI, the FTC, and DHHS), as well as influencing the courts (as with "expert witness" testimony).

However, the law also has limitations in this regard. Consider the following attempts to influence governmental action: directing the FDA onto alternative targets; passing laws against alternatives; influencing laws related to vitamins; giving testimony in courts against alternatives; submitting to government insurance programs "expert opinion" which results in suppressing competition, etc. These are nothing but harassment of a competitor, or a "mere sham." In such cases, the courts have found an unlawful combination in restraint of trade.

The antitrust laws indicate that such attempts to interfere directly with the business relationships of a competitor are actionable. If such activity is found to be a part of a conspiracy, a criminal conspiracy case can be brought.

Those involved in such a conspiracy would claim the defense that influencing governmental actions (which constitutes a high percentage of their activity) is their constitutional right. However, this is not the case if one can prove that what they have been doing is nothing but harassment, a "mere sham" perpetrated for anticompetitive purposes. *Sham* means "something false or empty that is purported to be genuine; the quality of deceitfulness, empty pretense." The following are some examples to which this term might be applied:

1. The AMA's fixed study on chiropractic. This was seemingly designed to influence Medicare officials against covering chiropractic services.
2. The Emprise NIH Grant Study and its reports and consensus from "expert panels." These were apparently designed to influence government agencies (FDA, DHHS, DOJ, etc.), insurance companies, medical boards, and government insurance programs against alternative health-care targets. These have been used to influence government investigation, enforcement, indictment, and prosecution of selected alternative targets.
3. The creation of a chiropractic group with purposes aligned closely with those of the anti-alternative Health Fraud/Quackery campaign. The presence on the Advisory Board of this chiropractic group the very same people who have been critical of chiropractic and others in the alternative health-care system.

4. The use of these same critics of chiropractic and alternatives to gain a foothold in the insurance industry. Acting in the capacity of "insurance consultants." Helping to suppress the competition, under the guise of "cost containment" within the insurance industry.
5. While acting in the capacity of an "insurance consultant," forwarding the policies and position of the anti-quackery/health fraud movement. This by itself appears to be anti-competitive and designed to restrain the trade of the economic competitors of the drug industry.
6. Testimony at Congressional hearings and the presentation of undocumented facts and figures designed to influence legislators against alternatives.
7. Identifying economic competitors as "quacks" or "health fraud." Forming an official agreement between the FDA and the pharmaceutical industry solely to pursue those economic competitors through governmental enforcement and prosecution actions, resulting in a conspiracy to restrain trade and unfair competitive activities designed to suppress and eliminate those economic competitors.
8. Insurance companies conspiring with anyone to refuse health insurance coverage for chiropractic services and to refuse payment of claims for services rendered by chiropractors. This is, in fact, a cause of action under the antitrust laws— especially if it can be proven that the purpose and effect of the alleged conspiracy was "to eliminate the competition of chiropractors [or any alternative profession]." (*Ballard v. Blue Shield*, 543 F. 2d 1075 [4th Cir. 19761).

There are many more activities that a good attorney could identify and use. Even this book, which is a good start for someone to begin the fight against the assault on health-care freedom of choice, does not cover the entirety of what is going on.

THIRD-PARTY LAWSUITS

A Third-Party Lawsuit is another legal remedy in certain circumstances. For example, consider a patient who was not reimbursed for a service paid to an alternative practitioner. Or perhaps a patient's insurance company refuses to cover a particular service provided for in an insurance policy. Or, consider the result if a government agency takes action against an alternative practitioner's clinic and it is closed as a result of that action; the patient in that case has been denied access to the treatment, modality, or service that he or she once used and now cannot use because the clinic has been closed down. In another situation, a customer could be denied a particular product as a result of the government taking that product off the market or as a result of a health-food store being raided and its products seized by a government enforcement agency. In such cases, a patient or consumer has the right to sue for having lost access to that alternative service, treatment, modality, product, or clinic. A Third-Party Suit could be filed by that patient/customer. The patient/customer (consumer) would sue the clinic, practitioner, store, or manufacturer for not making the subject alternative in question available to them anymore. The court would recognize that the Third Party—the FDA or the State Medical Board, or the insurance company involved—would have to be brought into the case.

The benefit of such a legal strategy is that it is not the practitioner, clinic, store, or manufacturer that is bringing the suit, but the consumer. It forces the alternative entity to join together with the consumer against the true cause of the problem and participate in the suit. An attorney should be consulted regarding using such a strategy to achieve success in the courts.

Consumer Suits Under Antitrust Laws

The power in this country is said to lie in the hands of the people. This is what the Constitution is all about. When one looks at the campaign against the alternatives, one can see that it is the individual consumer who stands to lose the most. If a patient, for example, goes to a practitioner of chelation therapy, or acupuncture, or chiropractic, or homeopathy, etc., and the insurance company refuses to cover the service, treatment, or modality that consumer had received, then that consumer (patient) has the right to sue the insurance company for not covering or paying for that service.

During the 1981-1982 term, the United States Supreme Court handed down two very important decisions involving the application of antitrust laws and how they relate to issues in the health-care industry. Both of these cases are relevant to the anti-alternative campaign outlined in this book and could help serve as legal remedies.

In *United Labor Life Insurance Company v. Pireno*, the Supreme Court addressed the important questions of antitrust defense, deciding whether the McCarren-Ferguson Act exemption for the "business of insurance" shielded activity which restricted competition between chiropractic groups. It was determined that an insurance company was not exempt under the McCarren-Ferguson Act, if the "business of insurance" was found to include antitrust violations. In other words, an insurance company cannot hide behind this law as a means to shield anti-competitive activity which restricts competition. It would certainly seem that this ruling would play a large role in seeing that any such defense put up by any insurance company or insurance group would be defeated. The specific acts of anti-competitive activity could then be addressed in a law suit brought against them.

The other case which plays a large role in possible remedies for a consumer is *McCready v. Blue Shield of Virginia.* In this case, the court was faced with the question of *standing,* that is, whether restrictions should be superimposed on the statutory language creating a private right of action for antitrust violations. The court basically ruled that a patient can sue an insurance company if that insurance company denies payment for a service the patient received from a practitioner. In this decision, the court assessed whether the requisite "physical and economic nexus" existed. In other words, was there a connection between the patient being denied and any physical or economic damage done as a result of anti-competitive activity by the insurance company?

The court quickly rejected Blue Shield's argument that a health-care plan subscriber (a consumer/patient) could not challenge the non-reimbursement policy of the insurance company as a conspiracy solely because the alleged conspiracy was intentionally directed at psychologists (or any similarly situated alternative practitioner) rather than patients.

The court held that the availability of Section 4 of the Sherman Antitrust Laws, ". . .is not a question of the specific intent of the conspirators. . ." The remedy cannot be restricted to the competitors (the pharmaceutical industry v. the alternative health-care industry, for example, or allopathic medicine v. alternative medicine) whom the defendants hoped to eliminate from the marketplace.

McCready was denied payment for her psychological therapy because the psychologist did not consult with a medical doctor/psychiatrist. It was important to the court that Blue Shield had allegedly sought to achieve its illegal ends through the denial of reimbursement to consumer-subscribers such as McCready. The injury to McCready in the form of increased net cost for psychotherapeutic services was "therefore both foreseeable" and "a necessary step" in effectuating the ends of the alleged conspiracy. The court finding could apply to an alternative patient denied payment or reimbursement for a number of reasons. For example:

1. An acupuncturist did not consult with a medical doctor, or a licensed medical doctor was not used in the performance of the acupuncture.
2. An alternative treatment, modality, or service was denied because it does not meet with the "medical standards," or was reviewed and denied by someone who is not trained in the alternative modality, treatment or service.
3. A Medicare claim was denied for more than 12 visits. This would in fact put a financial burden on a patient who would be forced to seek out medical care to address the same ailment that the patient's alternative practitioner was treating. It is probable that the secondary treatment would be more expensive (and perhaps require more than 12 visits). A medical doctor might recommend surgery or a regimen of drugs over a period of time to handle back pain, at a considerably higher cost to the patient.
4. A consumer cannot get a specific remedy because that product is not recognized by the insurance company. A vested interest says it is "quackery or health fraud."

There are many more examples where the principles of the McCready case could be applied by a patient/consumer in a consumer lawsuit.

The court noted that McCready's claim of injury was based on *a concerted refusal to reimburse her,* not on the allegation of restraint of trade in the market for group health plans. The Court characterized the injury to McCready as a patient as "inextricably intertwined with the injury the conspirators sought to inflict on psychologists and the psychotherapy market."

The most obvious and straightforward result of the McCready decision is that consumers who are covered by insurance company plans and policies now clearly have the right to sue insurance companies over payment and reimbursement issues where the insurance company, discriminating against targeted practitioners or procedures, has refused to pay or reimburse.

The disfavored (or targeted) practitioner has always had standing to sue under antitrust laws. Under *McCready,* the patient now has standing as well. Probably this point is the most significant of this

Supreme Court opinion as it relates to all of the alternative practitioners, clinics, treatments, and modalities.

The potential significance of this remedy can be best appreciated when the impact of the *Virginia Academy of Clinical Psychologists v. Blue Shield of Virginia* decision on the merits of such claims are considered. Under that decision, Blue Shield (or any insurance company) plans are vulnerable whenever they adopt reimbursement policies which affect competition between physicians and non-physicians, or between specialists using one procedure (bypass surgery for example) and specialists using other procedures (such as chelation therapy).

In view of the fact that access to insurance reimbursement is, as a practical matter, absolutely essential to the viability of any practice, including an alternative practice, the anti-competitive effect of such discriminatory policies must be readily acknowledged. The fact that some group of "experts" placed themselves into a position of acting as advisors to the insurance industry and in so doing have effected a plan to block payment, reimbursement, or coverage by policy definition of targeted alternatives is in itself, apparently, a *per se* violation of the antitrust laws of the United States.

Not only do the practitioners of the alternatives have a right to sue under these laws, but so do the consumers/patients who have been denied reimbursement for those services or procedures.

Other Consumer Remedies

The following remedies can be used by consumers, as well as practitioners, manufacturers, distributors, multilevel companies, sales outlets, clinics, and so on. These remedies have been used effectively in the past.

WRITING LEGISLATORS

A consumer or patient sending a letter to a Congressman or Congresswoman, senator or state representative carries a lot of weight. This is especially true if the person sending the letter is one of many writing about the same complaint. There are some rules that should be kept in mind to get action:

(a) Keep it to the point.
(b) Try to include a brief chronology of events.
(c) Attach any documentation that would help your complaint.
(d) Try and keep it a short letter.

(e) Anticipate that the politician you are writing will send your complaint on to the agency about which you are complaining, i.e., FDA or State Medical Board, etc. With that in mind, cut off their defense by showing that they have been *used* in this campaign or attack against the alternative practitioner, manufacturer, etc. about which you are writing.

(f) Always be polite.

(g) If possible, send in a typewritten letter. If handwritten, make sure it's neat and legible. Avoid form letters.

(h) Give a possible solution, such as asking the Congressman or legislator to support an investigation by a committee into possible monopoly hearings on this issue.

You should try to find out where your state or federal representative stands on the issue at hand. Before you send your letter, you should find out that representative's voting record on various issues that relate to what you are writing about. If your representative has taken a lot of Political Action Committee (PAC) money from vested interests such as the medical association or drug industry, you may want to educate him or her on the issues by sending a copy of this book. Inform him or her that siding with the vested interests is not always in the best interest of constituents such as you. You might add that you expect that person to rise above such interests and look into this matter in an objective manner. Remember, you have a vote that could be cast against that person in the next election. You have the power.

CONGRESSIONAL HEARINGS

The Congress has several committees and subcommittees that could be asked to look into these matters. One tool the voter/consumer has is to instigate a hearing to look into the monopoly that has been exposed here. Know where your representative stands on the issues.

If enough voters/consumers of the alternative health-care system were to successfully demand such hearings, they could effect a major change in what is going on. Such hearings could be the starting point of breaking up the monopoly that does in fact exist in the health-care marketplace.

A grass-roots movement can make a big difference. You might want to join an existing consumer-oriented group or more than one group. Start up a drive to call for a Congressional hearing into the monopoly. One person *can* cause a lot to happen by being really interested in seeing something change for the better. You could also start a chapter of a national consumer group. Get petition drives going demanding a Congressional hearing into the monopoly. It could be a letter-writing campaign. Whatever it is, if enough people get involved, then change can occur.

It is your Constitutional right to petition government. In fact, the power is in the hands of those who exercise that right. Your rights have been violated and are continually being assaulted. You can fight back. . .in numbers.

WHISTLEBLOWER GROUPS

A very effective tool of the consumer/people over the past few decades has been something called whistleblower groups. They have cropped up within government and also outside government. The following are examples of successful whistleblower activities:

1. Internal Revenue Service whistleblowers. These have shown up inside the IRS, as well as from groups outside of government.
2. Defense Department whistleblowers. Over the years many officials inside the Defense Department and the defense industry have blown the whistle on corrupt government defense contracts that have cost the taxpayer billions of dollars in overspending and waste.
3. Bounty-hunter laws have been applied to fraud and waste within government agencies. These laws usually apply to government workers, but can also be applied to those outside government who are aware that fraud is being committed. The Lincoln Laws have been among the laws that apply to this area. A person turning in someone found to be guilty of fraud is qualified to get a reward. Usually it is a certain percentage of the total amount saved or exposed.

Whistleblower laws usually apply to people who work inside government. However, someone outside of government who is aware of fraudulent practices within government may also apply for such rewards should the government succeed in prosecuting those involved in the fraud. Private groups are also doing this.

A recent development along these lines is outlined in this press release, issued December 5, 1993, by the National Commission on Law Enforcement and Social Justice.

Let's Clean Up the FDA!

The National Commission on Law Enforcement and Social Justice (NCLE) is announcing the establishment of the "FDA Whistleblowers" campaign.

As you may know, the Hatch "moratorium" was over on December 15th. While various safety measures are in the works by concerned groups and individuals, the FDA may start to infringe in our lives by attempting to increase regulation of vitamins, herbs, amino acids, etc.

The reason why our vitamins are being threatened, why poisonous and deadly drugs are "approved" by the FDA, but truly helpful substances like laetrile and L-tryptophan are banned is very simple. Power vested interests including pharmaceutical companies, control the FDA and have bought them.

There is corruption within FDA, which until exposed, will never unravel the problem that health conscious individuals are trying to solve—the free choice of vitamins and nutritional supplements without having them dictated by the FDA.

The "Whistleblowers Act" was enacted by the U.S. Congress to protect government workers who "blow the whistle" on corruption and unethical conduct within the workplace. Quite a bit of corruption of government employees has been exposed by whistleblowers.

NCLE's FDA Whistleblower program is designed to successfully weed out the corruption by offering rewards to those government employees who come forward with information that will lead to the criminal prosecution of unethical FDA employees, who are jeopardizing our safety and that of our children. Since FDA employees deal with regulating safeguards on our food and drugs, their corruption and vested interests are far-reaching and affect the lives of every American.

NCLE has a team of crackerjack attorneys who will review the documents, work out the legal handling, and get them implemented.

Until vested interests within the FDA are spotted and exposed, we will continue to have the same problem of repressive regulations on health care, and favoritism towards the large medical and pharmaceutical industries.

NCLE volunteers have been passing out fliers in front of the FDA buildings soliciting Whistleblowers to come forward. If they turn over evidence and documentation that leads to the prosecution of an FDA employee, they will be awarded up to $10,000. NCLE will also have volunteers doing events in front of the FDA, and getting broad media coverage. Additionally we want to place large full-page Whistleblower ads in major media across the country, especially in the D.C., N.Y. and L.A. areas.

Please join us in our fight for health care by exposing the corruption and vested interests within the FDA. Your assistance is needed to help clean up the FDA.

NCLE, 20929-47 Ventura Blvd., Suite 205, Woodland Hills, CA. 91364.

NCLE is incorporated as a public benefit corporation. You can call or write the NCLE (phone 818-955-5388) to get a copy of the survey they sent out with this press release and additional information on how you might be able to help. There are many other groups listed in the back of this book that you can contact to help as well.

MEDIA EVENTS

One source of help for consumers/patients who wish to bring about change for the better may be the media, both print and electronic (television and radio). Getting local daily newspapers, weekly newspapers, alternative newspapers, television news shows, and radio talk shows to cover stories related to the issues raised in this book is important. The media is very interested in controversy, especially if it involves something as big as the pharmaceutical industry or the government. If a story also involves large sums of money—which this issue obviously does—that too would pique their interest in what you might have to say. The fact that there is obvious harm done to the health-care system, and that the story would include orthodox medicine versus alternative medicine, makes for good copy.

If a story is presented with most of these above ingredients, the chances are good that this will interest the media. For example, the following incident took place in Minnesota in September 1987.

Blue Cross/Blue Shield of Minnesota had reportedly removed 350 chiropractors from its list of providers under their insurance plan. It happened that Dr. John Renner was scheduled to make a presentation to officials of BC/BS of Minnesota on September 8, 1987. According to one highly placed source in BC/BS of Minnesota, Dr. Renner was allegedly there to show the insurance executives how to better combat health fraud and quackery and help them set up a fraud unit. A group of chiropractic patients got wind of Renner's scheduled visit and planned to use the opportunity to picket BC/BS of Minnesota headquarters. Insurance companies absolutely hate bad press, let alone a group of activist patients picketing in front of their headquarters. What the group apparently planned was to rotate about 30-40 patients over a one- or two-day period, with placards and signs protesting what they felt were the issues.

These patient/picketers knew that Dr. John Renner had been a vocal opponent of chiropractic and other alternatives over the years. They also knew that he was a member of the National Council Against Health Fraud (NCAHF) and also the head of the Kansas City Council On Health and Nutritional Fraud and Abuse (KCCHNFA).

According to the newspapers that covered the event, these were among the picketers' signs and placards:

Keeping Consumers Confused on Health and Nutritional Facts in America (**KCCHNFA**)

Is Renner a FRAUD??

HEALTH FRAUD CAMPAIGN IS A <u>FRAUD</u>!!

RENNER EXPERT for VESTED INTERESTS?

The group of picketers had chosen one person to be their spokesperson with the media. When they gathered in front of the BC/BS building with their signs, they already knew what the issues were and who would best communicate these issues to the media. Each of their priorities, in the form of issues and protest, was worked out beforehand. In this way, the person speaking with the media knew exactly what to say and what answers to give when asked questions.

The group had its selected spokesperson inform all local television and radio stations and all local newspapers that a large picket was to take place in front of the BC/BS building the following morning. They gave this notice by phone to all the media contacts that they wanted to cover the event. These calls were placed in the late afternoon and early evening, after BC/BS offices had already closed for the day, to insure that BC/BS wasn't tipped off by any industry-sympathetic press.

The media was informed of the time the picketers would be there, the date, and the place. They were also advised that it was a controversial issue and that it involved one of the biggest names in health-fraud issues. It also involved the livelihood of hundreds of health-care practitioners (350 chiropractors), millions of dollars, and potential harm to thousands of patients. In this way the protestors effectively captured the interest of the media.

All of the signs and placards purposely said nothing about what the main issues were, causing the newspaper reporters to actively pursue information and to ask questions regarding the specific issues about which the protesters were there picketing. Some of the resultant story lines were:

> Protesters angry with Blue Cross/Blue Shield of Minnesota's recent insurance policy changes regarding chiropractors picketed outside the company's office on September 8, 1987.
>
> More than 30 sign-wielding chiropractic patients marched across the company lawn, to draw attention to their complaints and concerns.
>
> "Blue Cross/Blue Shield has cut their insurance benefit for chiropractic patients from full coverage to 15 services per year," complained group spokesperson, Dolly Newberg. "It's our belief that they're trying to eliminate coverage completely."

Strategically, the first one in the door with a story has an offensive advantage in the media. Secondary stories or comments usually appear to have the taint of a defensive statement or the ring of denial by the parties being accused. It has been said that the best defense is a good offense. It is also true that if you can get your opposition to only defend and not attack, you will have won that battle. To attack your opposition on their weaknesses, and on your terms, is good strategy. This is what was done here, as the following quotes from a resultant story show:

> Bill Jennison, vice-president of claims at BC/BS of Minnesota, dismissed Newberg's claim, stating "there is clearly a

distortion of facts leading to confusion among chiropractic patients."

Note that in saying this the spokesman made two tactical errors. He made an entire group of consumers angry by implying they didn't know what they were talking about, and he dismissed the claim of Ms. Newberg in a patronizing way, yet later proves her claim is true with his own words. The story went on to point out, "Jennison admitted that BC/BS changed its insurance in February."

The article explained how BC/BS justified cutting services down to 15 and that BC/BS stated that the majority of chiropractors could handle their patients within 22 visits. However, Jennison also stated that the 25% of patients who could not be adequately treated within 22 services must obtain pre-authorization before insurance would cover the costs. The article continued:

> This pre-authorization also angers the picketers, who said they feel it's just another way for the company to resist paying for chiropractic services.
>
> Rumors that Dr. Renner, who is affiliated with the National Council Against Health Fraud, was meeting to establish a similar group [fraud unit] at Blue Cross prompted Newberg to organize picketers.
>
> "He's publicly denounced chiropractors and has called them quacks," Newberg said. "We believe he wants to eliminate any health-care professional that does not actively use drugs as a mode of treatment."
>
> Blue Cross Public Relations Director Katherine Maza said the rumors that Dr. Renner will be hired as a consultant to Blue Cross's fraud committee are false. She said that he was invited to speak to senior staff and board members on fraud abuse in the health fields.

This article is a classic example of getting one's platform into an article. Note that the opposition had to defend, and in so doing they also gave the public more information to use to make their own minds up about Dr. Renner and why he was at BC/BS.

Making your cause interesting to the media is a very good tool, as this incident illustrates. The result of this particular picket was that the 350 chiropractors who had been suspended as providers of chiropractic services because they were delivering more than 15 services per patient per year were reinstated. There were two or three articles about this picket and the issues raised. Another result of that incident was that the State Insurance Commission opened an investigation into BC/BS of Minnesota and its policy on chiropractic coverage.

The best time to present a story to the media is when something happens that is timely to your issue. For example, when an insurance company raises a new policy coverage issue that cuts or in some way restricts the delivery of an alternative service, such as the above incident, or when a government agency takes an action against an alternative practitioner, clinic, manufacturer or outlet. A group of organized patients, consumers, or customers picketing in front of a government building will always get media coverage. Understandably, government agencies hate bad press. Remember, if you get in the first shot, carry your points through a spokesperson who knows the issues (but is not a professional practitioner or member of the office staff of a target), you have a better chance of presenting your case to the public. You may even gain their understanding and support. At the same time, you will put the opposition on the defensive. They will be making "klutzy" statements and issuing denials to your charges.

Another way to get press coverage is to hold a press conference and/or issue a press release. Again, time your presentation with the occurrence of a relevant event. Here are some points on holding a press conference:

1. The best place to hold a press conference is at the Press Club located in your city, if there is one. If not, rent a hotel conference room close to your local newspaper office or television station.
2. Contact the Press Club to secure a date and reserve a room.
3. The best time to hold a press conference should be determined by asking the Press Club officials. Usually lunch time is a good slot. Among the press it is said that Monday is a slow day for news. Check with Press Club officials on what day is best.
4. Have sandwiches and drinks for the media.
5. If you have enough advance time, send out a press release announcing the press conference. Promote the free lunch and drinks in the release.
6. Let the media know a little about why you are calling a press conference and that a complete press release and story, with documents, will be provided to them.

7. At the beginning of the press conference distribute a "press pack," which includes your press release and the documents to back your story. Hold the conference giving your verbal account of the story. Answer all questions honestly and to the point; never lie to the media. Always give them your main concern and repeat it as often as you can during the conference. If you are trying to get across that there is a planned campaign being financed by the drug industry against their economic competitors, then repeat that as often as you can within the framework of your story and in answering the media's questions.

The ideal situation would be to hold a press conference with advance notice to the media of anywhere from 48 hours to a week. Valid motivations for a press conference include:

1. A planned countersuit against the government and its allies involved in an attack against your business.
2. A "new find" you have now just come across which sheds new light on what is behind the government action.
3. A formal request to have a federal grand jury look into charges of a government campaign being directed against your business by your competitors in the pharmaceutical industry.
4. A major legal motion, including the filing of information or documentation that charges a conspiracy going on against your business.
5. The filing of a counterclaim involving a very large damage figure. When asking for damages, the larger the figure the bigger the draw. Whenever possible, in a class action suit or a RICO conspiracy charge against a government individual or outside-of-government vested interest, a large damage amount should be asked for and promoted in all media contacts and press releases and press conferences.
6. The gathering of a large number of patient signatures on a petition to the legislature. Patients demanding legislative hearings to investigate allegations of anticompetitive activity, conspiracy and a campaign against your practice, profession, business, etc.
7. A suit filed by a group of chiropractors (or other professionals) against the insurance industry for not covering a particular service.

Legal Victories

There are legal remedies that have been used or could be used successfully. These remedies are available to manufacturers, multi-level companies, sales outlets, and distribution companies involved with alternative products. They can also be used by practitioners, clinics, and others who have been targeted by this campaign. In all cases an attorney should be consulted, to determine the best remedy that would apply to your specific case.

With the FDA, U.S. Customs, U.S. Postal Service, Department of Justice, the FBI, the Department of Health and Human Services Inspector General for Investigations, Medicare Fraud Units, Medicaid Fraud Units, and others involved in the Health Fraud Campaign, one can get the feeling of being up against the entire government. Well, *all isn't hopeless.* There are many cases in which a manufacturer, store, sales company, distributor, practitioner, or clinic has taken on the system and has won.

The inescapable fact of the matter is that in many cases the government has overstepped its bounds. It has been shown to be involved in one or more of the following:

1. Selected Prosecution.
2. Selected Enforcement.
3. Abuse of Power.
4. Violation of Due Process.
5. Malicious Prosecution.
6. Party to Conspiracy to Restraint of Trade.
7. Party to RICO Conspiracy.
8. Violation of Civil Rights Laws.
9. Illegal Enforcement of Quota Systems.

Examples cases in which these abuses were recognized follow:

The Case of Leonard Licht, Ph.D. Dr. Licht was a practicing psychologist in Hawaii. The State Medicaid Program director secured an indictment against Dr. Licht in April 1985. He was charged with 14 counts of Medicaid fraud and one count of theft. He was accused of defrauding the Medicaid program of $1,600 over a three year period. Newspaper headlines charged Dr. Licht with fraud, he was indicted by a grand jury, and then went to court before a jury. In November 1985 he was *acquitted of all charges.*

During this case, the ACLU testified that ". . .the Medicaid Fraud Control Unit has abused the subpoena process and disregarded the privacy of people in this state." The ACLU also condemned the use of ". . .unchecked, unrestrained, and unlimited power" which ignored the due process rights of providers." The jury found that the Department of Human Services had disregarded its own procedures by the manner in which it conducted the investigation. It accused Medicaid Fraud Chief George Yamamoto of initiating an unwarranted criminal prosecution against Dr. Licht. The jury awarded Dr. Licht $600,000 in damages after they found that he was in fact a victim of malicious prosecution. The Medicaid Fraud Unit Chief was also deemed responsible for "intentional infliction of emotional distress."

The Case of Carol A. Brown, M.D. Dr. Brown, a psychiatrist, was charged with 134 counts of Medicaid fraud, which carried total penalties of 670 years imprisonment and $268,000 in fines. Dr. Brown was targeted for political reasons; she was outspoken about a newly planned hospital and the high estimated costs of the project. She also wanted to blow the whistle: finding that many of the children she was seeing for organic brain problems were linked to high levels of mercury poisoning, she identified this as being caused by high levels of mercury found in locally grown marijuana. She wanted to make this known, but it was suppressed by state health officials, and the state Medicaid Fraud Unit came after her.

On April 24, 1987, she was *acquitted on all counts.* The judge in the case even questioned why the state had brought charges against her. Following her acquittal, she filed a suit against the state of Hawaii, the Department of Human Services, and four state officials on the grounds of inflicting emotional distress, breach of contracts, negligent administration of Medicaid, invasion of privacy, tortious interference with contracts, and civil rights violations.

The plaintiffs appealed, and according to the record Dr. Carol Brown lost in Appeals Court. Although she was found innocent to begin with, she was up against too much politics on the issue of the mercury poisoning of children in the State of Hawaii. According to Howard Fishman, author of the series on Medicare/Medicaid investigation abuses, she ended up moving out of Hawaii and to Florida, where she lives today.

The Case of Kenneth Melashenlfo, M.D. A suit filed in the U.S. District Court in Fresno, California, by a family practitioner seeking to be reinstated into the Medicare program resulted in exposing a quota system within the Inspector General's Office in the Department of Health and Human Services (HHS). The quota system, which the court called a "merit pay/bounty system," required employees of Inspector General Richard P. Kusserow to increase sanctions and fines imposed on Medicare providers each year in order to qualify for pay increases. U.S. District Court Judge Robert E. Coyle of Fresno, California, ordered Kusserow to terminate this practice, ruling that it had deprived Doctor Melashenko of his Constitutional rights to due process. A former Assistant Inspector General of the HHS who was in charge of assigning quotas stated, "These agents know that their promotions are very much dependent on how many scalps they put on the wall. They are prone, therefore, to overly zealous enforcement which may, in fact, ignore some of the basic rights to which the physicians they are investigating are entitled." Other providers who were excluded from the Medicare program under similar circumstances may be able to base their appeals on Judge Coyle's ruling.

The Case of Eugeniu Liteanu, M.D. Dr. Liteanu was a Long Island, New York, psychiatrist who was charged with five felony counts of offering a false instrument for filing with knowledge and intent to defraud. His case went to the Suffolk County Criminal Court in New York in September 1990. After only one hour of deliberation, a jury *totally acquitted him of Medicare fraud charges.* Dr. Liteanu, who is from Romania, said of his acquittal, "The jury decision shows the triumph of our democratic system of justice in the United States."

After the trial, the jurors unanimously agreed that the case should have never been brought. They were outraged that the taxpayer's money was wasted on a case like this where—even if you agreed with the prosecution (which they did not)—the value of the case brought against the doctor was a grand total of $90.00 that the government claimed was fraudulently claimed.

The Case of A.O. Supply Company, Hebron, Ohio. A.O. Supply Company is a sales and distribution firm involved with alternative products. It is owned and run by the Michaelis family. The FDA conducted a search and seizure of products addressed to and shipped by Michaelis. The searches were conducted without a warrant at various common carrier terminals in Columbus, Hebron, and Cincinnati, Ohio. These included air freight cargo offices and United Parcel Service (UPS) depots. FDA investigators had conducted an undercover surveillance of the Michaelis' business for six months, and had

observed packages going to and being shipped from the Michaelis'
business at the offices of these common carriers. They also opened
up these packages without a warrant. Then on January 17, 1977, the
FDA conducted searches of the various packages at the air cargo
office and UPS depot.

The FDA presented its investigator's affidavit to a judge, who
then issued a search warrant authorizing the search of the Michaelis
home and business premises. They seized all records, products, and
other property that the government said was linked to their operation.
On July 14, 1977, the search-and-seizure warrant was executed.

The Michaelis family filed for a return of all of their property,
claiming they were the subject of an illegal search and seizure. The
court determined that the validity of the July 14, 1977, search-and-
seizure warrant depended on the validity of the preceding searches of
their packages at the various common carrier offices and depots. The
Michaelises argued that the searches were unconstitutional as warrantless criminal searches. The government argued that these searches were "regulatory and therefore conductible without a warrant"
and cited several cases to justify its position. The court ruling on this
point aptly pointed out, "Even assuming the searches were
regulatory, this Court does not find that they come within the *Bis-
well-Colonnade* exception to the warrant requirement. [These are
two cases the government cited to justify their warrantless searches.]
The court also ruled that the statute under which the FDA operated
(21 U.S.C. s 374) regarding its powers to search, where and when
and who they can search, didn't apply in this case. The court stated,
". . .the statute on its face would authorize the inspection of any place
thought by FDA agents to contain the regulated articles without
showing to anyone that the place bears a relation to the industries
subject to inspection under the Act, or it is reasonable to believe that
it is an establishment where drugs are held. This Court does not
believe that Congress intended to authorize so broad of a search."
Also, the court cited a case wherein it was ruled that "the mere fact
that common carriers are engaged in interstate commerce does not
make them establishments under the Act." So the U.S. District Court
for Southern District of Ohio, Eastern Division (Judge Robert M.
Duncan) ruled, "The provision does not authorize the warrantless
inspection of regulated articles in the hands of common carriers in
the absence of any showing that the carrier's business activity is such
that an investigator could reasonable believe that the carrier's
premises and vehicles are a place where drugs are held. Here there is
no proof that the investigator, before searching the carrier's

premises, knew it to be an 'establishment' where drugs were held for shipment in interstate commerce. . .The seizure of articles from Michaelis' home and business premises in Hebron, Ohio, was unlawful as undertaken pursuant to an invalid warrant. Finding Michaelis to be an aggrieved person under Rule 41 (e) and finding that possession of none of the articles seized is unlawful, the Court finds that Michaelis is entitled to return of the property under Fed. R. Crim. P. 41(e). The plaintiff's motion for a return of property is therefore granted."

The Case of Nutri-Cology. This case was detailed in Chapter 9. However, it is worth a second mention because it is a classic case that other manufacturers and distributors of alternative products need to know about. Some brief highlights of the court decision in that case are:

Defendants correctly noted that claiming that a product improves immune function is not identical to claiming that a product should be used to cure, prevent, mitigate, or treat a disease.

The government's position on the definition of "drug" appeared to be overreaching to say the least. It is apparently the FDA's view that if a company claims milk helps prevent rickets, milk suddenly becomes a drug.

The government's theory that Section 1845 permits it to recover restitution and disgorgement in civil proceedings on mail and wire fraud charges, smacks, again of overreaching, in this case.

Accordingly the government has failed to demonstrate that Germanium and Borage Oil are unsafe food additives and its motion for summary judgment on this issue is denied.

The bottom line is that the Nutri-Cology case was in fact a victory for every alternative product manufacturer, health-food store, clinic, or practitioner that either sells or distributes alternative health-care products. This victory by Nutri-Cology and owners Steve Levine and Susan Levine is a standard to hold high and one that should be quoted, used, and worked into other litigation whenever possible.

Conclusion

There are many ways in which you can exercise your rights in this assault on our medical freedom. The preceding are just some of the remedies that you can use to bring about a change for the better. Everyone who has been targeted by this campaign, or who has been a victim of it, should use whichever remedy that applies to the situation to fight back.

1. Know your rights.
2. Exercise them.
3. Fight back.
4. Unite.

We need to never forget the following statement, taken from a paper that was delivered by the former Deputy Director of the Federal Trade Commission's Bureau of Competition to the National Conference of Bar Presidents in New Orleans on February 4, 1983 (just about the time that the PAC/FDA Anti-Quackery Campaign started.)

Our goal, as in all our activities, is to encourage competition and informed consumer choice. As the Supreme Court stated. . . the basic premise of our economic systemas reflected in the antitrust laws—is that "competition will not only produce lower prices, but also better goods and services."

In extreme contrast to this reference to the Supreme Court's statement about the basic premise of our economic system and competition (the free-enterprise system), we must also remember the statement of Associate FDA Commissioner for Regulatory Affairs Gary Dykstra:

The Task force considered. . .what steps are necessary to ensure that the existence of dietary supplements on the market does not act as a disincentive for drug development.

We have seen to what lengths the private vested interests and their allies in government have gone in their attempts to deny the public access to a truly competitive free-enterprise system, which would bring down the price of health care, thus making it possible for more people to have good health care at a reasonable cost.

The opponents to alternative health care seem to be saying, "Our way is the only way. It is either your money or your life."

It is believed that the majority of the people in this country do not agree with that assessment, and that this assault on our medical freedom must stop. To exercise our rights is the American way; to take those rights away or deny them is something else.

Key Documentation by Chapter

The documents listed below are only the key *documents mentioned in the various chapters. These are, by no means, all of the documents referenced. There are thousands of pages of documentation; the following are the most important. In many instances a document, memorandum, letter, or report is mentioned more than once in this book. A document mentioned, for example, in Chapter 3 may also appear in several other chapters throughout the book. In these cases, a document is listed only the first time it is mentioned, in the chapter in which it first appears.*

Part One

Chapter 1: The Problem
1. Memorandum. September 21, 1967, from Robert A. Youngerman to H. Doyl Taylor, AMA Department of Investigation, Re: Meeting of Committee on Quackery, September 9, 1967. 5 pages.

Chapter 2: The Clash of Medical Philosophies
1. CCHI, Agenda. Friday May 2, 1975, Meeting. 1 page.
2. *Time* magazine article. August 18, 1976, "Sore Throat Attacks," page 54.

Chapter 3: Dirty Politics and Dirty Tricks
1. Memorandum. August 28, 1974, from H. Doyl Taylor to all members of the CCHI. Cover memo to 5-page package of minutes, goals, objectives etc.
2. Incorporation Papers of Lehigh Valley Committee Against Health Fraud, Inc. April 27, 1970. 13 pages.
3. *AMA News* article, "Profile: Stephen Barrett, M.D. Fighting Health Fraud." August 25, 1975. 2 pages.
4. Articles: Glances: "Forming a Group to Fight Quackery", by Stephen Barrett, M.D. Circa 1974-75.
5. CCHI Meeting Minutes. May 4, 1973. Page 5 of 8.

Chapter 4: The Current Campaign

1. DHHS Grant Application from Paul Chusid, Grey Medical Advertising, for PAC/FDA Public Service Anti-Quackery Program: amount $55,000. July 28, 1983. 2 pages of 2.
2. Letter of Agreement between PAC and FDA. Circa 1983-84. 3 pages.
3. PAC Letterhead "Public Service Anti-Quackery Program." Goals, Audience, Strategy, Tactics, Methodology, Evaluation, Key Personnel, Budget and Funding. 7 pages.
4. Letter from FDA Associate Commissioner Joseph Hile to Paul Chusid, re: expenditures of campaign. May 27, 1983. 1 page.
5. Letter to Advertising Agencies on Joint PAC/FDA letterhead, jointly signed by FDA Commissioner Frank Young and PAC President Roger O'Neill. October 22, 1984. 2 pages.
6. DHHS Memorandum from Roger Miller, Director of Communication Staff, to FDA Commissioner Frank Young, re: Jury Members Selected to review PAC/FDA ad proposals. March 20, 1985. 2 pages.
7. Roper Reports (Survey), re: Alternative survey. October 1984. 1 page of 51.
8. Typed memo to "Roger" from "Bruce" (Brown-FDA PR official), re: "Big Three." April 11, 1985.
9. "Health Fraud Products" list, attached to the overall Program and submitted by FDA for PAC/FDA campaign. Circa 1983. 4 pages.
10. FDA Compliance Policy Guides: Guide 7150.10. "Health Fraud-Factors in Considering Regulatory Action," Chapter 50—General Policy. June 5, 1987. 3 pages.

Chapter 5: The October Plan

1. Proposal for Funding for the Public Issues in Health Care Choices: A Project of the Ohio Council Against Health Fraud. October 9, 1986. 8 pages.
2. Grant Number CA41953-03, Progress Report Summary. June 1, 1988 to May 5, 1989. "Evaluative Database on Questionable Cancer Remedies," Applicant organization: Emprise. 5 pages.
3. Phase 1 Report on Study. October 1, 1986 to July 31, 1987. re: Expert Consensus Panels. 7 pages.
4. Grant Study data re: List of Major Questionable (Dubious) Remedies to Prevent or Treat AIDS. Subjects and Consensus Panels. Plans for use of Consensus Panel Report. 14 pages.

Chapter 6: Merchants of Misinformation
1. Cover letter from Associate Commissioner FDA, attached to Health Fraud Activities Status Report February 1988. February 26, 1988. 13 pages.
2. FDA Investigations Activities Report: From Division of Field Investigations (HFC-130) to FDA Directors, Investigations Branch. February 10, 1992. 18 pages.
3. Statement of Dr. John Renner, M.D., before Committee on Small Business, Subcommittee on Regulation, Business opportunities and Energy: "Recent Trends in Dubious and Quack Medical Devices." April 9, 1992.
4. *Medical Economics* article: "Insurance Fraud Cops Have a Whole New Set of Teeth," by Mark Holoweiko. March 7, 1988.
5. *Food Chemical News* article: "FDA Criminal Investigations Await OPM Clearance." September 23, 1991.
6. *Food Chemical News* article: "Ex-Secret Service Man to Head FDA Criminal Investigations." February 3, 1992.
7. Department of Justice, "Report to Attorney General On Enhanced Health Care Fraud Initiative," from George J. Terwilliger, III, Acting Deputy Attorney General. February 3, 1992.
8. *Food Chemical News* article: "Strong Enforcement to Continue, FDA's Dykstra Tells N.Y. Bar." February 10, 1992.
9. *The Psychiatric Times* series of articles on "Medicaid/Medicare Fraud Investigation Abuses," by Howard Fishman.

Chapter 7: Big Brother and the Insurance Industry
1. National Health Care Anti-Fraud Association confidential memo from Thomas Brunner and Kirk Nahra to NHCAA Board of Directors. August 3, 1990.
2. National Health Fraud Conference Program, Washington, D.C. September 11, 1985.
3. Articles of Incorporation, National Health Care Anti-Fraud Association, Washington, D.C. December 5, 1985.
4. NHCAA Third Annual Meeting, Phoenix, Arizona: program and panel sessions. November 13-16, 1988.
5. NHCAA 1988 Membership List.
6. Emprise NIH Grant Progress Report, June 1, 1988.
7. *Health Insurance News Digest* article: "First Computerized Network Designed to Combat Health Care Fraud Is Un-

veiled." December 5, 1987. (Originally announced November 12, 1987 in *Insurance Advocate*.)

8. RICO Conspiracy Law Suit: *Stanislaw Burzynski and BRI v. Aetna Life Insurance, Emprise, Grace Monaco.* June 29, 1990.

9. Aetna interoffice memo from D.C. Kellsey, M.D., Medical Directors, Medical Claims, to Russ Robertson, Senior Examiner, Group Claims, Aetna. October 14, 1980.

10. National Health Fraud Conference, Kansas City, Missouri: program and workshops. March 13-15, 1988.

Chapter 8: The Business of Drugs
1. FDA Dietary Supplements Task Force: Final Report. May 1992.

2. PAC/FDA Joint-letterhead cover letter from Paul Chusid, Coordinator PAC/FDA Anti-Quackery Program, to P.J. Lisa, with list of 26 pharmaceutical companies who are "Contributors to PAC/FDA Anti-Quackery Campaign." November 15, 1985.

3. U.S. Health Care Financing Administration Health Care Financing Review, Chart 135: "National Health Expenditures 1970-1986." Summer 1987.

4. _____, Chart 921: "Magazine Advertising-Expenditures, By Product Type 1970-1987"

5. 1992 *Physicians Desk Reference*.

6. *San Francisco Chronicle* article: "Vitamin Research Grows Up," by Natalie Angier. April 12, 1992.

7. *Time* magazine article: "The New Scoop on Vitamins," by Anastasia Toufexis. April 6, 1992.

Part Two

Chapter 9: The Nutri-Cology Case
1. Notes of Joint Investigation meeting with FDA and California Food and Drug. August 2, 1988.

2. Food and Drug, State of California, Fraud Branch, Operations Manual. July 11, 1978.

3. *L.A. Times* article: "Medical Quacks' Growing Threat Told," by Myrna Oliver. August 24, 1978.

4. Summary Intragency Health Fraud Meeting to discuss strategies on fraud investigations. May 23, 1984.

5. Anonymous typed noted to Sally 0. Lum (California Food and Drug Investigator) from "An angry public."

6. F&D Branch "Program Activity Report," note from Jim Eddington re: Nutri-Cology (Fraud) investigation. January 30, 1985.

7. Transcribed notes of Jim Eddington's phone conversation with F&D Branch Inspector Sally 0. Lum on Nutri-Cology.

8. Memo of call by Jim Eddington re: Sally 0. Lum's inspection of Nutri-Cology and refusal of entry. February 8, 1985.

9. Report of observations by Sally Lum re: Nutri-Cology. February 15, 1985.

10. Undercover letter sent to Steve Levine from F&D Branch, signed Dr. J. Jacobson and authorized March 21, 1985 by Jim Eddington.

11. Memo of call between Jim Eddington and FDA official Fischer, April 4, 1985.

12. Inspections Report, F&D Branch re: "Labels for products are relatively free of drug claims." July 1983.

13. Undercover letter to Dr. Levine from F&D Branch from D.M. Moore, F&D Branch Investigator. 12 May 1986.

14. Investigation Report. 7 August 1986.

15. Notice to Appear Summons to Mary Garcia, from Eddington, not issued, dated August 7, 1986.

16. Program Activity Report re: "Claims toned down." August 12, 1986.

17. Routing and Transmittal Slip from FDA to Eddington, re: "doubt whether our agency (FDA) will do anything. . ." September 23, 1986.

18. Memo of call from Dan Walsh re: Nutri-Cology and "felony conviction. . ." May 3, 1988.

19. FDA Notice of Adverse Findings Letter. May 6, 1988.

20. FDA Import Alert re: germanium products. June 29, 1988.

Chapter 10 : The Herbalife Story

1. "Chronology History of Food and Drug Branch Involvement in Herbalife Investigation" draft February 26, 1985. 8 pages.

2. Summary Interagency Health Fraud Meeting "to discuss strategies on fraud investigations." May 23, 1984.

3. *USA Today* article: "Herbalife Mogul Mark Hughes Addresses Weighty Issues," by Karen S. Peterson and Mark Mayfield. May 16, 1985.

4. *Nutritional Forum* (editor Stephen Barrett, M.D.) list of "Important Articles on the Way" and list of associate and contributing editors.

5. *Food Chemical News* article: "FDA Confirms Effective Date of Aspartame Clearances." March 7, 1988.
6. *Food Chemical News* article: "Wurtman Asks for Warning to Physicians on Aspartame-Epilepsy Link." April 28, 1986.
7. *Food Chemical News* article: "Searle Filing Aspartame Complaints With FDA Each Month, Young Says." April 28, 1986.

Chapter 11: The Conspiracy Against Chiropractic
1. Indiana Medical Association "Report on Chiropractic: The Chiropractic Dilemma." June 25, 1980. 15 pages.
2. National Council Against Health Fraud Position Paper on Chiropractic." February 14, 1985.
3. National Association for Chiropractic Medicine (NACM) By-Laws.
4. NACM Proposed NACM Advisory Board.
5. NACM Officers and State Directors List.
6. NACM Membership Benefits.
7. "Facts on Spinal Manipulative Therapy," presented to Ohio Association of Civil Trial Attorneys-Columbus, Ohio, by Charles DuVall. March 3, 1984, and April 14, 1984.
8. "How to Evaluate a Chiropractic Claim," presented to Intracorps Chiropractic Seminar by Charles DuVall. April 5, 1988.
9. "Specialty Criteria-Chiropractic" (list of chiropractic items to challenge, or not pay for), by Charles DuVall.
10. Chiropractic Claims Review Flow Chart, by Charles DuVall.
11. Intracorp *Forum* magazine article: "Chiropractic Bill Review: A Timely Idea for an Old-Time Treatment."
12. Deposition of Charles DuVall, Akron (Ohio) Court Reporters.
13. Articles of Incorporation, "National Association for Chiropractic Medicine."
14. Incorporation Papers for Ohio Council Against Health Fraud, April 17, 1987, filed May 4, 1987.
15. Department of Health and Human Services, Office of Inspector-General report on "Inspection of Chiropractic Services Under Medicare."

Chapter 12 : Chelation Therapy
1. Letter from Dr. R.W. Johnson, Minot, North Dakota, to Vernon Wagner, Executive Secretary, N.D. Medical Association re: Dr. Brian Briggs. September 29, 1978.

2. Letter from Rolf Sletten, Executive Secretary N.D. Medical Board of Examiners to Minnesota Medical Board re: Dr. Brian Briggs. February 7, 1983.

3. Letter from Dale C. Moquist, M.D., to Rolf Sletten re: his meeting with Dr. John Renner regarding Dr. Briggs. October 8, 1986.

4. Note (circa November 1986) re: Board official calling Renner.

5. Note from Dr. John Renner's office to "Lynette" (N.D. Dakota Medical Board Staff investigator) re: Briggs and the list of alternative practitioners. November 12, 1986.

6. Minutes of North Dakota Medical Board July 1987 secret meeting voting to revoke Dr. Briggs' license.

7. Note from ND Medical Board staff re: trouble finding MD to testify against Dr. Briggs.

8. ND Medical Board Findings of Acts, Conclusions, and order following July 16, 1988 public meeting on Dr. Briggs' license. July 21, 1988.

9. Letter from Boar attorney R.W. Wheeler to all Board members re: their "good job" on Dr. Briggs at "public meeting." July 25, 1988.

10. "Health and Nutritional Quackery, Fraud and Abuse" paper, delivered at St. Luke's Hospital Tumor Conference by Dr. John Renner. November 7, 1985.

11. Letter from unnamed D.O. of The University of Health Sciences to Marvin Meck, D.O., president of the American Osteopathic Association, re: Dr. McDonagh's defending chelation therapy and countering Dr. Renner on radio show. March 2, 1984.

12. Kansas Board of Healing Arts Notes and Summary in Chronological order from Feb. 25, 1984 to October 6, 1984.

13. Letter to Dr. John Renner from Dr. Richard Rubin re: chelation therapy. January 26, 1984.

14. Letter to Dr. John Renner from Riker Labs manufacturer of EDTA. January 26, 1984.

15. FDA Cover Note to Kansas Board of Healing Arts, with attachments on chelation therapy, from Julia S. Hewgley, Consumer Affairs Officer, FDA Kansas City, Missouri. February 27, 1984.

16. Kansas Board of Healing Arts hand-written note re: EDTA chelation and Dr. John Renner. September 28, 1984.

17. Copies of pages from Morton Walker's book *The Miracle Healing Power of Chelation Therapy*.

18. Kansas Healing Arts Board position statement on chelation therapy.
19. Letter from Dr. Uhlig, D.O., of the Kansas Board to Missouri Board of Healing Arts re: the Kansas resolution on chelation therapy. October 16, 1984.
20. Letter from Kansas Board to Charles Rudolph, D.O., inviting him to the December 7, 1984 meeting on chelation.
21. Letter from the Montana Board of Medical Examiners to the Kansas Board, asking about their resolution on chelation. December 3, 1984.
22. Reply from the Kansas Board to the Montana Board with a copy of their resolution on chelation attached. December 14, 1984.

Chapter 13: Naturopathy
1. Grand Jury Findings on Naturopathy re: 1950 Naturopathy Act. November-December 1955. Recommendations published January 2, 1956.
2. American Medical Association's Report on Naturopathy, circa 1950.
3. Letter from Postal Inspector W.F. Callahan, Chicago office, to John Kiser, Medical Association of Georgia. January 1954.
4. Letter from Oliver Field, AMA Department of Investigation, to John Kiser re: naturopathy. January 20, 1956.
5. Letter from John Kiser to Oliver Field. February 23, 1956.
6. Letter from Herman Jones, Director of Crime Labs, to John Kiser re: test case of naturopathy. March 13, 1956.
7. Letter from John Kiser to William Bartleson, Jackson County, Missouri, Medical Board re: obtaining records surreptitiously on naturopathy. September 24, 1956.
8. Letter from MAG attorney Frank Shackelford to Georgia State Solicitor General Jay re: helping the state's case against naturopathy. April 19, 1960.
9. Minutes of CCHI meeting re: Inspector Callahan putting together "quackery booklet" including naturopathy. November 20, 1964.
10. CCHI survey on homeopathic and naturopathic medicine by National Analysts, Inc.
11. Memo from Robert Youngerman to Doyl Taylor of AMA Department of Investigation re: rolling back licensure and the

"professional withering on the vine" of chiropractic (or naturopathy). September 21, 1967.

12. Letter from Andrew Watry, Georgia Medical Board, to Attorney General re: "increasing number of calls from the public about. . ." naturopathy. December 1981.

13. Letter from Andrew Watry to Marie Steinmeyer re: naturopathy. April 20, 1982.

14. Memo from Andrew Watry to Rusty Kidd, lobbyist for MAG re: naturopathy. March 2, 1983.

Chapter 14: Acupuncture and Holistic Dentistry

1. National Council Against Health Fraud's Position Paper on Acupuncture. Circa January 1991. 12 pages.

2. Statement from television-doctor Dean Edell, KGO-TV, San Francisco, on acupuncture. January 25, 1991.

3. *Andrews v. Ballard*, 498 F. Suppl.,1038 Southern District Court, Houston Division, 1980. Re: Acupuncture.

4. FTC Bureau of Competition Director Timothy J. Muris re: "sharing information between competitors." June 26, 1984.

5. NCAHF Resource Material List re: acupuncture. May 1986.

6. *Postgraduate Medicine* article: "The Health Fraud Battle: Education is the Best Defense." June 1989.

7. *Minnesota Medicine* article: "Patients Who Seek Unorthodox Medical Treatment." June 1990.

Chapter 15: Homeopathy

1. Fax Transmission from Dr. John Renner to Missouri Chiropractic Board and Missouri State Attorney General re: Dan Clark and reporting to FBI, FDA, AG and St. Louis Post. February 26, 1992.

2. Letter of resignation from Dr. Dan Clark. November 2, 1981.

3. Administrative Complaint by Department of Professional Regulation (DPR) against Dr. Dan Clark. March 31, 1982

4. DPR letter to Grace Monaco re: Dr. Clark's case records. April 2, 1984.

5. Letter from Grace Monaco to DPR requesting additional data on his case. April 16, 1984.

6. Letter from Grace Monaco to Florida Medical Board re: Dan Clark re: laetrile. June 20, 1984.

7. Letter from DPR to Grace Monaco re: orders and records on Dan Clark case. July 5, 1984.

8. DPR Consumer Complaints staff memo re: anonymous phone tip re: Dr. Dan Clark practicing medicine. August 20, 1984.
9. DPR Case # 0063702 brought by DPR against Dr. Dan Clark, Investigative Report summary including list of exhibits #14, 15, and 16 related to Florida Cancer Council's Confidential Report re: Dr. Clark.
10. Letter from FDA Investigator, Orlando office, to DPR requesting all files on Dr. Dan Clark. June 26, 1992.
11. DPR reply to FDA Investigator Melissa Hill re: Clark's case, and records. August 7, 1992.

Chapter 16: The Case of Dr. Willem Khoe
1. California Board of Medical Quality Assurance, Case #- D 2750—Willem Khoe, M.D., Respondent's Brief Before the Court (Board).

Part Three

Chapter 17: Solutions to the Problems
1. Associated Press article: "Court Rules State Officials May be Sued for Damages," by James H. Rubin: November 7, 1991.
2. *Barbara Hafer, Petitioner v. James C. Melo, Jr., et al.*, (1991 WL 221067 (U.S.). Syllabus of case, West. November 5, 1991. 7 pages.
3. Review and Analysis of *Hafer v. Melo.* 4 pages.
4. *Washington Post* article: "Court Clears Psychologist's Payment Suit," by Jane Seaberry. June 22, 1982.
5. "Recent Supreme Court Decisions: *McCready v. Blue Shield of Virginia*, by Timothy Bloomfield. 29 pages.
6. Department of Health and Human Services (HHS) Office of Hearings and Appeals, Medicare Case, Dr. E.M. Nash, D.C. Hearing Summary and Decision. August 22, 1989. 12 pages.
7. *Gilbert's Law Summaries*: "Antitrust." 1983.
8. National Commission on Law Enforcement and Social Justice, press release re: FDA Whistleblower Campaign. December 5, 1993. 2 pages.
9. *Burnsville Press* article: "Picketers Protest Blue Shield Policy Changes." September 14, 1987. 2 pages.
10. U.S. District Court, Southern District of Ohio, Eastern Div., Court Judgment Ordering FDA return of property seized

belonging to Steven Michaelis, owner of AO Supply. June 29, 1978. 5 pages.
11. *U.S. v. Nutri-Cology et al.* Case #C-91-1332 DLJ. Order by Judge D. Lowell Jensen, U.S. District Judge. 39 Pages.
12. Fax Statement from Stephen Levine, Ph.D., re: "Nutri-Cology Wins Cross Motions: On Summary Judgment in Federal Court." October 15, 1993. 2 pages.

Appendix I

Organizations and Resources for Information

The following are some organizations whose members can provide alternative therapies and help for those in need:

American Academy of Environmental Medicine
P.O. Box 16106
Denver, CO 80216
(303) 622-9755

American College of Advancement in Medicine
23121 Verdugo Drive, Suite 204
Laguna Hills, CA 92653
(800) 523-3688 or (714) 583-7666

American Holistic Medical Association
2727 Fairview East
Seattle, WA 98102
(206) 322-6842

British Holistic Medical Association
179 Gloucester Place
London, NW1 6DX
England
011-44-71-262-5299

Canadian Holistic Medical Association
491 Eglinton Avenue West, #407
Toronto, Ontario M5N 1A8
Canada
(416) 485-3076

Discovery Experimental & Development, Inc.
29949 SR 54 West
Wesley Chapel, FL 33543
(813) 973-7200 FAX (813) 973-7002

Great Lakes Clinical Medicine Association
Jack Hank, Executive Director
70 W. Haron
Chicago, IL 60610
(312) 266-7246

Foundation of Homeopathic Education and Research
Dana Ullmann, M.P.H., Director
5916 Chabot Crest
Oakland, CA 94618
(415) 649-8930

The following consumer rights groups are involved in activity directed at making change. Contact one about membership.

Cancer Control Society
2043 N. Berendo Street
Los Angeles, CA 90027
(213) 663-7801

Citizens for Health
Alex Schauss, Exec. Dir.
2722 Pioneer Way
East Tacoma, WA 98404
(206) 922-2457

National Commission on Law Enforcement
    and Social Justice (NCLE)
20929-47 Ventura Blvd. #205
Woodland Hills, CA 91364
(818) 955-5388

National Health Federation
P.O. Box 688
Monrovia, CA 91017
(818) 357-2181

National Nutritional Foods Association
150 East Paularino Avenue
Suite 285
Costa Mesa, CA 92626
(714) 966-6632 FAX (714) 641-7005

Publications of interest and as a source of information on alternatives:

Choice Magazine
Michael Culbreath, Editor
1180 Walnut Avenue
Chula Vista, CA 92011
(619) 429-8200

Freedom News Journal
6331 Hollywood Blvd.
Suite 1200
Los Angeles, CA 90028
(213) 960-3500

Health Consciousness Magazine
Roy B. Kupsinel, M.D., Publisher
1325 Shangri La Lane
Oviedo, FL 32765
(407) 365-6682

Health Freedom News
National Health Federation
P.O. Box 688
Monrovia, CA 91017
(818) 357-2181

Appendix II

Documentation Catalog Order Form

The documentation referenced in this book, along with many other documents, are available through a Catalog Order Form. There are over 4,000 pages of documentation in the categories listed below. These documents can and should be used in any or all of the following applications: (1) with the media; (2) for staff and patient education; (3) in legal counterclaims—civil, RICO, criminal suits; (4) in depositions, discovery procedures, documents, interrogatories, and examination and cross-examination; (5) in publications and articles about this campaign; (6) in the state and federal legislature, to either defeat legislation impacting the alternative health-care system, or lobby for legislation supporting it; (7) for reimbursement and payments from insurance companies for alternative services denied; and 8) in negotiating settlements with insurance companies, government agencies and state boards of examiners involved in passing judgments against alternative practitioners, products, services, treatments, or modalities.

These documents have been located, collected and assembled over a ten-year period. In all cases, they have been legally obtained from either the government, the insurance industry, or medical/pharmaceutical organizations. Knowledge is Power. Using these documents could result in adjudication of wrongs, increased income for practitioners and clinics, and very possibly jury trial settlements and/or awards or out-of-court settlements over issues that these documents reveal and uncover. They can also result in positive exposés in the media of the campaign that has been perpetrated against the alternative health-care system.

DOCUMENTS PACKAGES AVAILABLE

Package A - INSURANCE INDUSTRY - 260 pages
More than 250 pages of evidence documenting the tie-in between private insurers, government, and spokesmen for the vested interests. Includes the medical plan to create a front of chiropractors to carry

on the medical campaign against chiropractic, as well as the October Plan. Also includes court records, depositions, and incorporation papers linking together the massive web between government, insurance companies, and those outside of government adversely influencing the insurance industry against chiropractic, chelation therapy, holistic dentistry, DMSO, hair analysis, and other modalities used by alternative practitioners, but not covered by the insurance industry. These documents could open the door for reimbursement and payment from insurers, as well as other uses described above. This is a must for those interested in surviving in the 1990s.

Package B - MATERIALS ON HEALTH FRAUD - 103 pages
Includes incorporation papers on all of the key anti-health fraud groups mentioned in the book. Also included are lists of their affiliates and chapters, Conferences on Health Fraud programs and attendees, minutes of meetings with state and federal agencies, position papers, and more. This is a must to know who's who in this campaign and what they have been disseminating at conferences.

Package C - PAC/FDA CAMPAIGN MATERIALS - 79 pages
Includes all Campaign documents referenced in this book, and more—the PAC/FDA original plans, financing, letters, memos, and lists of targets named in the initial campaign plans, as well as documents showing involvement of anti-health fraud members, their roles, connection to the AMA, the FDA, the FTC, the U.S. Post Office, Better Business Bureaus in the campaign. This package is invaluable evidence of the pharmaceutical industries involvement and role in this campaign for legal and media purposes and for exposing their allied connections.

Package D - CCHI/AMA DOCUMENTATION - 309 pages
Includes minutes of the CCHI/AMA meetings held with the federal government between 1964-1975 (almost all meetings are included). Minutes clearly show a long-term pattern of the AMA dictating to government agencies such as the FDA, thee FTC, and the U.S. Post office to go after specific targets named by the medical vested interests. These documents are evidence of the extensive damage and activity directed against the economic competitors of medicine in the alternative health-care field. Tied into the current campaign, it could prove the long-term pattern needed to make a RICO case against those involved in the campaign.

Package E - LEGAL CASES AND DOCUMENTATION - 353 pages

This package draws on successful cases that have been won before the Supreme Court of the United States and Federal District Courts, on issues dealing with the FDA, U.S. Customs, and others; Administrative Hearings before Medical Boards; adjudications before Boards on Medicare cases; minutes of meetings of Medical Boards showing outside influence and involvement directed against chiropractors, and chelation therapists; government files on manufacturers showing possible illegal activity on the part of the government; a RICO suit filed against an insurance company,, as well as Emprise et. al.; and key testimony from a deposition of an insurance consultant on issues of importance to chiropractic and the use of themography. These could be used in formulating legal strategy, depositions, suits, counterclaims, defense, and other legal issues with the insurance industry, medical boards, and other areas. A must to have and use to benefit from others legal wins.

Package F - BACKGROUND ON KEY INDIVIDUALS IN CAMPAIGN - 170 pages

Includes bankruptcy file and documents on a key spokesman in the anti-health fraud movement; case documents from suits and counterclaims filed on another spokesman; affidavits and briefs filed against a VA doctor/spokesman; VA files, records, memos and letters, including data on a federal investigation into possible wrongdoing on the part of one of the key spokesman in the anti-health fraud movement. This data is good for background to law suit discovery and depositions of some of the key players in the campaign, as well as for media use. Know before you go.

Package G - LEGAL DEPOSITION/CROSS EXAMINATION - 2000 pages

This package contains about 2000 pages of depositions, cross examination, and direct examination of one of the key spokesman in this campaign. It can be used as a basis of depositions and discovery, as well as challenging expert testimony against alternative practitioners. It is full of valuable information and a must for anyone dealing with this "expert."

Package H - LISTS OF TARGETED ALTERNATIVES - 58 pages

Includes all of the documents which contain any named targets, including names of practitioners, products, treatments, therapies, modalities, and services. These lists are from the PAC/FDA campaign; the Emprise study (includes actual pages listing out the panelists and the items they studied); names of chelation therapists found in medical board files covering eleven different states; names of multi-level companies involved in alternative products; individual chiropractors named; and much more. If one wants to know what and who they're going after, then this Package is a must.

Package I - AMA/CCHI TARGET LIST - 134 pages

The lists of alternative targets that the AMA, the American Cancer Society, the Arthritis Foundation, the Better Business Bureau, the FDA, the FTC, the U.S. Post office went after for twelve years is included in this package. The list shows the long-term campaign against such targets as chiropractic, chelation therapy, homeopaths, naturopaths, acupuncture, and a long list of alternative cancer, heart, and arthritis targets. This package is a must to show the long-term pattern.

Package J - GOVERNMENT DOCUMENTATION - 353 pages

Includes memos, letters, reports, inter-governmental newsletters; policy on health fraud; quota system against alternative targets; government plans on health fraud "beef-up"; 11 fraud activities reports from the FDA, Field Investigation reports on health fraud; Congressional testimony with lists of alternatives turned into Congress; Department of Justice reports on health fraud; FDA Report on supplements; as well as the entire series of articles exposing Medicare/Medicaid fraud investigation abuse by the government against targeted practitioners. This Package is a must for anyone dealing with these government agencies.

Package K - ANTITRUST LEGAL PAPERS - 173 pages

Includes papers presented by experts on antitrust law which could serve as background research, as well as guidelines for future legal activity in this area. These papers also provide use for application in the insurance industry and in the area of medical professional groups, as well as what to do when government investigates and issues related to refusal to cover alternative providers and new technology and much more. Every practitioner and attorney representing alternative practitioners should have these at hand for use.

PRICE CATALOG ORDER FORM

Note: The Catalog lists every specific document that is included in each package.

You may request copy/copies of the Document Catalog Price List, at a cost of $5.00 each. Please send your NAME, ADDRESS (Street/P.O. Box), CITY/STATE/ZIP CODE, and PHONE (Daytime)(Weekends/Evenings. Enclose a check or money order payable to:

> DocUsearch
> P.O. Box 7199
> Stateline, NV. 89449

Please do not send cash. Please allow two weeks for your catalog to arrive. Thank you for your interest.

Index

A

A.H. Robbins (pharmaceuticals), 127, 131
A.O. Supply Company, 182, 353-355
ABC-TV, 91
abscisic acid, 82
Accupath 1000 (EAV machine), 82, 312
Acidophillas, 82
Acker, Stevens B. (M.D.), 252, 256
acupressure, 133, 227, 283, 285
acupuncture
  as treatment, 133, 135
  case victory for, 304-315
  targeted, 35, 36, 47, 80, 86, 151, 228, 282-287
ADS tea, 82
Aetna Life Insurance Co., 65, 109, 114, 116-118
African Bio-Mineral balance, 86
AIDS Buyers Clubs, 176, 177, 185
AIDS Health Fraud Conference (Orlan do, Florida), 99
AIDS treatments list, 86, 87
AL-721, 86
alfalfa, 251
algae, 58, 87
Aller-Aid (hypoallergenic product), 169
Allsafe Gel, 86
Allsafe Liquid, 86
aloe vera, 58
Alsleben, Rudolph, (D.O.), 251
AMA & U.S. Health Policy Since 1940, 22
AMA News, 42, 45, 46
American Academy of Family Physicians, 111
American Academy of Medical Acupuncture, 233
American Cancer Society, 33, 35, 55, 64, 65, 69, 119, 157, 158
American Chiropractic College of Thermography, 233
American Council on Science and Health (ACSH), 73, 74, 163,
American Council Science and Health (ACSH), 162, 163
American Heart Association, 157, 254
American Medical Association (AMA), 13-18, 22, 23, 26, 29, 32, 37-39, 206-211, 233-235, 265, 266
American Pharmaceutical Association, 33, 55, 64
American Society of Clinical Oncology, 111
amino acids, 86, 142
AMPAC (Politcal Action Committee), 32
Amygdalin, 83

anti-competitive network, 120-122
anti-Microbial treatments, 86
antineoplastins, 83, 117
antitrust laws
  use of, as a solution, 333, 334-337
  violation by AMA, 17, 30
applied kinesiology, 216
APR (Arthritis Pain Reliever), 131, 188, 189
Arizona Council Against Health Fraud, 76
Arthritis Foundation, 33, 35, 55, 64, 77, 157, 158, 189
arthritis products, 61
Arthur Amid Test, 82
Art of War, The, 8
Association of Food and Drug Officials (AFDO), 92, 98
auto-immune system, 86
auto-urine therapy, 83
autogenous vaccines, 83, 86
Aveloz, 82

B

Ballard v Blue Shield, 337
Barnett Technical Services, 92, 95, 111
Barrett, Dr. Stephen, 42, 45-47, 69, 74, 76, 85, 122, 163, 217, 219
Beard method, 84
Beaulieu, David (D.C.), 251
bee pollen, 163
Beecham Laboratories (pharmaceuticals), 126, 131, 133
benzaldehyde, 84
beta-carotene, 86, 139, 140
Better Business Bureau of Georgia, 266
BHT, 86
Billings, Dr. Frank, 25
Bio-Active Nutritional Products, 302, 303
bio-oxygen, 177
biofeedback, 85
Blonz, Edward R., Ph.D, 83
Blue Cross/Blue Shield, 65, 120, 148, 210
Blue Cross/Blue Shield of Michigan, 110, 323-326,
Blue Cross/Blue Shield of Minnesota, 346-349
Blue Cross/Blue Shield of North Dakota, 247
Blue Cross/Blue Shield of Ohio, 110
blue green manna, 82
Bogumill, Mike, 165, 190, 191
Bolen Test, 82
bone marrow aspiration, 86
botanicals, 85

orthomolecular therapy, 216
osteopaths/osteopathy, 28, 150, 181
osteoporosis tests, 147
Owens, Brenda, 251
Oxysport/PO 2, 177
ozone therapy, 87, 148

P

Palmer, Daniel David, 28, 206
Pardridge, Dr. William M., 202
Parker, James (D.C.), 219
Pau d'Arco, 83, 97, 174
pendulum divination, 216
pendulum testing, 148
penicillin, 87
Pennwalt Corporation, 126
Pharmaceutical Advertising Council
 (PAC), 52-61, 76, 77, 126, 127,
 130-137, 163, 164
polarity therapy, 87
primrose, oil of, 165, 251
priority targets, 34, 35, 57-61, 180-182,
 188-190, 194
Pritchett, Henry S. (president of
 Carnegie Foundation), 23
Propaganda Department (of AMA), 29, 30
Prophyle (EAV machine), 146
proteolytic enzymes, 83
psychic surgery, 35
psycho immunity, 87
psychological counseling, 56, 130
purified antigen, 87
pyramid power, 148, 216

Q

quota system (CFDB), 159, 160, 161,
 164, 169
quota system (DHHS-OIG/FDA), 62, 63,
 103-106

R

racism, 285
radon mines, 36
RDA (Recommended Daily
 Allowance), 137
Reams (treatment), 84, 216
ReBella (douche), 87
red blood cell transfusion, 87
reflexology, 87, 216
Rejuvelac, 87
Renner, John (M.D.), 73, 78, 175, 244,
 245, 258, 346-348
 and CHIRI, 48
 and Emprise, 67, 69, 76, 82
 and FDA, 91-93, 96, 122, 301
 and Kansas Board, 253-257
 and Kansas City (Mid-West) Council
  Against Health Fraud, 48
 and NACM, 220
 and NCAHF, 48

and NHCAA, 111
and North Dakota Medical Board, 245
appearance before Congress, 99, 100,
 107, 146-151
statements on chelation therapy, 252,
 256, 259-262
Tumor Conference, 248, 250-252
Retenzyme, 83
Revice's lipid therapy, 87
RICO (Racketeer Influenced and
 Corrupt Organizations Act), 37, 50,
 100, 114-118, 196, 333
Roche (pharmaceuticals), 130-135
Rockefeller Institute, 23-25
Rodaquin, 84
Roper Survey, 56, 57, 130
Rorer Group, 127
Rudolph, Charles J. (D.O.), 261

S

saliva analysis, 148
Sandoz (pharmaceuticals), 127, 131,
 133, 134
Sani-fone (protection from saliva), 87
Schalira, David V., 83
Schering Corp. (pharmaceuticals), 127,
 130-134
Schmidt, Ozzie (CFDB), 191
Schwartz, Ronald, 67, 70, 110
sclaraglyphics, 216
Searle, G.D., 196-199, 202, 216
Seelman, Robert C. (M.D.), 299
seizure actions by government, 7, 34, 59,
 88, 89, 97, 105, 169, 183, 193
Selenium (Sellinium), 87, 89, 97, 174
sexual rejuvenation products, 60, 133
Shaklee, 58, 134
Sheehan, Helen (American Cancer
 Society), 96
Sheehan, James (Assistant U.S.
 Attorney), 100
Shitake mushroom, 87
Siegel, Fred (D&F Industries), 193
Simmons, Dr. George, editor of *JAMA*, 25
Simonton, 85
Smith, Kay (Neo-Life), 251
Smith, Lois, 46
sodium selenite, 169
Somarin (Chinese mushroom extract), 87
SOO, 84
sound wave healing tapes, 87
Southern California Council Against
 Health Fraud, 47, 48, 158
spinal column stressology, 216
Spirulina, 58, 163
Squibb (pharmaceuticals), 127, 309
staphyloccus phase lysate, 84
starch blockers, 58
State Action Information Letter
 (SAIL), 98, 99
Sterling Drug Inc. (pharmaceuticals),
 127
Stuart Pharmaceuticals, 127, 134

Syntex (pharmaceuticals), 53, 127, 131, 188

T

Taheebo, 83
Tang, Dr. Katrina, 182
Tang, Dr. Yiwen, 182
Task Force on AIDS Fraud, 73, 98, 99, 183
Taylor, H. Doyl (AMA head of
    Department of Investigation/CCHI), 14,
    15, 17, 33, 39, 43, 45, 46, 157
teas, 85
The Guardian (insurance co.), 110
The Proprietary Association, 126
thermobaric treatment, 87
thermography, 148, 216, 228, 230-235
thermoscribe, 216
Thiemann, Alfred H. (D.O.), 256
Thymosin, 84
Thymus extracts, 87, 174
TMJ (temporal mandibular joint), 148, 313
Toftness device, 148, 216
trace elements, 83, 174
translinoleic acid, 87
Trevor, William, 17, 37
Turner, Jim (Swankin & Turner,
    attorneys), 197, 202, 204
Turner, Perry, 194

U

U.S. Attorney's office, 102
U.S. Postal Service (USPS), 33, 35, 36,
    37, 39, 55, 56, 72, 163, 184, 191
Unfair Trade Practices, 30, 120, 196
University of Pennsylvania, 76
    targeted in Emprise study, 35, 87
urine (use of in treatments), 84
urine amino acid tests, 148

V

Vega Machine (EAV machine), 146
Viralaid, 87
visualization, 85, 87, 134
vitamins, 50, 56, 135, 137, 344
    as treatments, 132-135, 137-141
    attacks against, 15, 35, 47, 48, 50,
    55, 57, 61, 77, 80, 83, 87, 97, 127,
    135-141, 147, 149, 150, 161, 163,
    164, 174, 182, 242, 250, 306-310
Volusia County Medical Society, 295

W

Waddell, Jim (CFDB-San Diego), 165, 189
    worked on Nutri-Cology case, 165
Walker, Dr. Morton, 255
Walsh, Dan (CFDB investigator), 176,
    190-194
Walters, Sam (D.C.), 251
Warner-Lambert Co.
    (pharmaceuticals), 127

water purification devices, 148
wheat grass, 83, 87
Whitaker, Dr. Julian, 182
Wigmore (diet, nutrition,
    detoxification), 83
Wilk v AMA, 218, 272, 331
Williams, Sid (D.C.), 37
Wilms, Heinz (Director of
    Federal/State Relations, FDA Office
    of Regulatory Affairs), 177, 183
Wilson, Dr. Benjamin, 76, 78, 82
Wilson, Ray (CFDB), 190
winter tea, 83
Wogee, Chris, 191
Women's Health Expo, 251
Workmen's (Worker's) Compensation
    Insurance, 148, 207
Wright, Dr. Jonathan, 182
Wurtman, Dr. Richard (MIT)197, 200,
    201

Y

yeast sensitivity diagnosis, 148
yellow and black salves, 85
yoga, 87
Young, Dr. Frank (FDA
    Commissioner), 53, 199
Youngerman, Robert (AMA
    Department of Investigation), 208, 209

Z

Zavertnik, Dr. Joseph, 299, 300
Zelner, Barbara (National Association of
    Medicaid Fraud Control Units), 110
Zerbo's Health Food Store (Michigan), 182
ZPG-1, 87

About the Author

P. Joseph Lisa has been a dedicated champion of civil and human rights since 1968. His exhaustive background includes work as a private investigator, investigative journalist, undercover operative, and health-advancement researcher. His published work includes many articles and scathing reports on abuses in the field of medicine, government mind-control experiments, illegal biological and chemical experiements on U.S. citizens, politics, psychiatry, and infringements on basic Consititutional rights of all American citizens.

Mr. Lisa is also the author of *Are You a Target For Elimination* and *The Great Medical Monopoly Wars*. He is currently working on a book exposing government abuses in psychiatric human experimentation (mind-control experiments), identifying its pre-World War II roots and tracing through the 1990s a conspiracy involving the U.S. Army Chemical Corps, the CIA, and illegal domestic intelligence operations directed against American citizens.

He is also involved with Native American culture; he serves as the Secretary to the Board of Trustees of the Stewart Indian Museum and is on their Pow-Wow Planning Committee and Community Relations Committee. He lives in Nevada with his wife and five children, three of whom he home-delivered.